OXFORD MEDICAL PUBLICATIONS

# MATERIALS IN
# CLINICAL DENTISTRY

GW00703255

# MATERIALS IN
# CLINICAL
# DENTISTRY

BY

## D. F. WILLIAMS
Senior Lecturer in dental materials, University of Liverpool

AND

## J. CUNNINGHAM
Lecturer in operative dental surgery, University of Liverpool

OXFORD NEW YORK TORONTO
OXFORD UNIVERSITY PRESS
1979

*Oxford University Press, Walton Street, Oxford* OX2 2DP

OXFORD LONDON GLASGOW
NEW YORK TORONTO MELBOURNE WELLINGTON
KUALA LUMPUR SINGAPORE JAKARTA HONG KONG TOKYO
DELHI BOMBAY CALCUTTA MADRAS KARACHI
IBADAN NAIROBI DAR ES SALAAM CAPE TOWN

© *D. F. Williams and J. Cunningham 1979*

**British Library Cataloguing in Publication Data**

Williams, David Franklyn
  Materials in clinical dentistry.—(Oxford medical
  publications).
  1. Dental materials
  I. Title    II. Cunningham, J
  617.6'95     RK652.5     79–40148

ISBN 0–19–267006–9 Pbk
ISBN 0–19–267007–7

*Filmset in Great Britain by Northumberland Press Ltd,
Gateshead Tyne and Wear
and printed and bound by William Clowes (Beccles) Limited,
Beccles and London*

# Preface

There is no doubt that materials science makes a significant contribution to the practice of dentistry. The majority of dental procedures utilize materials at some stage, and it can be argued that the properties and manipulation of these materials control to a large extent the clinical success of many dental operations. Not so many years ago, the use of dental materials could be more accurately described as an art. The materials were usually derived from other applications and adapted for dental use, most often on an empirical basis. More recently, technology has caught up with their practical use and many current products have been developed specifically for dental use. As their requirements are so stringent, products are often based on very sophisticated materials.

Increasing technological input has meant that the dental practitioner now requires a greater awareness of the products he is using. This, in turn, has led to a change in the dental curriculum, and now most dental schools have material scientists to teach students the concepts involved and to relate these concepts to the clinical behaviour of dental materials. Undoubtedly the practitioners of the future will benefit considerably from the scientific approach.

*Materials in clinical dentistry* is largely aimed at the undergraduate dental student who is studying the science and clinical uses of dental materials. The emphasis is on the relationship between these two aspects, so that the student can appreciate the basic structures of the materials and how the effects of clinical variables are related to these structures. The concepts of materials science and the very important subject of adhesive dentistry are covered in the early chapters of the book. The remaining chapters deal with the clinical applications of these materials. Included here are not only the traditional areas of conservative and prosthetic dentistry usually covered in books of this nature, but also the subjects of endodontics, preventive dentistry, orthodontics, periodontology, and oral surgery. The scientific content of the book has been aimed at a level which will provide an understanding of the clinically significant properties of the materials without giving too much unnecessary detail.

It is also hoped that dental practitioners will find this book of some use as a source of reference or for postgraduate study, including preparation for further examinations. It should also be of value to dental technicians undergoing their training.

Many colleagues have given assistance during the preparation of the manuscript. We would particularly wish to record our gratitude to Professor

F. E. Lawton, Mr D. Adams, Mr J. Brady, Mr D. Horsefield, Mr G. T. R. Lee, Dr J. M. Mumford, Mr A. V. Newton, Mr D. G. Smith, and Miss E. M. Theil for their valuable comments on individual chapters in the book.

D. F. W.
J. C.

*April 1979*

# Contents

# 1

# Introduction to dental materials science

In this book the term 'dental materials' refers to those materials that are used in the dental treatment of patients, where they are either placed permanently or semi-permanently in the mouth or, alternatively, used in the laboratory during the preparation of an intra-oral appliance. Included, therefore, are all the filling, cavity lining, luting, endodontic, crown and bridge, prosthetic, preventive, orthodontic, and periodontal materials as well as the impression, investment, and modelling materials used in the laboratory. Although some materials may have a number of different applications, a very wide range is required to cover the diverse requirements. The materials used range from ceramics, which give a very realistic appearance to crown and bridge restorations, to metals used to restore teeth and make the framework of dentures and appliances for orthodontic treatment, and polymers, from which denture bases, filling materials, and impression materials are made. Some of these, such as stainless steel and acrylic resin, are relatively simple materials, well known and used by engineers in completely different situations. Most, however, are complex structures, using unconventional substances in their constitution and having few uses other than those in dentistry. The amalgam and composite filling materials, the zinc oxide/eugenol cements, the periodontal dressing materials, and some root-canal filling materials, all of which are described in this book, come into this latter category.

In order to understand why different types of material should have different properties, and indeed, what these properties mean in relation to their use, it is necessary to understand a little about the science of materials. It is clearly inappropriate to discuss all aspects of materials science, or to cover any one aspect in great depth. Instead, those areas that are most relevant to the uses of dental materials have been chosen, the discussion of which will serve as the basis for ensuing chapters.

All properties of materials can be related to their structure. This chapter therefore begins with an introduction to basic structures, which leads conveniently to a classification of materials that explains the origins of metals, plastics, ceramics, and composites.

One of the more important aspects of the science of dental materials is the manner in which they are prepared. Dentistry is virtually unique in that the user of the materials also controls, in most cases, the chemical reactions or thermal processes that are involved in their preparation for use. It is necessary to describe in general terms the nature of these processes and reactions in the context of dental materials.

The properties of dental materials can be described under four broad headings.

**a** Mechanical properties, such as strength and toughness.

**b** Physical properties, such as thermal conductivity and thermal expansion.

**c** Chemical properties, which control solubility, water absorption, corrosion and so on.

**d** Biological properties, which relate to the effects of the materials on oral tissues.

In the sections dealing with these properties, the basic terms will be defined, observed phenomena explained, and the significance discussed in the context of clinical applications.

## THE STRUCTURE OF MATERIALS

The atoms that make up a substance determine its properties, both by virtue of their nature and the way in which they are arranged. These two aspects combine to determine the structure of the substance, which, as noted earlier, controls the properties. If the structure is such that the substance is useful for making objects, then it is called a material.

The expression 'properties of materials' refers to the behaviour of materials in use; that is, how they react to mechanical forces and excesses of temperature, for example, and how they behave in different environments. It is important to understand the structure of dental materials both to know how and why properties vary from one type to another and also to appreciate how small, intentionally introduced changes in structure can have a significant effect on the properties. It will be seen in Chapter 8, for example, that gold alloys may be used for dental castings, and that their strength can be greatly increased by including the right amount of copper and heating the casting, which produces a subtle change in the structure. Similarly it will be shown in Chapter 10 that structural changes in some kinds of silica prove very useful in controlling dimensional changes in the moulds used for these castings. Other important structural changes are those that produce the setting reactions of impression materials for, as described in Chapter 6, these changes provide the basis for a change in properties that is necessary when taking an impression.

There are several different organizational levels in the structure of a material and it is very important to consider all of them. A useful analogy is that of the behaviour of a wall when it is subjected to a force. If the wall is built from a number of blocks that are joined together by cement, and the whole wall is secured to some firm external structure, the strength of that wall will depend on (a) the strength of the blocks themselves, (b) the strength of the bond between them due to the cement, and (c) the strength of the fixation to the external support. The wall will collapse when subjected to a force if any one of these components is weak. If the building blocks are comparatively weak, the strength of the cement and external fixation become largely irrelevant; and similarly if either the cement or external fixation is weak, the wall will be easily destroyed irrespective of the strength of the blocks.

Thus a weakness at any one point in the structure of a material will ultimately control its properties in response to external stimuli, such as a mechanical force. The building blocks in this case may be considered to be the atoms, which are held together by inter-atomic forces, often resulting in the formation of molecules. These molecules may aggregate to form crystals or amorphous particles which themselves combine to constitute the sample of the material. The structures of the atoms, molecules, and crystals, and the forces holding them together are all important in determining the strength of a material.

## Atomic structure

This complex subject will only be discussed here at a level adequate to form a basis for the remainder of the chapter.

Each atom consists of a nucleus, which contains a large number of sub-atomic particles, including neutrons and protons. The former are electrically neutral while the latter carry a positive charge. Around each nucleus move a number of electrons whose negative charge exactly balances the positive charge of the protons.

An atom is characterized by the number of electrons it possesses. There are as many protons as there are electrons and the number of neutrons is between 1 and 1·5 times the number of protons. A combination of atoms of identical electronic structure form an element. There are 92 naturally occurring elements, each of which is composed of atoms with a unique number of electrons. This number is known as the atomic number of that element. Hydrogen has the smallest atom with one electron and just one proton in the nucleus, without any neutrons. The largest is uranium which has 92 electrons in each atom and a correspondingly large nucleus. In between are all the other elements, which are listed in Figure 1.1. They are arranged as the Periodic Table in which vertical columns contain elements of basically similar structure and hence similar properties.

The majority of electrons of any one atom are strongly attracted to the positively charged nucleus by electrostatic forces. These 'inner electrons' are considered firmly bound to the nucleus and have low energy. The outer electrons, called the valence electrons, are not so firmly bound and have higher energy. It is these outer electrons that primarily control the relationship between one atom and another. An atom may have between 0 and 7 valence electrons and this number controls the group of the Periodic Table to which that element belongs. The structure of lithium is shown in Figure 1.2a. Sodium, potassium, and the other elements of this group have similar structures, with the same single valence electron, but with an increasing number of inner electrons. Similarly, beryllium, shown in Figure 1.2b, has two outer electrons, the same as magnesium, calcium, and other elements of group 2. The inert

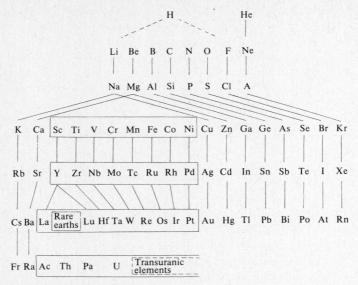

**Fig. 1.1** Periodic Table of elements.

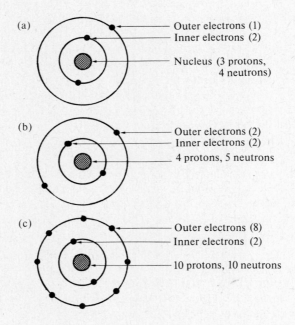

**Fig. 1.2** Atomic structures of (a) lithium; (b) beryllium; (c) neon.

gases, such as helium and neon (Fig. 1.2c), have no electrons in an outer group. This arises because eight 'outer' electrons form a stable, low-energy configuration to which no further electrons can be added. All the electrons are therefore effectively 'inner' electrons. This stable, inert gas structure is extremely important, as described below.

## Inter-atomic bonds and molecular structure

The one factor which, above all others, controls the behaviour of a material is its internal energy, for it is a fundamental law of nature that the components of any substance will attempt to adopt the structure that has the lowest possible energy. In the case of the interactions between atoms, each atom would prefer to have the structure of an inert gas, which, as just noted, is of minimum energy. Therefore, in the interactions between atoms that result in their aggregation into molecules, the atoms try to adopt this minimum energy configuration. There are, in fact, three principal ways in which this may be done, which give rise to the three main classes of material, the plastics, metals, and ceramics. The bonds produced between individual atoms in these classes are called primary valence bonds.

PRIMARY VALENCE BONDS

Those elements on the right-hand side of the Periodic Table require only a small additional number of electrons to achieve a full shell of electrons, with no valence electrons. Chlorine atoms, for example, have seven valence electrons and need only one further electron to achieve minimum energy. If two chlorine atoms approach each other, two electrons, one from each atom, are shared, both participating in the structure of the individual atoms, so that each acquires the stable structure (Fig. 1.3a). The two atoms are naturally attracted to each other by this mutual sharing of electrons. The bond produced in this way is called a covalent bond. The covalent bond, as shown in the next section, is the primary valence bond of polymers, upon which plastics are based.

Atoms of elements on the left hand side of the Periodic Table have only a small number of valence electrons. A stable structure is achieved here simply by loosing these outer electrons with the formation of a 'cloud' of free electrons. In lithium, for example, each atom releases one valence electron, whilst beryllium atoms lose two and so on. Electrically unbalanced atoms are produced, bearing a net positive charge. These atoms are more strictly referred to as ions although it is often more convenient to continue with the term atom. Materials made up of positively charged ions and a cloud of free electrons, shown in Figure 1.3b, are called metals and the general electrostatic bond that exists between the ions and electrons, and which therefore holds the structure together, is known as the metallic bond.

Atoms from one side of the Periodic Table may also combine with atoms from the other side to form chemical compounds. In this case the bond is usually established by the transfer of electrons from the atoms with a small

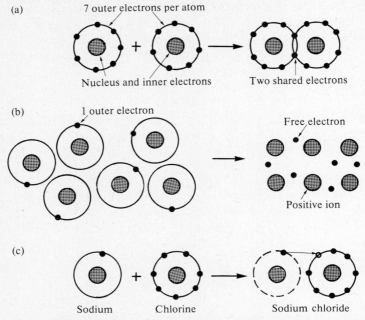

**Fig. 1.3** (a) Covalently bound chlorine structure; (b) metallic structure; (c) ionic structure of sodium chloride.

number of valence electrons (i.e. of the metallic element) to those which need only a few to complete a full shell (i.e. the non-metallic element), both thereby gaining the stable low-energy structure. For example, sodium atoms donate their sole valence electrons to chlorine atoms yielding positive sodium and negative chloride ions, held together by electrostatic forces (Fig. 1.3c). The bond produced is called an ionic bond and this is the basis of materials known as ceramics.

In each of these three cases, strong forces of attraction, the primary valence bonds, hold individual atoms together. If two or more atoms are joined by these forces, the resulting collection is called a molecule. Thus the two atoms of chlorine form a diatomic molecule. Small discrete molecules such as these are not conducive to the production of strong, useful materials, as described in some detail below. The exact manner in which a structure is built up from large numbers of atoms or molecules is, therefore, very important.

## Inter-molecular bonds and macromolecular materials

There are, broadly speaking, three states in which substances can exist, gas, liquid, and solid. In a gas, the individual molecules have little affinity for one another; they are free to move about so that a gas has no boundary but will fill any available space. Similarly in a liquid the molecules are free to move about, but not to such a great extent. A liquid again has no shape but it does have a surface and is far more dense than a gas. Neither gases nor liquids can be considered structurally useful substances.

Solids, on the other hand, have a distinct shape because the atoms or molecules are tightly bound. They are generally able to retain this shape without external support. A substance clearly has to exist as a solid at mouth temperature if it is going to be useful as a structural dental material.

A very important factor controlling the state of matter which a substance will adopt is the nature of the inter-molecular forces and, more specifically, the strength of these bonds compared to the thermal energy that the molecules possess by virtue of the temperature. Thus, in a gas the molecules are free to move about because their thermal energy is greater than the inter-molecular bond energy whereas in a solid, the inter-molecular forces are too large to allow random movement. For this reason, most substances transform from solids to liquids and then to gases as their thermal energy is increased by raising the temperature.

## Covalent bonds and polymers

Although the inter-atomic bond may be strong in covalently bound substances, there is usually very little attraction between the molecules. The primary valence bonds are solely associated with the atom–atom relationship and are not involved with the inter-molecular bonding. There are some inter-molecular forces of attraction which are also of electrostatic origin and are collectively called Van der Waals, or secondary valence, forces. These are considered in some detail in Chapter 2 because of their importance to adhesion phenomena.

Van der Waals forces are very weak in comparison to primary valence forces. Covalent substances therefore often exist as gases at room temperature because the thermal energy of the molecules easily exceeds the energy of the Van der Waals bonds. The bonds themselves are dependent on the size of molecules, tending to be stronger in bigger molecules. Thus in any group at the right hand side of the Periodic Table, elements of low atomic number tend to be gases while those of high atomic number are often liquids or even weak solids. The halogens provide a good example, fluorine and chlorine being gases, bromine a liquid, and iodine a weak solid.

Covalently bound substances, therefore, do not usually provide useful solids. There is one very important group of exceptions, however, which involve the carbon atom and, to a lesser extent, the silicon atom. Carbon, with a valency of four, has the well known and virtually unique capability of bonding to itself, covalently, to form long chains. A wide variety of other atoms and groups of atoms may be attached to the carbon atoms so that there is an almost infinite series of large molecules based on carbon atoms. The substances containing these molecules are called polymers. Two features combine to make many polymers useful materials. First, in very large molecules the secondary valence forces are high. Secondly, since the molecules are very long, they become entangled and their movement is restricted, favouring their existence in the solid state. Thus, whereas methyl methacrylate, $CH_2=C.CH_3.COOCH_3$, is a liquid, polymethyl methacrylate, $+CH_2.C.CH_3.COOCH_3+_n$, where $n$ may be several thousands, is a relatively strong solid. For reasons discussed later, pure polymers are rarely used but they form the basis of the plastics, which include rubbers, resins, and fibres. Occasionally polymers may be based on silicon, which also has a valency of four.

## Metallic bonds and metals

The covalent bond is spatially directed; that is the bond is specifically established between the two atoms that are involved in the electron sharing process so the line of action of the inter-atomic force is directed between the two atoms. In contrast, the metallic bond is not spatially directed as it does not specifically join any one atom with its neighbour. It is, instead, formed by the general attraction between the diffuse electron cloud and the aggregate of positively charged ions. There are, therefore, no molecules in a metallic structure as there are in a covalent struture and consequently there are no weak inter-molecular bonds. Metals usually exist, therefore, as strong solids. The metallic bond is generally strong so that high temperatures are necessary to melt metals. Mercury, of considerable importance in dentistry, is the one exception and exists as a liquid at normal temperatures.

## Ionic bonds and ceramics

Strong bonds also exist between the negative and positive ions in an ionically bound substance. If there are only two elements involved, all the positive ions will be identical, as will all the negative ions. Each positive ion will therefore be attracted with equal force to the negative ions and repelled by an equal force from all similar positive ions. This results in the arrangement of the ions in a lattice with oppositely charged ions occupying alternate sites. The classical example, the structure of sodium chloride, is shown in Figure 1.4. This again results in a continuous structure with no weak inter-molecular bonds since each atom is attracted to all its immediate neighbours by electrostatic forces. These ionic substances, typified by chlorides, nitrides, and oxides of metals, are usually solids, often of even greater stability than the metals. More than two elements can be involved and sometimes covalent bonding contributes to the structure as well as ionic bonding. Solid materials produced by this combination of metal and non-metal are often called ceramics.

## Crystalline and amorphous solids

In the case of all the inter-atomic forces discussed above, forces of attraction hold the atoms close together. However, because of the mutual repulsion of the positively charged nuclei there is a limit to the proximity of the atoms.

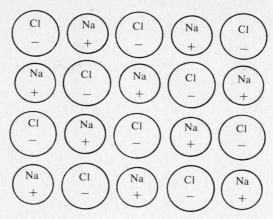

**Fig. 1.4** Lattice of sodium chloride.

They are, therefore, held at the equilibrium spacing at which the forces of attraction and repulsion balance. This is the configuration of minimum energy: external energy is needed to force the atoms either closer together or further apart, and if the atoms are in some way forced into different spacings the internal energy of the substance will rise. This is a very important concept, for it controls the physical manner in which the atoms are arranged. In other words, there is a tendency to adopt a regular, highly close-packed arrangement of atoms. This may be visualized by considering the problem of packing as large a number of ball bearings into a box as possible. Clearly this is best achieved if they are packed in a regular manner rather than haphazardly,

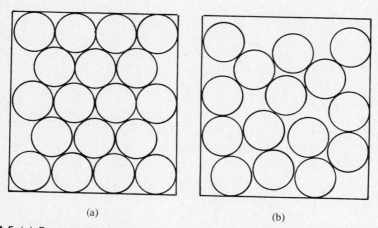

(a)                                        (b)

**Fig. 1.5** (a) Dense packing with ordered arrangement of atoms; (b) less dense packing with random arrangement.

as Figure 1.5 shows. When atoms are arranged in a regular, symmetrical manner, the solid is said to be crystalline. Metals and ionic substances are usually crystalline at room temperature. Any solid which is not crystalline and where there is no symmetry of the atoms, is said to be amorphous.

In amorphous solids there may be many different types of atom, with a number of differently directed inter-atomic bonds, so that the atoms cannot be arranged in a regular form. These solids are usually called glasses, as discussed later.

Some degree of symmetry is also possible with the large molecules of the polymers, if the side groups on the chains are small and well organized. Many polymers exist with partly crystalline and partly amorphous regions where areas of ordered molecular chains will be dispersed among disordered areas.

There are many different ways in which atoms can be arranged in a crystalline form. Even when simple metallic structures are considered, a number of different possibilities exist, with different energies and spacings. Not all crystal structures are of optimum close-packing and some exist in a slightly less dense arrangement. In Figure 1.6a, atoms in one plane, are arranged to give the greatest density of packing. If a second plane of atoms is arranged on top of this, again to achieve the closest packing, the atoms will be placed in the 'valleys' between the existing atoms, as in Figure 1.6b. When a third layer is added, however, the atoms can either be placed directly above the atoms of the first plane or in the 'valleys' of the second layer, as in Figure 1.6c. There are, therefore, two ways in which the optimum close-packed structure can be arranged. In the first case there are just two repeating units, whilst in the second case there are three. These two forms are very common in metals. The first is called the hexagonal close-packed (h.c.p) structure and the second is the face-centred cubic (f.c.c.) crystal structure. The arrangement of the atoms in space in these two structures can be seen in Figure 1.7 (a) and (b) where the derivation of the names becomes obvious. The basic units of the crystals shown in Figure 1.7 are repeated in all three directions to produce a space lattice. Amongst the other types of crystal structure found in metals are the body centred cubic (b.c.c.) structure, shown in Figure 1.7c and the body-centred tetragonal structure, which is very similar to the b.c.c. structure but with tetragons rather than cubes comprising the space lattice.

The majority of metals exist in either h.c.p., b.c.c., or f.c.c. form, but some can adopt more than one crystal structure, depending on the conditions. Iron is the classical example of this where it is b.c.c. up to 916 °C, f.c.c. from 916 to 1389 °C, and b.c.c. again above 1389 °C.

Whereas it is easy to visualize the arrangement of atoms in a metallic crystal, where all atoms are the same, it is more difficult in the case of ionic crystals where two or more ion species may be present. However, the same types of crystal structures may be produced, often with groups of atoms occupying the sites on the space lattice rather than single atoms. More will be said of this later.

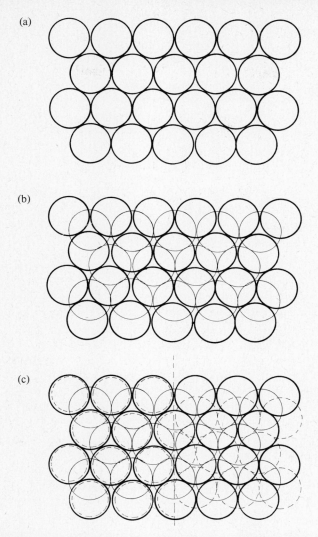

(a)

(b)

(c)

**Fig. 1.6** Atoms in a close-packed crystal structure showing the relationship between successive layers (a) first layer; (b) second layer; (c) third layer; indicating on left- and right-hand sides the two alternative positions of atoms.

## CLASSIFICATION OF MATERIALS

From the above description, three main classes of material can be identified:

**a** *Polymer-based materials*, in which large chain-like molecules are held together by secondary valence forces and physical entanglement. It does not take very much energy to overcome the forces of attraction between chains and so these materials are relatively weak and have low melting-points.

**b** *Metals* are held together by strong primary valence forces arising from the

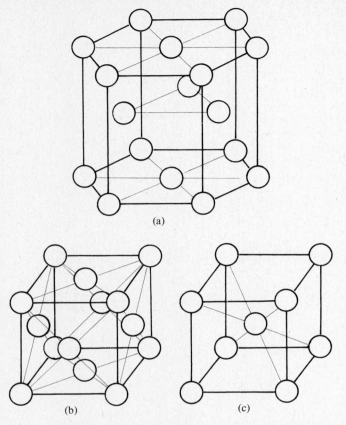

**Fig. 1.7** (a) Hexagonal close-packed; (b) face centred cubic; and (c) body centred cubic crystal structures.

electrostatic interaction between positive ions, arranged in a very symmetrical crystalline form, and a cloud of free electrons. The metals are usually strong with high melting-points.

**c** *Ceramics* are also materials with strong and uniform primary valence bonds, in this case of an ionic nature. Often ceramics are crystalline but they may exist as amorphous glasses. The bonding is very strong, usually resulting in very high melting-points. However, the arrangement of atoms results in a brittleness that betrays the high bond strength, as explained later.

**d** In addition there is a fourth type of material which exists as a combination of two or three of the basic types of material (a–c). Such materials are called composites. They may combine a metal with a ceramic, or a polymer with a metal, or, more usually, a polymer with a ceramic. They will naturally display some of the properties of both components but, as discussed later, the secret of a successful composite lies in the ability to retain the good properties of its components whilst eliminating their undesirable characteristics.

These four classes of material will now be discussed in a little more detail.

## Polymer-based materials

Polymers are materials containing long-chain molecules. Carbon atoms usually, although not always, comprise the backbone of the chains. If they are carbon-based, the materials are called organic polymers. The only other type of polymer that can be prepared with a similar structure has a backbone of silicon, which, like carbon, has a valency of four. Many organic polymers occur naturally, including polysaccharides, proteins, and polyisoprene (natural rubber). An almost infinite variety have also been produced synthetically by a process known as polymerization in which small molecules are made to react and link together.

POLYMER STRUCTURE

The simplest organic polymer considered from a molecular point of view is polyethylene, shown in Figure 1.8, which is based on the ethylene molecule $CH_2{=}CH_2$. The small molecule that comprises the repeating unit in a

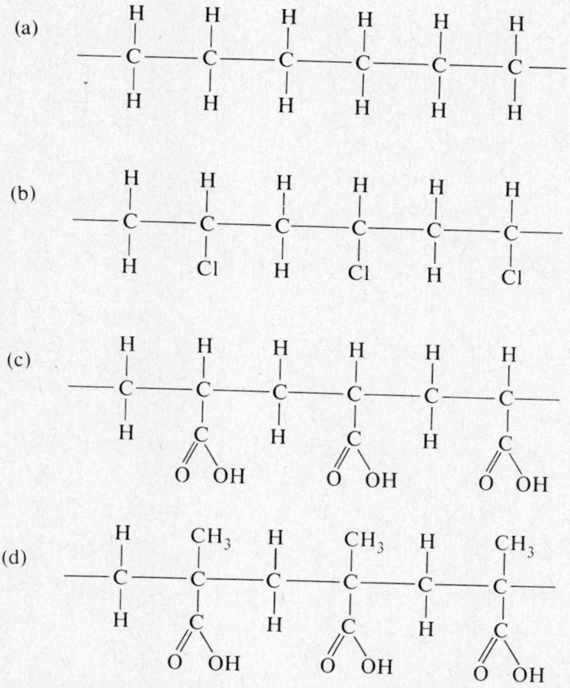

Fig. 1.8 Structure of some vinyl polymers (a) polyethylene; (b) polyvinyl chloride; (c) polyacrylic acid; (d) polymethacrylic acid.

polymer chain, in this case the ethylene, is known as the monomer. A large number of polymers can be derived from monomers that are very similar to ethylene, except that one or more of the hydrogen atoms is replaced by another atom or group of atoms. Thus polyvinyl chloride (PVC) is produced from vinyl chloride $CH_2{=}CH.Cl$ and polyacrylic acid from acrylic acid $CH_2{=}CH.COOH$. These are called the vinyl polymers and monomers respectively and other selected examples are given in Figure 1.8.

Since these polymers are actually formed by the repeated addition of monomer units to each other, they are known as addition polymers. Quite frequently addition polymers are highly crystalline since they have a very regular structure. Polyethylene, $-(CH_2.CH_2)_n$, and polytetrafluoroethylene, or PTFE, $-(CF_2.CF_2)_n$ are the simplest possible types and are usually 95–100 per cent crystalline. Where the side atoms or groups are larger, however, crystallization becomes more difficult, so that polyvinyl chloride $-(CH_2.CHCl)_n$ with a large chlorine atom, is only partially crystalline. When there are two large side groups per vinyl monomer, such as $-CH_3$ and $-COOCH_3$ groups in polymethyl methacrylate, and especially when these groups are not on the same side of the molecule, crystallization may be impossible. Polymethyl methacrylate, $-(CH_2.C.CH_3.COOCH_3)_n$, a very important dental polymer, is therefore amorphous.

Polymers may also be produced by chemical reactions involving more than one species. Some very important industrial polymers, such as the polyamides (commonly known as nylon) and polyesters (including polyethylene terephthalate, known as 'Terylene' or 'Dacron') are of this type. These polymers are known as condensation polymers since there is a reaction by-product, usually water or an alcohol. Polycarbonates provide a good example of condensation polymers that have been used in dentistry; they are synthesized by the reaction between bisphenol-A and a substance such as diphenyl carbonate, as shown in Figure 1.9.

In all the polymers mentioned so far, there is just one repeating unit in the chain. This occurs even in the condensation polymers where there are two reactants, as illustrated in Figure 1.9. These single-unit polymers are called homopolymers. It is possible, however, to produce polymers with more than one repeating unit. If these are addition polymers this may simply be regarded as the production of a polymer from two different monomers. These polymers are called co-polymers. They often give much better properties than homopolymers because of the combination of features derived from each monomer. Quite often small amounts of co-monomers are included in dental polymers to refine the properties.

CROSS-LINKING: PLASTICS, RESINS, AND ELASTOMERS

## Plastics and resins

Several terms are in common use to describe the various types of materials based on polymers. The term 'plastic' is rather difficult to define. As will be

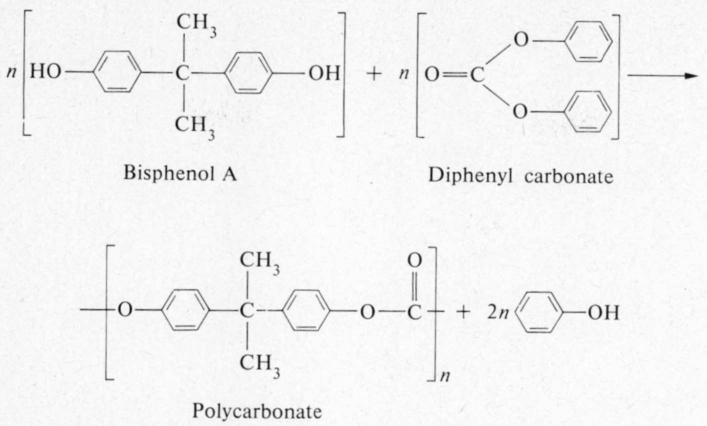

$$n \left[ HO-\text{⬡}-\underset{\underset{CH_3}{|}}{\overset{\overset{CH_3}{|}}{C}}-\text{⬡}-OH \right] + n \left[ O=C\left\langle\begin{array}{l} O-\text{⬡} \\ O-\text{⬡} \end{array}\right. \right] \longrightarrow$$

Bisphenol A                    Diphenyl  carbonate

$$\left[ -O-\text{⬡}-\underset{\underset{CH_3}{|}}{\overset{\overset{CH_3}{|}}{C}}-\text{⬡}-O-\overset{\overset{O}{\|}}{C}- \right]_n + 2n\,\text{⬡}-OH$$

Polycarbonate

**Fig. 1.9** Condensation polymerization reaction to give polycarbonate.

seen in a later section of this chapter, the word itself implies that the material can be easily and permanently deformed. It is normally used, therefore, to denote organic polymer-based materials that can be readily moulded.

There are two different types of plastic in this context, distinguished by the relationship between the polymerization and moulding characteristics. The first type, known as the thermoplastics, are characterized by their ability to become viscous fluids when they are heated, which allows them to be moulded very readily. The second type do not have this ability but are prepared in a partly polymerized form, usually as a very viscous fluid, moulded in this form and then hardened by further polymerization. Materials used in this way are usually called resins. The latter type are particularly useful to the dentist as they allow easy shaping and subsequent handling, often under the conditions prevailing in the mouth.

The difference between these thermoplastics and resins arises largely through one very important structural feature. Polymers have so far been represented as substances consisting of long-chain molecules which are attracted to one another only by secondary valence forces and physical entanglement. This is indeed the situation that exists in thermoplastics (Fig. 1.10a) and accounts for the ease with which they soften. As the temperature is raised, the thermal energy of the molecules is increased and since there are no primary valence bonds holding them together, the molecules can flow past each other very readily during moulding. The main problem with such materials in the dental context is that, although the moulding temperatures are not very high, often in the region of 200–300 °C, the need to use both elevated temperatures and pressure to force the polymer into the mould necessitates the use of fairly complex equipment and processes which are far more suitable to the mass production of components rather than the preparation of an individual dental restoration or appliance.

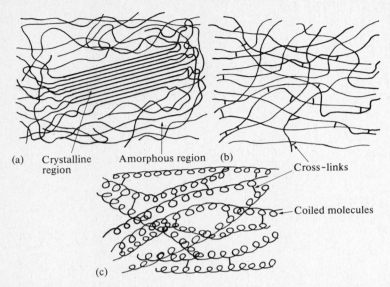

(a)   Crystalline    Amorphous region   (b)
      region                                          Cross-links

                                                      Coiled molecules

(c)

**Fig. 1.10** (a) Molecular arrangement in non-cross-linked thermoplastic; (b) cross-linked resin; (c) molecular arrangement of elastomer.

In contrast, however, fully polymerized or cured resins also have some strong primary valence bonds between the molecules, as in Figure 1.10b. Such a structure is said to be cross-linked and the presence of these strong inter-molecular bonds imparts a greater hardness and rigidity to the material and inhibits the softening on heating. Highly cross-linked resins are called thermosetting resins because, once formed or set, they will not soften; heating tends to decompose rather than soften these resins.

In practice the distinction between thermoplastics and resins is not as clear as this description suggests, for there are different degrees of cross-linking. It is possible with many thermoplastics to add some chemical species which introduce cross-links into the structure. One basic type of polymer may therefore exist as either a flexible, mouldable thermoplastic or a rigid thermosetting resin, depending on the precise molecular structure and whether cross-linking agents have been specifically added.

The vinyl polymers already mentioned are thermoplastics. Typical thermo-setting resins are the epoxy and unsaturated polyester resins, widely used as adhesives. Although polymethyl methacrylate is a vinyl thermoplastic, it can be moulded and cured in much the same way as these resins. It is, in fact, widely referred to as acrylic resin although it does soften on heating. The dental applications of this material are numerous and are discussed in detail in Chapter 11.

*Elastomers*

One final type of polymeric structure that has to be considered is the elastomer. In the polymer structure shown in Figure 1.10a the molecules are not always arranged in a straight line but are curved in places. Such a geometry allows the molecules to be straightened when a force is applied with the result that these plastics deform quite readily. Some polymers, however, have molecules that are even more curved and they may, in fact, be coiled, as shown in Figure 1.10c. In this case the molecules can be stretched very large amounts by a simple uncoiling. This gives a classical rubbery behaviour and these materials are known as rubbers or elastomers. Polyisoprene is the basis of natural rubber and a number of synthetic polymers may also adopt this molecular configuration. A certain degree of cross-linking may be achieved in these elastomers and the properties can be varied very significantly by the addition of cross-linking agents. Natural rubber provides a very good example of this as polyisoprene exists as a liquid. This may be cross-linked by the use of sulphur atoms in the vulcanization process to give rubber with its characteristic elastic properties, but further addition of sulphur produces less elastic but harder solids as the molecular uncoiling and sliding is inhibited, yielding ebonite and vulcanite.

COMPOSITION OF POLYMER-BASED MATERIALS

Polymers are very rarely used in pure form. Instead they are usually compounded with various other substances which confer specific properties to the end-product. Thus the plastic, resin, or elastomer may consist of:

**a** the polymer, either as a homopolymer or co-polymer,

**b** some residual monomer. Most curing processes do not go to completion so that a small amount of the monomer may remain unreacted. These traces of monomer may have a significant influence on the properties, as noted later,

**c** catalysts and other species involved in the polymerization process,

**d** additives to confer resistance to degradation, such as antioxidants, ultra-violet light absorbers, and heat stabilizers,

**e** additives such as plasticizers to improve mechanical properties,

**f** fillers, either to improve the strength or simply to reduce costs.

The additives mentioned above will be discussed at the appropriate places later in this chapter.

## Metallic materials

Metals, as already noted, consist of aggregates of positive ions, called atoms for convenience, regularly arranged in a crystalline structure permeated by a cloud of free electrons. A piece of metal very rarely exists as a single crystal but rather as an aggregate of very small crystals. Although the structure within each crystal is the same, the orientation of the layers of atoms in each case is different. The size and shape of these individual crystals, or grains as they are usually called, may vary considerably and can have a profound influence on the mechanical properties. There is no upper limit to their size as one grain may theoretically constitute the whole solid, giving a single crystal. Sometimes metals such as zinc and aluminium can have grains quite visible to the naked eye, and often several centimetres in diameter. More usually the grains are much less than a millimetre in diameter. The grain structure of a metal is illustrated diagrammatically in Figure 1.11. Naturally all the grains have to meet up with their neighbours and this places some restriction on their form. At sites where the different orientations meet, called grain boundaries, there is an inevitable loss of atomic order.

ALLOYS

For reasons discussed later, pure metals, consisting of the atoms of one element only, are rarely used as structural materials. Instead, materials are used that contain more than one element. The additional elements are usually, although not always, metallic themselves. Provided metallic elements constitute by far the greatest proportion of the aggregate, the structure will still be metallic in nature. Such a material is called an alloy. Most of the metallic materials in common use are alloys, for example brass (copper and zinc), bronze (copper and tin), and steel (iron and carbon). Several alloys are used in dentistry, including the amalgams, produced by alloying mercury with some other elements, alloys of gold with silver and copper, and alloys of cobalt and chromium. Frequently alloys will contain many different elements, each of which is added for a specific reason, usually concerned with the mechanical properties.

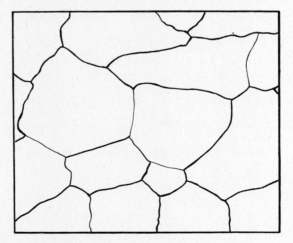

**Fig. 1.11** Grain structure of a metal.

The addition of a second element to a metal will naturally affect the structure, to an extent that will depend on the difference between the elements involved. Considering first the situation with two metals which are very similar in terms of their position in the Periodic Table, their crystal structure, and especially their atomic size, the atoms of one element may simply 'dissolve' in the lattice of the other element by a substitution process. Thus gold and silver, very similar elements, are mutually soluble over the whole range of composition from 100 per cent gold to 100 per cent silver. In an alloy of 90 per cent gold, 10 per cent silver, for example, 10 per cent of the sites in the gold lattice will be occupied by silver, as illustrated in Figure 1.12a. When atoms dissolve in a crystal lattice the result is called a solution and if, as in this case, atoms simply replace each other in the lattice, it is said to be a substitutional solid solution. In nearly all cases the distribution of the different atoms in a solid solution will be entirely random. There is a very important exception to this rule which is of great significance in dental gold alloys and is discussed at some length in Chapter 8.

Sometimes alloys are formed between elements of grossly dissimilar atomic size, for example when a non-metal of small atomic size, such as carbon or nitrogen, is added to a metal of larger atomic size. In this case, instead of the small atoms substituting for the large ones in the space lattice, they occupy the small spaces or interstices between the atoms (Fig. 1.12b). If all of the atoms are held in solution the structure is called an interstitial solid solution.

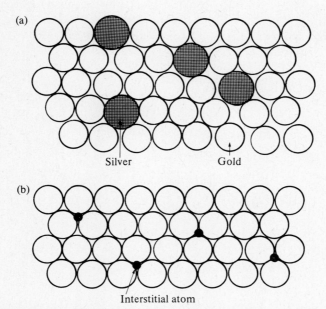

**Fig. 1.12** (a) Substitutional solid solution (note the distortion of the lattice caused by the few larger atoms); (b) interstitial solid solution.

PHASE DIAGRAMS AND MULTI-PHASE SYSTEMS

When there is complete solid solubility over the whole range of composition in an alloy, the microstructure, which is that structure discernable under a microscope, is the same as for a pure metal. This means that only one type of structure is seen, the solid solution of one element in the other. It is, however, relatively rare for two elements to display complete mutual solubility and more usually they show only partial solid solubility. This arises because the different atoms added must inevitably disrupt the lattice and increase its internal energy. This happens when (a) the atoms are of quite different sizes, (b) when the crystal structures of the two elements are different, or (c) when the elements are from different groups of the Periodic Table. Under these circumstances, different structures may be formed. In this context, structures within a material which are characterized by their composition and crystallographic form are called phases. In the case of complete solid solution, only one phase is stable across the whole compositional range, the crystal structure being the same irrespective of the alloy composition. When there is only partial solid solubility, two or more phases may be present.

The easiest way to understand which phases are stable in an alloy is to study the phase diagram for that system. Phase diagrams, otherwise known as constitutional or equilibrium diagrams, are plans which have temperature plotted on the vertical axis and composition plotted on the horizontal axis and which show the conditions under which phases may be stable.

Figure 1.13 shows the phase diagram of an alloy system such as gold–silver (labelled A and B) which forms a complete solid solution. This is a very simple phase diagram and it shows that only one phase, which may be called

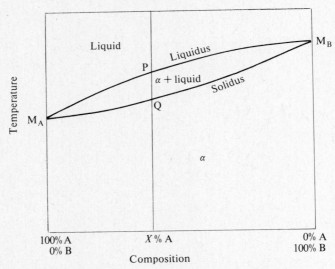

**Fig. 1.13** Phase diagram of alloy system showing complete solid solution.

the α phase, is stable over the whole compositional range at all temperatures below the melting-point. The other important feature shown by this diagram is the range of temperature over which an alloy melts. Two curved lines join the melting-points of the individual elements ($M_A$ and $M_B$), the upper line being called the liquidus and the lower the solidus. Above the liquidus, the alloy is completely liquid. For the composition indicated by the vertical line through $[A] = X$ per cent, the alloy, on cooling, will start to solidify at the point labelled P but will not be completely solid until the temperature has reached Q. In between these points, the alloy is partly liquid and partly solid. Thus alloys melt over a range of temperature whereas pure metals have a well-defined melting-point. This is important in the behaviour of alloys on casting.

If two metals displayed complete insolubility on alloying, the phase diagram would be as shown in Figure 1.14. Below the horizontal line EFG, the alloy consists of a mixture of two phases which are quite simply the elements A and B. This structure is exactly analagous to the dispersion produced when two immiscible liquids, such as oil and water, are mixed, for the two phases are quite separate and easily identified. In this situation the solidus is a straight line. The liquidus, on the other hand, drops from each of the melting-points and actually coincides with the solidus at point F. This point is called the eutectic point. It is important to note that this eutectic composition has the lowest melting-point of all alloy compositions and is often much lower than the melting-point of either of the constituent metals. This has an important practical value in the consideration of solders used for joining metals together, where melting-points lower than those of the metals to be joined are needed.

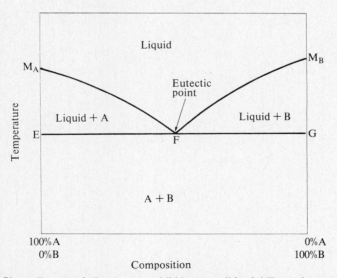

**Fig. 1.14** Phase diagram of alloy system exhibiting no solid solubility and a eutectic point.

In general terms it is also important to note that adding one element to another often, although by no means invariably, lowers the liquidus temperature and this is often the sole reason why small quantities of some metals are added to casting alloys, as noted in Chapters 8 and 10.

In the case of partial solid solubility a slightly more complex phase diagram results since, as shown in Figure 1.15, there are areas showing stability of the two different solid solutions, usually called $\alpha$ and $\beta$, adjacent to the vertical axes. However, all other features are the same, a composition in the middle of the range having a mixture of $\alpha$ and $\beta$ phases just as an alloy in the previous example consisted of a mixture of pure A and B. In this case the $\alpha$ phase represents the lattice of A with just a few atoms of B in solution, while the $\beta$ phase is the lattice of B atoms with some A atoms in solution.

One final type of phase diagram must be discussed, and that is for alloys in which intermetallic phases are formed. It will be obvious from the above examples that the phases exist over a range of compositions where there are no specific proportions of the individual elements. In some cases, this is not so and a phase which approximates to a very specific chemical formula may exist over a very narrow range of composition. Such a phase is called an intermetallic compound. The silver–tin system provides a good example of this kind of alloy, the phase diagram being shown in Figure 1.16. This alloy is particularly important since it is used to react with mercury to form dental amalgam. In practice the composition of the alloy is chosen such that it exists largely as the intermetallic phase $Ag_3Sn$, known as the $\gamma$ phase. This is discussed fully in Chapter 4.

In all the examples given so far, only two elements have been involved.

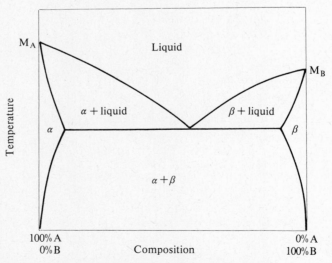

**Fig. 1.15** Phase diagram of alloy system with partial solid solubility.

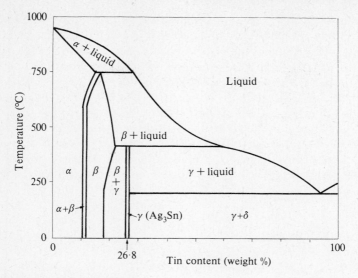

**Fig. 1.16** Silver–tin phase diagram.

Such two-element systems are called binary alloys. In practice, as mentioned earlier, alloys often involve many more elements. Clearly it is not possible to draw phase diagrams in the same way, but assessments can be made of the phases that will be stable under various conditions. Since the alloying additions are often present in small amounts they usually modify only the limits of the compositions over which the various phases are stable. Steels provide a very good example of alloys that often contain more than two elements. Steels are, by definition, alloys of iron and carbon. Carbon forms an interstitial solid solution with iron but the limit of solubility is very low and iron carbide, $Fe_3C$, an intermetallic compound, is readily produced. Very many different steels are available depending on the other elements present. Chromium, molybdenum, nickel, vanadium, and niobium are all important alloying additions. Chromium and nickel are especially important in the context of the stainless steels used in dentistry, as discussed in Chapters 10 and 13.

### Ceramics and glasses

Ceramics are compounds of metallic and non-metallic elements. They are primarily based on the ionic bonds formed between the two quite different types of atom. As noted earlier, some ceramics also display covalent bonding, especially if carbon, silicon, or other elements near the centre of the Periodic Table are involved. Silicon is a major constituent of many important ceramics.

Ceramics are usually crystalline solids; some exist in nature as minerals of single crystal form where the crystallinity is manifest by a highly regular external form. However, the internal crystal structure is not so simple as in the metals where atoms are either of identical or very similar size. A ceramic has negatively charged ions (anions) and positively charged ions (cations) which are often of significantly different size. Thus, although crystal structures similar to the f.c.c. and b.c.c. structures observed in metals are formed in ceramics, often more than one atom occupies each site on the lattice. If each atom of the sodium chloride lattice shown in Figure 1.4 is considered individually, the structure is a simple cube. If, however, the sodium and chloride ions are considered together, a close-packed f.c.c. lattice can be visualized with the anions at each lattice point and the smaller cations occupying the interstitial positions (Fig. 1.17). Many simple ceramics, including zinc oxide which is widely used in dentistry, have this type of structure.

SILICA AND SILICATES

As noted above the element silicon forms the basis for many ceramics, some of which are important in dental materials.

Silica, $SiO_2$, has a simple chemical formula, but is complex in terms of its crystal structure since it can exist in at least four different forms, quartz, cristobalite, tridymite, and fused silica. Silicon has a valency of four and the covalent bonds that it forms are directed towards the corners of a tetrahedron. Combination with oxygen, for example, gives the $SiO_4$ tetrahedron shown in Figure 1.18a. Since oxygen has a valency of two, each oxygen atom in this structure has an unpaired electron, only one of the two being required for sharing with the silicon. Each oxygen atom is, therefore, free to combine with another atom. In doing so, macromolecular structures

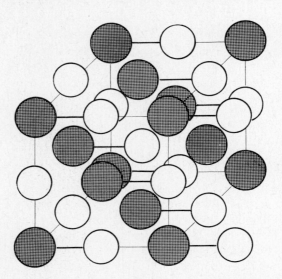

**Fig. 1.17** Face centred cubic lattice of sodium chloride with anions at each lattice point and cations in interstitial spaces.

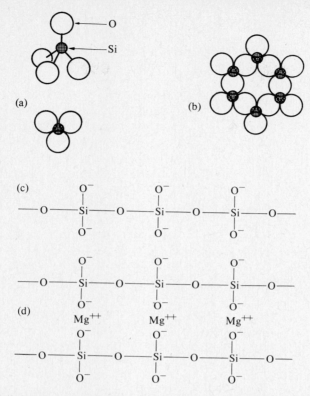

**Fig. 1.18** (a) SiO$_4$ tetrahedron showing side and plan view; (b) formation of SiO$_2$ by linking of tetrahedra; (c) SiO$_4$ chain structure; (d) silicate structure.

may be produced, the nature of which depends on the type of atom reacted with the oxygen. Silica represents the simplest case as each oxygen atom combines with another silicon atom, which itself will be the centre of another tetrahedron, as shown in Figure 1.18b. Since these tetrahedra may be arranged differently in space, different crystalline forms of silica are possible. This is important for the use of silica in materials used for the preparation of moulds for casting metals, as discussed in Chapter 10.

Not all the oxygen atoms need be coupled to two silicon atoms in this way and various anions may also be involved. If half of the oxygen atoms join two silicon atoms then an SiO$_4$ chain structure is produced, the structure of which is repeated two-dimensionally in Figure 1.18c. This is clearly quite similar to the organic polymeric structure except that there is a facility for ionic bonding to take place at each of the O$^-$ points. The type of structure produced in this way, called a silicate, is shown in Figure 1.18d, where cations form the ionic bonds with the oxygen anions. One or more cations may be involved, giving rise either to simple silicates, such as sodium silicate and magnesium silicate, or more complex compounds such as lithium aluminium silicate.

Several silicates are important in dentistry, and they are usually very complex structures. Dental porcelain, for example, as described in Chapter 9, is made by fusing silica with feldspars, which are substances based on the silicate structure but with some of the silicon ions replaced by aluminium ions, the difference in charge of these ions being balanced by the incorporation of sodium, calcium, or potassium ions. Thus feldspars are of the form $NaAlSi_3O_8$ or $CaAl_2Si_2O_8$. As discussed in Chapter 5, silicate cements used as filling materials are based on aluminosilicates, which consist of a network of $SiO_4$ and $AlO_4^-$ tetrahedra, with cations such as $Al^{3+}$, $Ca^{2+}$, and $Na^+$ incorporated to balance the negative charge.

### GLASSES

Not all ceramics are crystalline and, indeed, some ceramic structures may exist as either a crystalline or amorphous solid depending on the conditions. Silica provides a good example of this. It has already been mentioned that the $SiO_4$ tetrahedra may be arranged differently to give the various crystalline forms of quartz, crystobalite, and tridymite. A regular arrangement of these tetrahedra to give a crystalline form is shown in Figure 1.19a. If these tetrahedra are arranged randomly, as shown in Figure 1.19b, there is no regular structure and the material is amorphous. Such materials are called glasses. Most silicate structures can be prepared as either crystalline ceramics or glasses, the latter state usually being achieved by incorporating large cations into the silicate structures to prevent their ordered arrangement. Strictly speaking, dental porcelains are glasses rather than crystalline ceramics.

### Composites

As outlined earlier, composite materials are made up from two or more

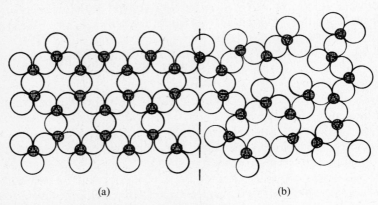

(a)                                    (b)

**Fig. 1.19** (a) Crystalline silica; (b) amorphous silica.

substances with quite different structures and properties. The ceramic–polymer composite is the most widely encountered although there is no reason why any other combination should not be used. Usually one component is prepared as a powder or as thin fibres and dispersed in the other component. The structure and properties of the individual components are not altered and the properties of the composite reflect those of the individual substances. Ceramic–polymer composites are extensively used as filling materials as described in Chapter 5. Since composite materials are usually developed in order to improve mechanical properties, they will be considered in more detail later in this chapter.

## PREPARATION OF MATERIALS FOR DENTAL USE

Although it is not necessary here to describe processing techniques in detail, some very important principles relating to the preparation and clinical handling of dental materials need to be discussed at this point.

There are two main types of preparation technique in dental technology. In the first a material has to be applied to some part of the mouth, where it has to adapt very closely to the tissues and then set. In all cases, the material has to be sufficiently fluid on insertion into the mouth to allow its ready adaptation to the tissues. It must then set, in a clinically acceptable time under intra-oral conditions, to give a solid, the desirable characteristics of which depend on the application. The main examples here are the materials used for fillings, linings, impressions, and cementation.

Secondly, processing may take place in the laboratory where an appliance or restoration has to be fabricated for subsequent intra-oral use. In these cases, more generalized construction techniques, often using high temperatures and mechanical forces may be used. High dimensional accuracy of the product is essential whatever the method chosen.

### Plastics, resins, and rubbers

Some of the principles of polymer processing have already been mentioned in the discussion of polymer structures. Thermoplastics are usually shaped by moulding processes performed on the fully polymerized material. These processes generally require the application of heat and pressure so that they are relevant only to the second category defined above. Even then, the techniques require relatively complex equipment which is not generally available in dental laboratories. This is discussed further in Chapter 11.

Techniques of moulding that can be carried out before curing the polymer *in situ* are far more applicable to dentistry. In between the extremes of a low molecular monomer, which is often a low viscosity fluid, and a high molecular weight polymer which is a solid, there is an intermediate stage, the 'dough stage', at which the material behaves as a very viscous fluid which is easily mouldable. The ideal situation is, therefore, to have a polymer system which can be easily prepared in this viscous fluid state and which then allows

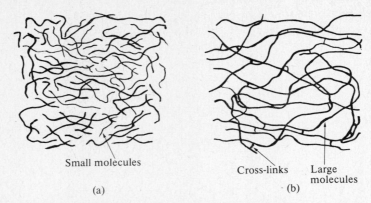

Small molecules

Cross-links   Large molecules

(a)   (b)

**Fig. 1.20** Processes of cross-linking and further polymerization in curing of a resin (a) low molecular weight polymer; (b) after cross-linking and further polymerization.

suitable time for manipulation before curing. This is usually done by producing a polymer of relatively low molecular weight (Fig. 1.20a) and, by the appropriate use of catalysts and cross-linking agents, inducing further polymerization and cross-linking. This gives the higher molecular weight solid, as shown in Figure 1.20b. The elastomeric impression materials provide a good example.

It is possible to achieve the same results with the few thermoplastic materials that polymerize at, or near, mouth temperature, such as methyl methacrylate. In this case the dough stage is achieved by the mixing of a powder of high molecular weight with some monomer, when the curing takes place by the polymerization of the monomer phase. This type of process is widely used, both for the *in situ* curing of filling materials (Chapter 5) and the laboratory preparation of dentures (Chapter 11).

One very important point to remember concerning the polymerization or cross-linking of a polymer within a mould or cavity is that these processes are usually accompanied by a degree of shrinkage. This polymerization contraction arises from the transition from a collection of individual small molecules to much larger, tightly knit structures; primary valence bonds bring molecules closer together than do secondary valence bonds. This means that if a material is placed in a cavity or mould and cured *in situ*, it may shrink away from the cavity walls. As discussed in Chapter 5, this is of great clinical significance and attempts have to be made both to reduce the total shrinkage by appropriate choice of the polymer system and to minimize its effect.

### Ceramics

Ceramics are difficult materials to fabricate. Moulding of fused ceramics is virtually impossible because of their high melting-points, and mechanical methods, such as machining or forming, which are so suitable for many metals, are inapplicable because ceramics are hard and brittle.

As with plastics, two types of preparation technique may be used, one in which the ceramic structure is prepared first and then shaped and the second where the final structure is produced *in situ* after shaping a relatively fluid form of the material. In the first case, the ceramic particles, usually held together by an appropriate binder, are heated, to bond them together. If this bonding is achieved by diffusion processes, where there is no fusion of the ceramic at all, the method is called sintering. Often some degree of fusion takes place to assist the bonding; usually this is achieved by heating to a temperature between the solidus and liquidus shown on the appropriate phase diagram. The process of heating the ceramic to do this is termed 'firing'. Dental porcelain is used in this way, as described in Chapter 9.

In the second technique a ceramic may act in its capacity as a basic or amphoteric substance and react with an acid. In this way a new type of composite ceramic structure is produced and, by careful choice of constituents, this can be achieved under the conditions within the mouth. Thus certain types of lining, filling, impression, and cementing materials are prepared for intra-oral use by this method. The ceramic used is either an oxide, such as zinc oxide, or an aluminosilicate glass, while the acids are usually weak solutions of phosphoric acid, organic polyacids such as polyacrylic acid, or eugenol and related compounds, which behave as acids. Details of these materials are given in the appropriate sections, but it is important to note that the function of the reaction product in all these cases is to act as a binder for the unreacted portions of the original ceramic particles, which are usually very much stronger. Thus the ideal reactions are those that do not go to completion but rather are confined to the surfaces of the ceramic particles and, as shown in Figure 1.21, allow the formation of just sufficient reaction product to bind the surfaces together in the required shape.

### Metals and alloys

There are only two situations in which a metal or alloy is prepared directly in the mouth. The first and most important of these concerns the use of dental

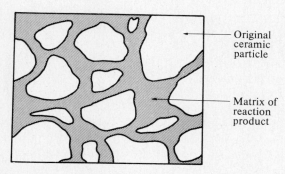

**Fig. 1.21** Structure of ceramic produced by acid–base reaction.

amalgam, primarily as a filling material. This relies on the fact that mercury is liquid at room temperature and is able to react with various metal particles to produce a solid alloy. The whole of Chapter 4 is concerned with this application; it should be noted here, however, that the principle of the reaction is the same as that for the ceramic–acid reactions just described, for the function of the reaction product is again that of binding strong particles together. The second method of preparation relies on the fact that pure gold foil can be made to bond to itself at mouth temperature so that a cavity may be filled layer upon layer with this metal. This is a very special example of the welding processes that are described below. Cohesive gold, as this material is generally called, is used only rarely now and is discussed briefly in Chapter 8.

Metals can be fabricated outside the mouth in numerous ways although again these may be divided into two categories, the casting and the forming methods. Quite frequently it is also necessary to join separately fabricated parts of an appliance and this is achieved by either welding or soldering.

CASTING

Casting involves pouring molten metal into a mould to produce the required shape. The technical details of casting are covered in Chapter 10. The quality of a casting, as judged from its shape, size, surface appearance, freedom from porosity, and so on, is largely governed by the technical expertise. The microstructure is determined by the composition of the metal or alloy and the manner in which it is cooled. Several features of this microstructure have an important influence on the resulting properties.

The process of solidification in a metal, that is the transition from liquid to solid state, requires the presence of nuclei of solidification (or nuclei of crystallization). It is possible for a metal to exist as a liquid well below its melting-point if no nuclei are present. Chance collisions of atoms within the metal itself may provide these, but far more commonly particles of extraneous matter act as nuclei. In Figure 1.22a, a section through a molten metal with just one or two nuclei is shown. Once nuclei are present and the temperature drops below the melting-point, then atoms will be deposited onto the nuclei, forming their normal crystallographic structure (Fig. 1.22b). These solid areas grow into the liquid phase until all the liquid has frozen (Fig. 1.22c), each nucleus of solidification, therefore, giving rise to an individual grain.

It will be appreciated from this discussion that the larger the number of nuclei present, the greater will be the final number of grains and hence the smaller will be the grain size (Fig. 1.22d and e). This is very important for, as noted in the section on mechanical properties later, a casting with a small grain size tends to be stronger than one with a large grain size. This can be particularly significant in dental appliances, where cross-sections are thin and may be cast with just one or two grains. It is possible to add components to the alloy specifically to act as nuclei of crystallization. For example,

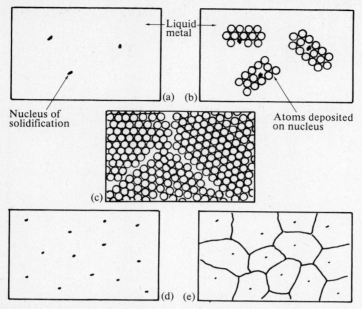

**Fig. 1.22** Solidification of a metal (a) few nuclei; (b) crystal growth into liquid phase; (c) complete solidification; (d) large number of nuclei in liquid; (e) corresponding small grain size.

molybdenum is added to the cobalt–chromium alloys used for partial denture construction for this purpose, as discussed in Chapter 10.

A binary alloy system in which the two metals are mutually soluble over the whole range of composition, but which have very different melting-points, is shown in Figure 1.23. As an alloy of 50 per cent A, 50 per cent B, cools from the liquid phase, it will start to solidify when the temperature drops below the liquidus at L. At this temperature, metal B would, if pure, be solid, while metal A would still be completely liquid. The first solid to form therefore consists largely of metal B. The composition of this first solid is represented by the intersection between the horizontal line drawn from L and the solidus, that is at S. As solidification proceeds, the solid gets less and less rich in B, and proportionately richer in A until the last liquid to freeze is largely A. Thus the casting may have a very heterogeneous structure. Since the solid forms a crystal, the atoms tend to be deposited along close-packed lines in the space lattice so that a partially formed crystal will have the appearance shown in Figure 1.24a, the arms of the crystals being termed dendrites. It is these first dendrites that are rich in B, whilst the last liquid to freeze will be located in the interdendritic and intergranular spaces, as shown in Figure 1.24b. This heterogeneous structure is said to be cored, and it is relevant to both the mechanical properties and the corrosion aspects

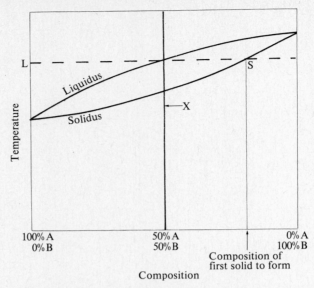

**Fig. 1.23** Phase diagram of alloy showing complete solubility, demonstrating origin of coring.

as discussed later. Clearly alloy systems that have a large temperature difference between the solidus and liquidus are most susceptible to coring.

It is possible to remove a cored structure by a simple heating process. Coring normally arises when the cooling is relatively quick so that the atoms do not have time to diffuse through the lattice to form a homogeneous or uniform structure. If, after casting, the alloy is heated to a point X just below the solidus (Fig. 1.23), this diffusion will take place. Heat treatment processes are normally referred to as annealing and this particular process is called an homogenizing anneal. They are encountered quite frequently in the discussion of dental alloys.

FORMING

Forming processes involve the permanent deformation of standard shapes by an appropriate mechanical method. The shapes normally encountered in dentistry are wires and sheets and their use is largely confined to the construction of orthodontic appliances (Chapter 13) and stainless steel denture bases (Chapter 10). These methods depend entirely on the mechanical properties of the metals and are, therefore, discussed later in this chapter.

JOINING OF METALS

Metals are usually joined by the application of heat or pressure, or both. Sometimes the temperature used may be sufficient to melt, or partially melt the metals or alloys to be joined, light pressure between the surfaces causing

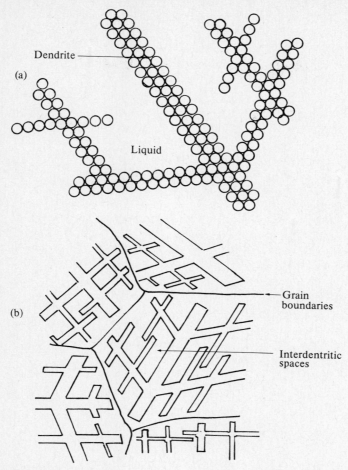

**Fig. 1.24** (a) Formation of dendrites; (b) last liquid freezing in interdendritic and inter-granular spaces.

fusion. Such techniques that involve the direct bonding of metal surfaces without the use of a low melting-point intermediary compound are called welding processes. Sometimes, as mentioned earlier, pressure between two surfaces at low temperature may be sufficient to give welding, but this is rare.

Alternatively, metals may be bonded by soldering. In this, a special alloy called a solder is used as an adhesive (as discussed in Chapter 2). A solder has a lower melting-point range than either of the metals to be joined and the application of heat fuses the solder, causes it to wet the metal surfaces and, on solidifying, bonds them together. Clearly different solders have to be used for different metals. Quite frequently they are eutectic alloys with correspondingly low melting-points. Soldering is discussed in Chapters 8 and 10 in relation to gold and in Chapter 13 in the context of orthodontic appliances.

## MECHANICAL PROPERTIES OF MATERIALS

The mechanical properties of a material relate to its behaviour under the influence of forces. They show how much a material will deform, how and when it will break, what happens when it is dropped, how hard it is, and so on.

Earlier in this chapter, the concept of equilibrium spacings between atoms in a solid was introduced. If a material is at rest, as shown for a perfect array of atoms in Figure 1.25a, the atoms will be in their equilibrium positions. The application of a mechanical force will tend to displace these atoms from the low energy positions. In Figure 1.25b, for example, the atoms are being pulled apart by a force. The energy put into the system by the mechanical force is used to move the atoms to higher energy positions. The mechanical properties indicate to what extent this displacement can occur.

### STRESS AND STRAIN

There are two fundamental parameters associated with the behaviour of materials subjected to mechanical forces that must be clearly defined at this stage. These are stress and strain. Figure 1.26a shows a uniform rod of cross-sectional area $A_1$ and length $L_1$. If a force $F$ acts along the rod, then the rod will extend to a length $L_2$ and the area will be reduced to $A_2$, as in Figure 1.26b. Stress is a measure of the force acting per unit of cross-sectional area.

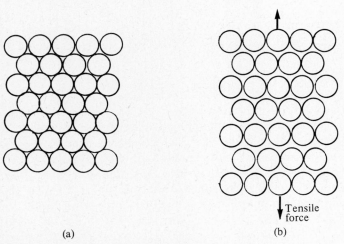

(a)                                                    (b)

**Fig. 1.25** (a) Atoms at equilibrium spacing; (b) atoms pulled apart by force.

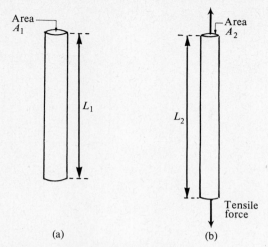

**Fig. 1.26** Extension of rod when acted upon by a force $F$.

That is:

$$\text{Stress} = \frac{\text{Force}}{\text{Cross-sectional area}} = \frac{F}{A_1}.$$

The unit of force is the newton and area is measured in square metres so that the units of stress are newtons per square metre, or $N/m^2$.

Strain is a measure of the amount of deformation that takes place when a force is exerted. It may be measured in terms of the change in length, or cross-sectional area and is related to the original dimension, and expressed as a percentage. Thus:

$$\text{Strain} = \frac{\text{Change in length}}{\text{Original length}} \times 100\% = \frac{L_2 - L_1}{L_1} \times 100\%.$$

Stress and strain are related to unit dimensions and can therefore be used to define the mechanical properties without referring to the actual size of the specimen.

In the example given, the force acts along the length of the rod and is, therefore, a tensile force, giving rise to a tensile stress in the material. This is a very simple stress system and is rarely encountered in dentistry. Figures 1.27(a) and (b) illustrate two other simple stress systems, compressive and shear. In practice stress systems are far more complex and have components of all three types of stress at the same time. It is, however, most simple to consider mechanical properties in terms of one or other of these simple systems, as materials can be more easily compared in this way.

ELASTIC DEFORMATION

In the example shown in Figure 1.25, atoms are pulled apart under the

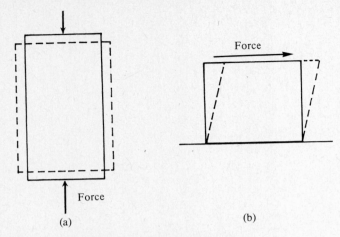

**Fig. 1.27** (a) Compressive and (b) shear stress systems.

influence of a tensile stress. The atoms do not move their positions relative to one another but merely become displaced from their equilibrium position by virtue of the applied energy. Under these circumstances, if the force is removed, the atoms will return to their original positions. This deformation is therefore reversible or elastic. All materials deform reversibly on the application of low loads. If a graph of stress against strain is plotted, the initial part of the curve corresponding to this elastic deformation is a straight line (Fig. 1.28a). Thus, as the stress on a material increases, the strain increases in proportion. The slope of the curve in this region numerically equals the stress divided by strain and is referred to as the modulus of elasticity or,

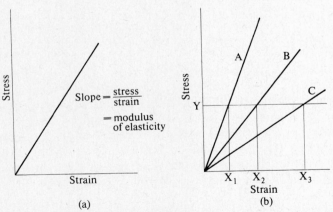

**Fig. 1.28** (a) Elastic region of stress–strain curve; (b) slopes of stress–strain curve for materials of different moduli.

in the case of a tensile stress, Young's modulus. Since this is a measure of the amount of energy needed to pull atoms apart, which will depend on the nature of the atoms in the material, the modulus is an inherent property or a constant for a material. Each material will have its own elastic modulus and it is important to note that this refers to the ease with which a material deforms elastically. It has nothing to do with the strength of the material. In Figure 1.28b the elastic region in the stress–strain curves for three materials are shown. Material A has a high elastic modulus. This means that for a given value of the stress $(Y)$, the strain $(X_1)$ is only small. Ceramics usually have very high moduli and are, therefore, very rigid. Material B has a slightly lower modulus, giving a larger strain $(X_2)$ at stress $Y$, and is less rigid. Metals generally have slightly lower moduli than ceramics. Material C has a low elastic modulus, displaying high strain $(X_3)$ at the stress level $Y$, and is very flexible and easily deformed. Polymeric materials come into this general category although their behaviour is a little different from this simple model, as explained later. Examples of the elastic moduli for some materials are given in Table 1.1. Since a modulus is defined as stress/strain and since strain has no units, the modulus is given in units of stress, that is $N/m^2$.

**Table 1.1** Elastic moduli of various materials ($GN/m^2$)

| | |
|---|---|
| Tungsten carbide | 690 |
| Alumina | 350 |
| Cobalt–chromium alloy | 220 |
| Stainless steel | 210 |
| Titanium | 120 |
| Gold alloys | 100 |
| Enamel | 48 |
| Dental amalgam | 21 |
| Silicate cement | 21 |
| Dentine | 14 |
| Polymethyl methacrylate | 3·5 |
| Polyethylene | 0·4 |
| Elastomers (typically) | 0·001 |

PLASTIC DEFORMATION

The atoms shown in the example of Figure 1.25 cannot be pulled apart indefinitely and a stage is reached when no further elastic deformation can take place. One of two things may happen at this point. First, the material may fracture; that is the bonds between the atoms are broken completely, the energy applied to any one inter-atomic bond being greater than the energy of the bond itself. Alternatively, the material may deform irreversibly or plastically. In this case some of the atoms have to move to entirely new positions, as indicated in Figure 1.29. In this way there is an overall shape change but inter-atomic distances are kept within the limits experienced

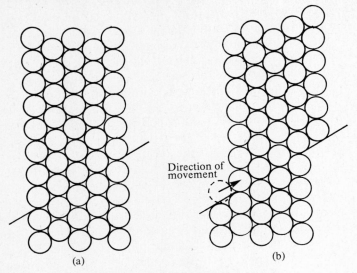

**Fig. 1.29** Atomic movements to give plastic deformation.

during elastic deformation. Typical stress–strain curves showing elastic and plastic deformation are shown in Figure 1.30(a) and (b). Once plastic deformation starts, the strain increases faster than the stress and the plot is no longer linear. There may be either a gradual or abrupt change of shape. In curves of type (a), which is typical of many metals and alloys, the change is gradual and it is often difficult to decide where the change starts to take place. The terms 'elastic limit', which is the stress level at which elastic deformation is no longer possible, and the 'limit of proportionality', which is the point at which the curve ceases to be linear, are used in this context. Although these points need not be exactly the same, they are usually taken to be identical and are therefore used synonymously to mean the point at which plastic deformation starts. The elastic–plastic transition is defined in terms of the 0·1 per cent proof stress. This is the stress at which 0·1 per cent plastic strain is achieved and is determined as the point of intersection of the stress–strain curve with the line, parallel to the initial slope of the curve and passing through the 0·1 per cent point on the strain axis, as shown in Figure 1.30a.

The point on curve (b) which corresponds to the sudden onset of plastic deformation is called the yield-point. This is seen in materials where it is difficult for plastic deformation to start but where, once atoms have started to move to new positions, they do so very readily and produce a large plastic strain all at once. Steels commonly display a yield-point.

Plastic deformation was represented in Figure 1.29 as the simple moving of atoms from one position to another. The process is, of course, more complex

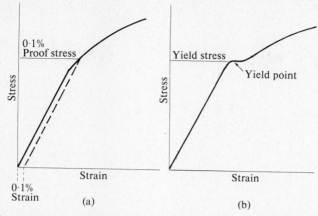

**Fig. 1.30** Stress-strain curves for elastic and plastic deformation showing (a) gradual transition; (b) yield-point.

than this. Considering a fairly symmetrical crystalline structure, for example one of the close-packed structures of Figure 1.6, the atoms under stress tend to slide over one another along the planes of densest packing. In any one crystal there will be several of these planes. However, this slipping does not take place all at once, but instead, first one atom moves to a new position and this movement is then carried along the layer such that one atom moves at a time, as shown in Figure 1.31. This means that there is a local disruption of the crystal lattice around the atom that is moving. This disruption is called a dislocation which is said to move along the crystal to produce the plastic deformation.

If many dislocations moved along the same plane in the same direction in a single crystal, then the situation shown in Figure 1.32a would result. In practice, however, single crystals are rarely encountered and crystal lattices are rarely perfect. The movement of dislocations is, therefore, hindered by the presence of grain boundaries and phase boundaries. If dislocations moving along a 'slip plane' meet some barrier, they tend to pile up at this barrier until the stress concentration produced becomes large enough to start new dislocations moving on the other side. Similarly, dislocations moving on planes that intersect interfere with each other. Thus plastic deformation in a polycrystalline material involves the movement of many dislocations, few of which travel far, and the generation of a distorted internal structure, as shown in Figure 1.32b.

FRACTURE: BRITTLENESS AND DUCTILITY

Whether a material is able to deform plastically or not, the ultimate fate on increasing the stress level is fracture, or the separation of the specimen into two or more fragments. In the case of a material that cannot deform

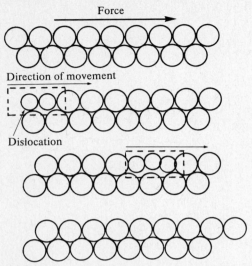

**Fig. 1.31** Dislocation movement along slip plane from left to right, producing plastic deformation.

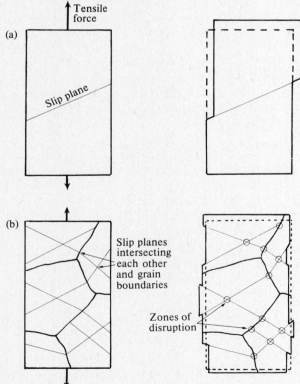

**Fig. 1.32** (a) Slip in a single crystal; (b) distorted structure arising from dislocation movement in polycrystalline aggregate.

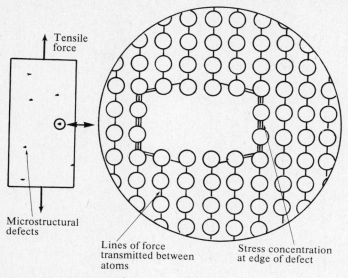

Tensile force

Microstructural defects

Lines of force transmitted between atoms

Stress concentration at edge of defect

**Fig. 1.33** Imperfections in a material leading to stress concentrations.

plastically, fracture takes place when the stress placed on inter-atomic bonds exceeds their own strength. In practice this stress level is far lower than the theoretical bond strength. This arises because no material has a perfect structure and imperfections occur on the atomic scale (Fig. 1.33). These imperfections may be cracks on the surface or flaws in the interior. Since the stress cannot be transmitted across the area of discontinuity, the atoms around the edge are subjected to a stress much higher than the nominal stress. Therefore bonds are easily broken at the site of stress concentrations around defects. Once a few bonds are broken in these materials, fracture propagates catastrophically since the stress concentration gets progressively worse. A material which fractures in this way without exhibiting any plastic deformation is said to be brittle.

The presence of small defects in a material that can deform does not have the same effect since the atoms near the edge of the crack tip can move and actually lower the stress concentration. However, as more and more plastic deformation takes place, the structure becomes increasingly congested with dislocations. This means that, as deformation proceeds, further deformation becomes more difficult; this is the reason for the upward slope on the stress–strain curve rather than a continuous horizontal line from the elastic limit. It also means that eventually the structure becomes so distorted that further deformation is not possible and that the material will fracture.

A material which is capable of deforming plastically is ductile. Ductility can be quantified in terms of the strain produced at fracture. Brittle materials essentially have zero ductility and their stress–strain curve is similar to that of Figure 1.28a. A very ductile metal may have 50–70 per cent ductility whilst some polymers have ductilities in excess of 500 per cent.

The ability of a material to deform plastically is determined by its structure. Considering highly crystalline ionic or metallic substances first, this is largely controlled by the characteristics of the atoms in juxtaposition and the nature of the inter-atomic bonds. Thus, in a pure metal, any one atom has identical near neighbours and there is no directional bonding. There is, therefore, no restriction on the position of any one atom in the lattice and so pure metals tend to be very ductile. The situation with alloys is more complex and this is discussed in the next section. In the ionic solids, there are two or more ionic species present and these are held together by strong, directional ionic bonds. Movement of ions here is far more difficult, and usually impossible because it would result in a large number of similar ions being forced too close together. Ceramic structures, therefore, usually display no ductility.

Polymers, of course, are held together largely by secondary valence forces between molecules. Applied stress may easily disrupt these inter-molecular bonds so that sliding of molecules over each other can give large plastic deformations. It is here that the concept of the strength of a solid being controlled by the weakest link is readily seen. A spectrum of behaviour can still be seen with polymers, however, for as well as these highly ductile materials there are polymers, such as polymethyl methacrylate, which have large side groups and are unable to crystallize. These groups of atoms also inhibit the molecular sliding so that the materials may be relatively brittle.

STRENGTH

The term 'strength' refers to the stress that is necessary to produce either plastic deformation or fracture in a material. Thus the yield stress, elastic limit, and limit of proportionality are all measures of the strength of a material in relation to its ability to resist permanent deformation. This is a very important parameter for in precision dental work an appliance or restoration that deforms permanently during use, and therefore takes up another shape, will not usually perform its desired function to maximum effect. The maximum stress a material can sustain before fracturing is called the ultimate tensile strength, which is measured in units of $N/m^2$. Generally alloys have the highest strengths of all materials, ceramics being too brittle and polymers deforming too extensively to give high values.

RESILIENCE, TOUGHNESS, AND IMPACT STRENGTH

The discussion of the mechanical properties so far has assumed that a material is subjected to a slowly increasing force. As usual, the situation in practice is not so simple. In particular stresses may be applied very suddenly and it is necessary to characterize the behaviour of a material under these conditions. The critical factor in determining this behaviour is the ability of the material to absorb energy. A material that can absorb a large amount of mechanical energy will be able to resist a force that is applied to it suddenly. Such a material is said to have a high impact strength, which is measured as the amount of energy that is absorbed before fracture.

The two terms 'resilience' and 'toughness' are related to this absorption of energy. Resilience is a measure of the amount of energy a material can absorb elastically. To be resilient a material must be capable of large amounts of elastic deformation whilst retaining a high elastic limit. Resilience is required in some denture linings, as discussed in Chapter 11. Toughness, on the other hand, refers to the total amount of energy absorbed before fracture and is measured by the total area under the stress–strain curve. A tough material is one that is able to resist both large strains and stresses without fracturing. Clearly the area under both curves 1 and 2 in Figure 1.34 is small even though the former material can withstand high stress and the second displays high ductility. The area under curve 3, and hence the energy to fracture, is the highest and such a material is relatively tough.

The significance of toughness is that it indicates the behaviour to be expected from a material when subjected to high rates of loading. Even some normally ductile materials may fracture at a low load if it is applied suddenly. Under these conditions cracks may open up and propagate through the material faster than plastic deformation can occur. A tough material is one that has the capacity to stop these cracks propagating by absorbing their energy. More will be said of this later in the context of composite materials.

HARDNESS

The hardness of a material is a measure of its resistance to abrasion, indentation, and scratching. It is generally indicative of strength since strong materials usually tend to be hard although hard materials need not necessarily be strong (especially in tension) if they are also brittle. There are many ways

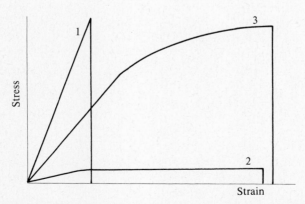

**Fig. 1.34** Toughness. The areas under curves 1 and 2 are relatively small. A material with stress–strain curve 3 is tough.

of measuring hardness but the most usual is by making an indentation on the surface with a standard-shaped diamond, using a standard force, and measuring the extent of the indentation. The hardness is calculated from the indentation geometry and expressed on one of several scales. The most commonly used scale is the Vickers scale in which the hardness is quoted as a Vickers Hardness Number: the higher the number the harder the material.

FATIGUE

If a stress is applied to a material, it may deform or fracture, as outlined above, and a given material may be characterized by typical values of strength and ductility. These values, however, refer to a single application of stress. If a material is subjected to repeated stresses then it may fracture at a value of stress much lower than the normal ultimate tensile strength and often lower than the proof or yield strength. This arises because cracks are able to open up at sites of stress concentration. Initially these cracks may be very small, too small to be of any significance under normal conditions, but the repeated application of the stress causes them to open up and eventually produce failure.

There are several quantities which define the fatigue behaviour of materials. Testing is performed by applying cyclic stresses and noting the number of cycles to failure and repeating this for several different stress levels. A graph of stress (that is, the difference between the highest and the lowest stresses in one cycle) against the number of cycles to failure is plotted, an example being given in Figure 1.35. With some materials (curve (a)) there is a stress below which there is no fatigue failure, whatever the number of cycles. This is often between 30 and 50 per cent of the ultimate tensile strength. Other materials exhibit no fatigue limit (curve (b)). Their behaviour is characterized

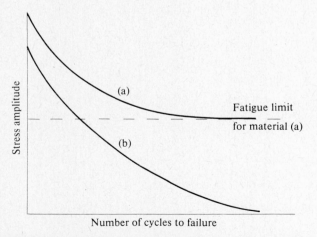

**Fig. 1.35** Fatigue curves, showing the relationship between the stress amplitude and the number of cycles that gives failure for two different materials, (a) and (b).

by the endurance limit which is the stress level that gives failure in a specific number of cycles, usually $10^8$.

Fatigue is important since any dental appliance or restoration is subjected to repeated rather than single stresses. It is also important to note that the stress concentrations that initiate the cracks usually occur at surface defects and that many fatigue fractures are associated with poor surface finish.

TIME-DEPENDENT DEFORMATION

The discussion of stress and strain has implied that if a stress is applied to a material, the associated strain is produced instantaneously. While this is true for many materials it is not always the case and time-dependent deformation may take place.

There are two phenomena to be considered here, which although related, concern different types of material. The first is called viscoelasticity and relates to polymers. This is the slow response of a material to an applied stress such that the strain lags behind the stress. It may take a polymer several seconds to attain the strain that is associated with a stress level that is applied. The term is used because the material is displaying characteristics of a viscous fluid as well as an elastic solid. Viscoelasticity may be relevant to the use of elastomeric impression materials (Chapter 6) and denture soft linings and tissue conditioners (Chapter 11).

Secondly, the phenomenon of creep, or flow, may be observed in some materials. Under the right conditions most materials will continue to deform if the stress is maintained but not increased, after the instantaneous value of the strain has been reached. With metals this is usually apparent only at temperatures close to the melting-point so it is not normally observed at room temperatures. One of the exceptions here is amalgam which has a low melting-point and therefore does display creep behaviour at mouth temperature. The term 'flow' is often used to denote this behaviour, which is discussed in Chapter 4. Dental polymers, and especially waxes, may also flow since they are near to their softening points at mouth temperature. The resulting dimensional changes that take place can cause problems in the preparation of accurate shapes.

## Mechanical properties of dental materials

In this section some of the mechanical properties of different types of dental material are reviewed in order that their behaviour in clinical practice can be related to composition and structure.

METHODS OF TESTING

It is first necessary to mention very briefly the way in which the mechanical properties of dental materials are measured.

Tensile properties may be determined in the same way as that described in the above discussion; that is a specimen is elongated and the simultaneous stress and strain recorded and plotted on a graph. It is often neither convenient nor relevant to perform this type of test and others have been developed.

With materials which are brittle and used in practice only in very small amounts, such as filling materials, it is inappropriate to construct the relatively long tensile specimens and in addition it is very difficult to grip them in the manner shown in Figure 1.36a without fracture occurring in the grips. An alternative test is the diametral compression test (Fig. 1.36b) in which a compressive load is applied across the diameter of a small cylindrical specimen. The compressive stress in the specimen induces a tensile stress at right angles to the loading axis, as shown. In this way the tensile strength of brittle materials may be calculated from the load at which fracture occurs. The test cannot be used for very ductile materials which merely flatten out. The compressive strength itself is determined simply by applying compression along the axis of a longer cylinder. It is important to measure both compressive and tensile strengths for a material as they can often be quite different.

Dental restorations and appliances are, of course, subjected to complex

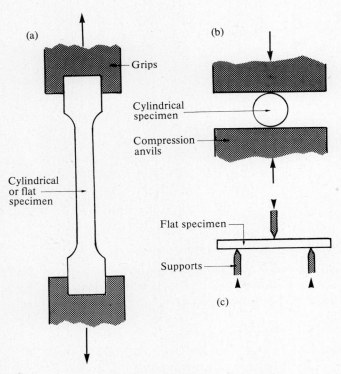

**Fig. 1.36** (a) Tensile test specimen; (b) diametral compression test specimen; (c) flexural bend test.

stress systems and the flexural or transverse strength test attempts to measure properties under a more realistic situation. In this a flat specimen, resting on two supports, is loaded in the middle (Fig. 1.36c). The load and deflection can be monitored and the flexural strength calculated.

## DENTAL METALS AND ALLOYS

As a class of material, metals are strong, ductile, tough, reasonably hard, and of relatively high elastic modulus. There are, of course, variations of properties within this group and in any application of metals, including those in dentistry, the structures are modified to achieve the optimum.

### Alloy hardening

Pure metals, as noted earlier, tend to deform plastically at fairly low stresses since there is very little restriction on the movement of atoms. For this reason pure metals are rarely used, except in situations which demand some of their unique properties. Pure gold is occasionally used in dentistry but far more common is the use of gold alloys. Alloys are invariably stronger than the pure metals from which they are made and thus alloying provides one way of increasing the strength of metallic materials.

The main reason for this increase in strength is the disruption of the crystal lattice that is produced by the alloying element. In the simplest case of a substitutional solid solution, as in Figure 1.12, since some of the atoms are of slightly different size to the majority, sliding of atom planes over each other is more difficult. Thus a higher stress level is necessary to initiate plastic deformation and so the alloy is stronger. This is called solid solution hardening. For obvious reasons an interstitial solid solution (Fig. 1.12b) will produce even greater strengthening, the interstitial atoms producing more disruption.

If more than one phase is present, the strengthening effect is enhanced since the phase boundaries intersect the slip planes and restrict the movement of dislocations, as already illustrated in Figure 1.32b. This effect is increased when the second phase is finely dispersed in the matrix of the major phase, in the form of a precipitate, and this strengthening process is known as dispersion or precipitation hardening.

Most alloy systems rely on either solid solution or precipitation hardening, or both, for their strength and examples will be found in Chapters 8 and 10 of gold alloys, cobalt–chromium alloys, and steels where such effects are used in dental alloys. Amalgam is a special case (Chapter 4) since it is made by a reaction between mercury and a silver–tin alloy. Amalgam is a complex structure and relies for its strength on the predominance of the strong silver–tin phase.

Whenever a metal is strengthened by alloying, there must be a decrease in ductility since the strengthening, by definition, is achieved through the inhibition of plastic deformation. Often this is no great problem since many metals are very ductile and can tolerate a considerable reduction in ductility before they can be classed as brittle. However, with some alloys which are based on relatively brittle metals, this can bring difficulties. The reduction in ductility of cobalt–chromium alloys by the presence of too many carbide precipitates is a good example.

### Work hardening

There is another way of strengthening metals which is used in some prosthetic and orthodontic appliances. The stress–strain curve for a ductile metal is shown again in Figure 1.37. It will be recalled that, above the elastic limit, continually increasing stress is needed to produce further plastic strain because of the increased difficulty of moving dislocations. If the metal is stressed to a point corresponding to X on curve (a), a large number of dislocations will be introduced into the structure. If the stress is removed, since this is plastic deformation, the disruption in the structure produced by the dislocations will remain. If the stress is applied again, it will have to reach this same level of X before further plastic deformation can take place. Thus the elastic limit has been increased to X and the material is therefore stronger. This phenomenon is known as work hardening. The forming processes used to produce wire and sheet-metal work harden the structures.

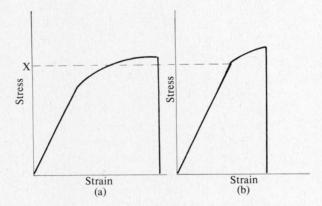

**Fig. 1.37** Stress–strain curve for ductile metal showing work hardening. Curve (a) shows behaviour when metal is first stressed to X. If the stress is removed and then reapplied, curve (b) results, the elastic limit now being X.

As with alloying, the work hardening process reduces the ductility. This may be a serious problem as the material may loose virtually all of its ductility during the forming process and start to crack. Fortunately this situation can be remedied since heating the metal, in an annealing treatment, may give the atoms sufficient thermal energy to move to lower energy equilibrium sites from their high energy positions around dislocations, thus restoring some ductility. By an optimum blend of work hardening and annealing, metals can be produced which are strong but also retain some ductility. This is discussed further in relation to orthodontic wires in Chapter 13.

### PLASTICS, RESINS, AND RUBBERS

Polymer-based materials, as already noted, tend to have low elastic moduli, display viscoelastic behaviour, and are relatively soft and weak but ductile. They are usually stronger in tension than in compression.

The mechanical properties of these materials are controlled by their composition; there is no equivalent of work hardening. The basic polymer itself is obviously very important. High molecular weight, highly crystalline polymers tend to be tough while amorphous polymers are often brittle, with low impact strength. These properties can be modified in the following ways.

*Co-polymerization.* This is the equivalent of alloy hardening although the effects are not usually so great. Co-polymerization is often used to increase the toughness of a plastic rather than the tensile strength. This may be achieved by the incorporation of rubbery polymers into a more rigid resin, as described in Chapter 11 for some denture base materials.

*Cross-linking.* Cross-linking often has a far more significant effect than co-polymerization on polymers by virtue of the replacement of secondary by primary valence bonds. The example of cross-linking natural rubber has already been quoted. Cross-linking is widely used in dental polymers as a way of controlling the mechanical properties as a polymer cures.

*Plasticizers.* It is sometimes desirable to improve the resilience or flexibility of a polymer and this may be achieved through the use of plasticizers. These are low molecular weight compounds which can be incorporated into the polymer. Their molecules reside between the much larger polymer molecules and, by separating them, allow them greater freedom of movement, facilitating deformation. The common household plastic PVC provides a good example since normally this is a rigid material but incorporation of up to 50 per cent plasticizer yields the well-known flexible product. In dentistry plasticizers are used in some resilient linings on dentures and in several other materials.

It should be noted that either unintentional loss or addition of plasticizers can radically alter the properties of a plastic. The seepage of a plasticizer by a process referred to as 'leaching' may cause a material to harden whilst the presence of water, residual monomer, or other such species can increase the flexibility of a material.

*Fillers.* Many commercial products based on polymers contain large amounts of fillers. These are inert substances that are sometimes used to lower the cost of the product or, more usually, to modify either the strength of the material or its viscosity. Fillers are widely used in dental materials for the latter purpose when the polymers are presented as fluids or pastes for application in the mouth. Their strengthening effect in the set polymer is due to much the same mechanism that is involved in precipitation hardening.

It must be realized, however, that the presence of fillers in an already brittle material may cause an unacceptable lowering of impact strength. This is a problem with the brittle polymethyl methacrylate used for denture bases and will be discussed later.

## CERAMICS

Ceramics are characterized by their excessive brittleness. This is mainly due to the restriction on plastic deformation as already discussed, and is further aggravated by the presence of defects in the ceramic structure. It will be recalled that brittle materials have a low impact strength since cracks are able to propagate through them very readily. Unfortunately the methods of ceramic preparation, that is sintering or acid–base reactions, tend to result in the presence of microcracks which propagate only too readily. This type of porosity may be controlled to a certain extent by the processing technique but it is largely an inherent feature of ceramics and, apart from incorporating the ceramic into a composite, little can be done to overcome the problem.

Ceramics are much weaker in tension than they are in compression since a tensile stress tends to open up cracks whereas compressive stresses have the opposite effect, continuing until the stress reaches a critical value at which the material shatters.

Since many dental ceramics, and especially those produced by acid–base reactions, are multiphase structures, it is important that the final structure contains as much as possible of the strongest phase. Usually it is the original ceramic phase that is the strongest and, as pointed out before, only just sufficient of the weaker reaction products should be formed to hold the original particles together.

## COMPOSITES

Generally, metals can be considered to have good mechanical properties. Plastics are not so good, largely because they deform too easily. Ceramics, on the other hand, are poor because they do not deform easily enough. Composite materials, usually although not necessarily consisting of a mixture of a plastic and a ceramic, are designed to overcome these weaknesses and produce strong, tough solids.

The brittleness of solids has been explained in terms of the ease with which cracks propagate through the material. One way of improving the ductility should be to put obstacles in the path of the cracks. Ductile materials deform easily because dislocations propagate readily through the material. Equally, one way of increasing the strength should be to put obstacles in the path of the dislocations. Putting these two requirements together, a structure consisting of alternate layers of ceramic and plastic should give the required combination of strength and toughness, the plastic phases acting to stop the cracks and the ceramic phases stopping the dislocations, as shown in Figure 1.38a. This is the type of structure found in fibre-glass.

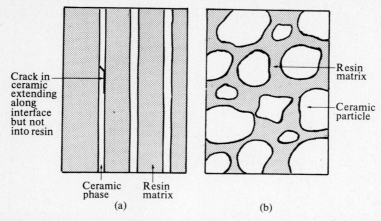

**Fig. 1.38** (a) Plastic–ceramic composite structure showing cracks arrested at interfaces; (b) dispersion of ceramic particles in resin matrix.

Although this type of composite may have good mechanical properties it is not fabricated very readily. It is far easier, and more appropriate to the moulding of materials used in dentistry, to use a fine dispersion of one phase in another. Invariably the plastic (or resin) phase is chosen as the matrix, which contains a dispersion of the ceramic particles, as in Figure 1.38b. This type of structure is widely used in filling materials as discussed in Chapter 5. By incorporating a ceramic, such as quartz which has a reasonably high compressive strength but low tensile strength, with a resin which has a very low compressive strength, a composite with good tensile and compressive strengths is achieved.

It is also possible to produce a significant improvement in the impact strength of ceramics by using ceramic–ceramic composites in which particles of a second ceramic are introduced into a matrix of the first, the improvement being largely due to the presence of the interfaces between them. This method is used in dental porcelain, as described in Chapter 9.

## PHYSICAL PROPERTIES OF MATERIALS

The important physical properties of a dental material are its electrical, thermal, and optical properties and radiopacity.

### Electrical properties

It is necessary to consider these only briefly. An electric current is the result of the passage of electrons through a material under the influence of a potential difference. The passage of an electrical current therefore requires the availability of free electrons. In ionic and covalent solids, the electrons are usually tightly bound to the atoms and are not free to move. Thus ceramics and plastics do not normally conduct electricity and are insulators. On the

**Table  1.2** Electrical  conductivity,  thermal  conductivity,  and  coefficient of expansion of various materials

|  | Electrical conductivity ohm/cm | Thermal conductivity W/m·°C | Coefficient of expansion m/m·°C × 10⁻⁶ |
|---|---|---|---|
| **METALS** | | | |
| Dental amalgam | 70 000 | 23 | 25 |
| Cobalt–chromium alloy | 80 000 | 70 | 20 |
| Gold | 400 000 | 300 | 15 |
| Stainless steel | 100 000 | 80 | 11 |
| **POLYMERS** | | | |
| Inlay wax | | | 350 |
| Impression compound | | | 250 |
| Silicone rubber | $10^{-15}$–$10^{-20}$ | 0·2–0·5 | 200 |
| Polysulphide rubber | | | 150 |
| Polymethyl methacrylate | | | 81 |
| Composite filling material | | | 30 |
| **CERAMICS** | | | |
| Porcelain | | 1·5 | 8 |
| Silicate cement | $10^{-12}$–$10^{-14}$ | 0·8 | 8 |
| Dentine | | 0·59 | 8·3 |
| Enamel | | 0·83 | 11·4 |

other hand metals have, by definition, many free electrons and thus make good conductors of electricity, as seen from Table 1.2. Electrical conductivity has only minor relevance in dentistry. As discussed in the next section, the corrosion of metals involves the generation of small electrical currents. Under some circumstances, current may flow from one restoration to another and through the tooth, producing pain. To avoid this, it is desirable in some situations to place an electrical insulator as a lining beneath a metallic restoration. As discussed in Chapter 3, various types of ceramic are used for lining purposes and, although several other requirements of lining materials are more important, they do also satisfy this requirement.

## Thermal properties

These will be considered under two headings, the transfer of heat through a material, or thermal conductivity, and thermal expansion.

### THERMAL CONDUCTIVITY

The conduction of heat involves the transfer of thermal energy from one part of a material to another. In order to conduct heat efficiently, a material must have particles which are free to move and carry the energy with them and also a very regular lattice which allows this movement to occur. Again metals are the only solids that possess the right structure for the transmission of thermal energy. Both plastics and ceramics are thermal insulators although here the difference between conductors and insulators is small compared to their difference in electrical conductivity, as shown in Table 1.2. When materials are placed as restorations near to vital dental pulp, it is desirable that they should not transmit heat directly to the pulp because of the trauma induced. In the case of amalgams, which are good conductors, a lining material is generally necessary to provide insulation. On the other hand, when a material is placed over normal mucosal surfaces, as with denture bases, for example, it is desirable to transmit some thermal energy to the tissues so that they can experience the sensation associated with different temperatures produced by hot or cold food and drink.

THERMAL EXPANSION

Except at the absolute zero of temperature, all atoms vibrate, their position on a space lattice in a crystalline solid representing the central point of the vibration. As a material gets hotter, that is, as its thermal energy increases, so the amplitude of the vibration increases. This causes the material to expand. The phenomenon is reversible and materials contract on cooling. Different materials expand by different amounts for a given temperature rise, depending on the freedom of the atoms or molecules to vibrate. The increase in size is usually proportional to the temperature rise and the rate of expansion is defined by the coefficient of expansion, values of which are given in Table 1.2. There is little difference between metals and ceramics, the former having slightly higher values on average, while polymers have much higher coefficients. As expected this behaviour is the inverse of that seen with elastic moduli, since both phenomena represent the ease with which atoms can be elastically displaced.

The thermal expansion and contraction of materials is of great significance in dentistry since many precision-fit restorations and appliances are fabricated at elevated temperatures, the resulting contraction on cooling to mouth temperature providing a source of dimensional error. This is especially significant with polymers and waxes, as predicted from the values in Table 1.2 and allowances have to be made during manufacture for subsequent contraction. This is discussed at several appropriate points in the book.

## Optical properties

The appearance of any dental material that is used in the mouth is of vital importance. Several features contribute to the overall appearance of a restoration. The colour and shade of a material are dependent upon its atomic structure. The mechanisms involved in this are beyond the scope of the book, but it is worth remembering that very few structural materials are highly coloured. All metals except copper and gold are silvery-grey in appearance. Most ceramics are white or off-white whilst plastics are also white, or occasionally yellow or brown. Little can be done to alter the colour of metals except by surface treatments, such as gold plating. Changes in the appearance of ceramics and plastics are achieved by the use of pigments.

The other main feature controlling the appearance is the translucency of the material. The majority of materials are opaque; that is they do not allow light to pass through them. All metals, most ceramics and most polymers, especially in thick section, are opaque. Very few materials are translucent, allowing the transmission of some light. In a translucent material, some of the incident light is absorbed, some is scattered, and some is transmitted directly through it, as shown in Figure 1.39. The absorption of light is controlled by the electronic structure of the atoms. The scattering of light is also controlled to a certain extent by the atomic structure but also by the microstructure. Generally, highly crystalline materials are opaque because the regular lattice causes the incident light to be reflected. On the other hand amorphous materials, with no regular atomic arrangement, offer no resistance to the passage of light and are usually quite transparent. Glass and amorphous polymers provide good examples. A critical factor in dental restorative materials for anterior teeth is that they should have some degree of translucency so that they can simulate the appearance of the surrounding hard tooth substance. Most of the ceramics and polymer-based materials used are able to do this, their slight translucency being adequate in the thin sections used. Some otherwise good materials, however, have been limited in this type of application because of a lack of translucency.

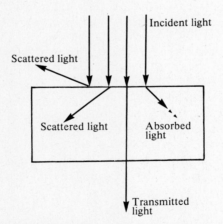

**Fig. 1.39** Absorption, scattering, and transmission of light by a solid.

### Radiopacity

There are several situations in dentistry where it is useful to be able to distinguish a material from the surrounding tissue radiologically. It may be desirable to identify the margin of a restoration in order to assess its condition, or alternatively it may be necessary to locate an appliance if it is accidentally swallowed. When a beam of X-rays impinges on a material only a part of the energy is transmitted in an unmodified form directly through the material.

In addition to the unabsorbed primary ray, modified and unmodified scattered rays, fluorescent X-rays, $\beta$ rays, and several other types of radiation will be produced. The amount of energy absorbed depends on the nature and thickness of material and the energy of the radiation. Under given conditions, the effect of the material is seen largely as a density effect, there being a logarithmic increase in absorption with increasing density. Light metals are therefore only moderately radiopaque while heavy metals strongly absorb X-rays and produce good contrast. Since polymers largely contain the small atoms of carbon and hydrogen they are very light structures and radiolucent. The behaviour of ceramics is dependent on the cations involved.

Since dental resins are, therefore, radiolucent, attempts have been made to incorporate dense substances into them. Compounds of heavy metals, such as barium sulphate, have been most commonly used for this purpose.

## CHEMICAL PROPERTIES OF MATERIALS

Dental materials come into contact with many chemicals and physiological fluids during preparation and use and it is desirable that there should be no reaction between them that would adversely affect the properties and, therefore, the usefulness of the materials. This means that no component of a dental material should dissolve or corrode in any of the fluids with which it is in contact, nor should there be an unacceptable level of absorption of constituents from these fluids. These aspects will be discussed in relation to the different types of material.

### Plastics, resins, and rubbers

Under some conditions polymers may degrade, usually by a depolymerization process that is the reverse of addition polymerization. However, these processes normally require excesses of heat, ultraviolet light, or other radiations and oxygen and are not relevant to the dental situation. High molecular weight polymers can, therefore, be considered inert with respect to the aqueous solutions they are likely to encounter when used as dental materials.

On the other hand, polymers are often dissolved by many types of organic solvent, such as chloroform, acetone, or alcohol. Care may have to be taken, therefore, to avoid contact with such materials during processing or cleaning.

Although the structure of polymers is not usually affected by water, there is a tendency in many cases for polymers to absorb water. This may have several effects. First, absorption of water tends to swell a polymer. Where accuracy is concerned this could be a disadvantage, although it is often thought of as beneficial if it can compensate for the contraction that occurs on polymerization. This is discussed further in Chapter 5. Secondly, as mentioned earlier, water in a polymer may act as a plasticizer, giving the polymer greater flexibility and resilience. Thirdly, the polymer may contain water-soluble additives, such as plasticizers which can be leached out at the same time as the water is being absorbed. Finally, excessive water absorption may facilitate contamination of a polymer with micro-organisms and make the surface more difficult to clean.

## Corrosion of metals and alloys

With a few exceptions, pure metals do not occur naturally. They are usually bound with non-metals in the form of minerals, such as oxides and sulphides, and these have to be refined to produce the pure metal. A great deal of energy has to be used in these processes and the pure metal that results exists at a higher energy level than the mineral. Since all materials will adopt the lowest energy state available to them, metals attempt to reconvert to the combined state. The processes by which this takes place are called corrosion phenomena.

### ELECTROCHEMICAL ASPECTS OF CORROSION

Corrosion is an electrochemical process; that is it involves the movement of electrons and positive ions. An aqueous environment is usually necessary to facilitate this movement and this is why metallic corrosion is a significant problem in the mouth where the saliva constitutes a very effective electrolyte.

If a metal M is placed in an electrolyte, as shown in Figure 1.40, metal ions will tend to go into solution, where they have a lower energy. The loss of ions results in an excess of free electrons in the metal, the reaction in effect being

$$M \longrightarrow M^+ + e^-.$$

This process cannot go on indefinitely since the lowering of energy is eventually balanced by the increased energy associated with the build-up of a negative charge on the metal due to the excess free electrons. At equilibrium, the solution of metal ions ceases, a potential difference having been established between the metal and the electrolyte. This potential difference is characteristic of the metal and the value obtained under standard conditions of

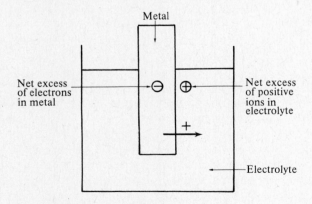

**Fig. 1.40** Metal electrode in electrolyte, showing transfer of ions and establishment of electrode potential.

temperature and electrolyte concentration is known as the electrode potential. In general, the greater the reactivity, the more ions will go into solution before equilibrium is reached and the greater will be the negative electrode potential. Thus the metals can be placed in a table, known as the electrochemical series, which is an order of their reactivity based on electrode potentials. These potentials are measured with reference to the hydrogen electrode, the more reactive metals giving increasing negative values and the more noble metals giving increasing positive values, as shown in Table 1.3.

**Table 1.3** Electrochemical series

|        | Element | Voltage |
|--------|---------|---------|
| Noble  | Au      | +1·68   |
|        | Pt      | +1·19   |
|        | Pd      | +0·99   |
|        | Hg      | +0·86   |
|        | H       | 0·0     |
|        | Fe      | −0·04   |
|        | Co      | −0·28   |
|        | Cr      | −0·81   |
|        | Ti      | −1·63   |
|        | Al      | −1·66   |
|        | Mg      | −2·37   |
|        | Na      | −2·70   |
| Active | Li      | −3·05   |

The electrochemical series is of limited value in predicting the susceptibility of metals to corrosion. This is partly due to the fact that some metals are protected by an oxide layer and are therefore far less susceptible to corrosion than their position in the series would suggest, and secondly because specific mechanisms are required to upset the equilibrium that has been reached between the metal and the environment and these may be unrelated to their intrinsic reactivity.

OXIDE FILMS AND PASSIVITY

With the exception of the noble metals such as gold, all metals react with oxygen on exposure to the atmosphere to produce an oxide. Again this happens because the oxide represents a lower energy state. The nature of the oxide film is extremely important and two general types of behaviour can be distinguished.

In most cases the oxide that forms on the surface of a metal is not totally coherent with the metal. Instead it forms as either flaky deposits or as an uneven, porous layer that is easily dislodged, as shown in Figure 1.41a. With some metals, however, the film is coherent, uniform, and non-porous, as in Figure 1.41b. In such cases the film is self-limiting since it can itself act as a barrier to further transport of oxygen and metal ions. The important point

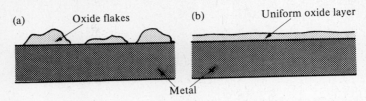

**Fig. 1.41** (a) Flaky, porous, non-protective oxide layer; (b) uniform adherent, protective oxide.

is that not only will the oxide film prevent further oxidation but it may also protect the metal from attack in corrosive environments. A metal that is protected in this way is said to be passivated. Generally it is the fairly reactive metals that become passivated, which leads to the paradox of the more inherently chemically reactive metals being the most corrosion-resistant. The formation of the first type of oxide film, of course, offers no similar protection.

Three metals are primarily noted for their ability to become passivated. These are titanium, chromium, and aluminium. Of these, titanium is probably the most corrosion-resistant metal available and is widely used for surgical implants, as discussed in Chapter 14. Aluminium is infrequently used in dentistry but chromium has widespread applications. Fortunately this element carries its passivating effect with it when alloyed with other elements so that alloys containing, say, a minimum of 12 per cent chromium are reasonably corrosion-resistant. Thus stainless steels containing about 18 per cent chromium and a variety of cobalt–chromium and nickel–chromium alloys are used in dentistry. Several other metals display some degree of passivity but are not as good as the three mentioned because the oxide film is more easily broken down. Cobalt and mercury are two examples.

Since, as discussed below, the oral environment is so corrosive, only noble metals such as gold and platinum and good passivating metals or alloys such as the chromium alloys and titanium are resistant to corrosion.

CORROSION MECHANISMS

Corrosion of metals can occur quite readily in the mouth as the discussion of amalgam in Chapter 4 will show. Before describing the mechanism by which this takes place it is necessary to distinguish between tarnish and corrosion. These two terms are frequently used interchangeably and indeed there is no universally recognized absolute distinction between them. However, tarnish is generally taken to mean the discoloration of a metal surface due to deposition of substances onto the surface, which may take place with little or no involvement of the metal itself. This could arise from the deposition of plaque and calculus in the mouth or from the formation of films of oxides, sulphides, or other species. Although tarnishing is often the precursor of a more significant form of attack on the metal, this need not necessarily be the case and a tarnished surface may, in fact, protect the metal from further attack in the same way as the oxide film does in a passive metal. Corrosion, on the other hand, is the specific and continued reaction of a metal with its environment, leading to the formation of specific corrosion products.

### GALVANIC CORROSION

In the situation described earlier for a metal in an electrolyte, equilibrium is reached when the potential difference between the two equals the electrode potential. If the excess electrons were to be removed from the metal then the potential difference would no longer exist, there would be no equilibrium and the metal would continue to dissolve. This consumption of excess electrons provides the mechanism for corrosion. There are several ways in which the electrons can be consumed. In the first, which gives rise to galvanic corrosion, the electrons are removed via a second metal. If two different metals are placed, in isolation, in the same electrolyte each will develop its own potential with respect to the electrolyte, say $V_A$ and $V_B$ for the metals A and B. If these metals are now joined together by an electrical conductor, as in Figure 1.42, there will be a potential difference between them, equal to $V_A - V_B$. Whenever two metals of different potential are coupled, a current will flow from the metal with the highest potential. Therefore, the excess electrons in A will flow in the external circuit to B, allowing more ions to be lost from A, and at the same time, causing ions to be redeposited on B. The metal A, known as the anode, therefore suffers accelerated corrosion. This is the origin of the galvanic cell that is used to produce electrical current and is also the reason that corrosion occurs

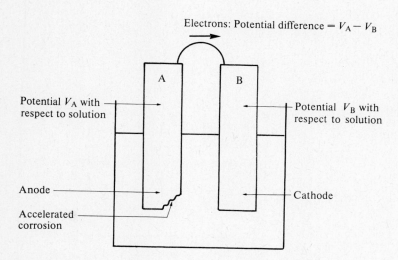

**Fig. 1.42** Galvanic cell, with two different metals placed, in contact, in an electrolyte.

whenever two metals (that are not passive) are coupled together in an electrolyte.

One further important point to note about this phenomenon is that galvanic cells may be quite small and may, in fact, be established between different places in one alloy. Thus if an alloy system is multiphase where the electrode potentials of some of the phases are significantly different, corrosion of the more electronegative phase will take place preferentially. This is one of the main causes of corrosion of amalgam.

### CREVICE CORROSION

The electrons may also be consumed by a chemical reaction. The dissolution of the metal which takes place at the anode has been described by the equation

$$M \longrightarrow M^+ + e^-.$$

This is known as the anodic reaction. A number of different reactions may consume the electrons at a cathode, the equation

$$O_2 + 2H_2O + 4e \longrightarrow 4OH^-$$

representing the most common cathodic reaction. If both these reactions can take place then corrosion will occur, the metal and hydroxyl ions reacting to give the metal hydroxide as the corrosion product in this case. It should normally be possible to choose an alloy system for use in a particular environment that does not allow this cathodic reaction to take place. However, there are some situations in which, even in reasonably corrosion-resistant alloys, the equilibrium can be upset and the reactions take place.

One such situation arises when there are crevices on the surface, such as the pit shown in Figure 1.43. Within a crevice the amount of oxygen dissolved in the fluid will slowly be depleted and a time is reached when the cathodic reaction can no longer take place in the pit because of the lack of oxygen. However, there is still sufficient oxygen over the remainder of the surface to allow the reaction so that a small cell of anodic area in the pit and a cathodic area surrounding it is established. Further dissolution of metal in the anodic area, that is, within the pit, can therefore occur, and this is a self-

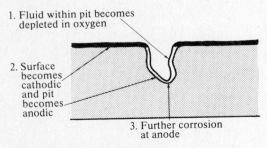

1. Fluid within pit becomes depleted in oxygen

2. Surface becomes cathodic and pit becomes anodic

3. Further corrosion at anode

**Fig. 1.43** Crevice corrosion initiated at a surface pit.

perpetuating phenomenon. This again is important in the corrosion of amalgam, as crevices can either be produced when one phase is preferentially corroded or alternatively when plaque is deposited on part of the surface, leaving other areas exposed.

## Ceramics

Ceramics are generally very stable structures. This is not surprising when one considers that the corrosion processes of metals just described lead to the formation of metal compounds, which are basically ceramic structures, as the low-energy corrosion products. Some ceramic structures are soluble in water, however, and those used in restorative dentistry may be divided into two categories.

First, there are the materials prepared by the sintering or fusion techniques, dental porcelain being the prime example. These can be considered totally insoluble in the oral fluids. Secondly, there are the materials prepared by acid–base reactions. These structures consist of aluminosilicate-type glass particles bound by a matrix of reaction product. The glass itself has to be soluble in an appropriate acid, which may be of pH 1 or 2, to take part in the reaction but it is unlikely such a low pH will be experienced in the mouth. The solubility of the cement matrix in acid solutions is largely due to its ionic structure, which has intrinsically low resistance to acids. Cements which are produced with matrices involving covalent as well as ionic bonds are far more resistant to attack. The matrix may also be soluble at a higher pH. The silicate cement used as a restorative material (Chapter 5) has a matrix which is slowly soluble at around pH 5 and since this level can under some conditions be attained on the surface of teeth, the cement itself is liable to erosion.

# BIOLOGICAL PROPERTIES OF DENTAL MATERIALS

Any material used in the mouth should ideally produce no adverse effects on the oral tissues. Moreover, no dental material, whether used in the mouth or laboratory should have any adverse effect, local or systemic, on patients or the dentists, assistants, and technicians, who will be handling it. Since dental materials can all be classed as foreign bodies, and since many are reactive chemicals at some stage in their preparation, the requirement of totally inert behaviour towards the tissues is very difficult to achieve. The phenomena associated with these effects arising from the use of dental materials are collectively called their biological properties. The term 'biocompatibility' is also used in this context although this includes all aspects of the interactions, including the effects of the tissues and oral fluids on the material.

It is very difficult to relate the biological properties of materials to their structures since so many different mechanisms can result in toxicity. It is only possible, therefore, to make a few general statements about the subject and leave more detailed discussion to the sections on the individual materials.

The biological properties may be classified first by the type of tissue involved and secondly by the type of material.

## The tissues

It is necessary to consider the oral mucosa, gingival tissues, hard tooth substances, the dental pulp, and finally the rest of the body.

### ORAL MUCOSA

The oral mucosa comes into contact with a number of materials for varying periods of time. There is, for example, short-term contact with impression materials, medium-term contact with periodontal dressings, and long-term contact with dentures.

Impression materials rarely produce any really harmful effect but they can irritate the mucosa for reasons mentioned later. Periodontal dressings should ideally promote healing after oral surgery but, as discussed in Chapter 14, they often have an adverse effect on the oral mucosa.

Long-term contact with the oral mucosa may result in more significant effects. In denture sore mouths, for example, the mucous membrane under a denture becomes inflamed. This may be due to direct irritation produced by the material, although this is unlikely, or there may be a hypersensitivity response to one of its components. Several dental materials can act as sensitizers and examples are found in both denture and impression materials. Dentists and their assistants may become sensitized to some products through repeated handling. These materials are usually readily identified, and the only remedy is to avoid contact with them.

Irritation of the mucosa may also be due to factors not directly related to the material and, in fact, denture sore mouth is usually caused by the traumatic effects associated with ill-fitting dentures and superimposed infection, as discussed in Chapter 11.

### GINGIVAL TISSUES

The dental materials used in many restorations and devices come into contact with gingival tissues. It is very unlikely that they produce any chemical or mechanical irritation in these tissues but their presence can have a most significant influence due to the ease with which plaque accumulates on some restorative materials, especially those which have rough surfaces. This plaque will cause inflammation of the gingival tissue which, if not treated, may progress to involve the whole of the periodontium.

The effects on tissues that surround and support dental implants are discussed in Chapter 14.

### HARD TOOTH SUBSTANCE

Dental materials are not normally considered to have an adverse effect on dentine or enamel. In some situations acids may be used to etch the enamel surface to enhance bonding between a material and the tooth but this is not a direct effect of the material itself (Chapters 2, 5, and 13). Dentine may allow the passage of substances that are harmful to the pulp, but is itself not affected by them. However, the presence of a restoration in a tooth or of an appliance attached to the tooth generally leads to an increased susceptibility of the adjacent tooth substance to caries. Secondary caries around a restoration is common. Although the restorative material itself cannot be said to contribute to the incidence of caries from a biological point of view, its physical characteristics are clearly very important. Occasionally restorative materials can have a therapeutic effect by increasing the resistance to caries if they are able to release fluoride into the adjacent enamel where it decreases the acid solubility of the tooth substance. This effect is discussed in the context of silicate cement in Chapter 5.

DENTAL PULP

Harmful effects on the dental pulp are probably clinically the most important. Pulp is a very sensitive tissue and is easily damaged by irritants which may gain access to it when restorative materials are placed in contact with a prepared tooth. The detailed histological changes that can take place are beyond the scope of this book but range from mild hyperaemia to pulpal necrosis, which usually follows a period of acute or chronic inflammation. If the source of irritation is removed early enough, resolution may occur accompanied by secondary dentine formation. On the other hand, loss of pulpal vitality may lead to the production of a periapical lesion (see Chapter 12).

It is important to bear in mind when considering the effect of restorative materials on the pulp that the process of cutting cavities in teeth also has a significant effect and that the observed response may be due to the combination of these two aspects, very often in addition to changes induced by the carious process itself. The effect on the pulp will depend not only on the nature of the material but also its ability to pass through the dentine. Therefore, the thickness of dentine between the cavity and pulp chamber and its structural characteristics, especially the presence of sclerotic dentine, influence the extent of the pulpal response. Since all restorative materials are potentially damaging, although to differing extents, lining materials are normally used to minimize the transport of the irritant to the pulp, as discussed in Chapter 3. It is, of course, desirable that lining materials themselves have little or no adverse effects.

If a vital pulp is exposed a material may be placed in direct contact with it. Here it is desirable that the material should not only have no harmful effects but should have a positive beneficial effect, preferably an antibacterial action and also stimulating secondary dentine formation to seal off the pulp chamber. This rather special situation is covered in more detail in Chapter 3.

SYSTEMIC EFFECTS

It is possible for a dental material, or more importantly a component of a dental material, to produce systemic toxic effects. The classical example here is mercury used in the preparation of amalgam (Chapter 4). However, these effects are not significant in patients; no substance that could produce significant acute systemic effects is used in dentistry. The problem of systemic effects becomes manifest only in dental personnel who are exposed to airborne vapour over a long period of time. The remedies are either to stop using the material or to adopt strict codes of practice to minimize the absorption of the toxic substance.

## The materials

The biological properties of specific dental materials are discussed at the appropriate points in the text. It is worth considering here, however, the general ways in which toxicity or irritancy can arise.

Dental materials come into contact with the tissues in a number of different forms.

**a** Some materials are mixed and applied to the tissues in an unset state. The individual components may therefore reach the oral tissues or contaminate the laboratory.

**b** The set material that has been prepared in this way must also be considered.

**c** Materials may be fabricated and applied to the tissues in finished form.

**d** A material may degrade or corrode *in situ* so that the products of the reaction are released into the tissues.

COMPONENTS OF DENTAL MATERIALS

This is by far the most important category. By definition, components of a dental material that have to combine to give the set product are reactive chemicals that are potentially irritant. In resin preparations, low molecular weight monomers, which are usually quite volatile, and cross-linking agents may be present. In the ceramic preparations, acids, sometimes of around pH 1, are used to react with the basic oxide or glass. Amalgam, as noted above, requires mercury for its preparation. In all these cases, the reaction between the components is still proceeding as the material is presented to the oral cavity and diffusion of low molecular weight species through the dentine is easily achieved.

SET STRUCTURES

Usually the irritation produced by the reactants in the setting process can be regarded as a transient phenomenon since they are eventually utilized in the reaction. Fully cured resins, for example, are rarely toxic. In the case of ceramics, it may take some time for the pH of the material to rise to an acceptable level, so that the source of the irritation remains a little longer in this case. Care must always be taken to ensure that the reaction has proceeded to a sufficient extent. The residue of free monomer in partially polymerized resin also provides a potential source for continued irritation.

PREFABRICATED MATERIALS

Fabrication of structures outside the mouth usually results in a more uniform product and no problems should arise from toxicity. The only exceptions are those materials, such as alloys containing nickel, which may produce the occasional hypersensitivity response.

DEGRADATION PRODUCTS

Within the oral environment the effect of corrosion, solution, or degradation on the restoration or appliance is usually more important than that on the tissues. Degradation products may be harmful to tissues if they gain access to them but more usually they will be washed away in the oral fluids. The main exception is that corrosion products of implants which are buried deep in tissue may have a direct influence on the response of the tissue.

If the corrosion or degradation takes place at the margin of a cavity, the loss of material may allow the ingress of oral fluids resulting in secondary caries. These processes may, therefore, indirectly affect the tooth structure.

# 2
# Adhesion

Restorative dentistry may be defined as the provision of functional and aesthetic replicas of parts of the dentition that have been lost. It can be readily appreciated that one of the most important aspects of this is the attachment of the replica to the remaining part of the dentition or, in the case of full dentures, the retention of the prosthesis in intimate contact with the mucosa. Marginal apposition between a filling material and the walls of the prepared cavity is essential if leakage of oral fluids is not to result in recurrent caries. Fixed appliances intended to produce tooth movements also have to be firmly attached or linked to the teeth, if the necessary forces are to be transmitted to them. Similarly, the pit and fissure sealants currently popular in preventive dentistry will not reduce caries unless the sealant is permanently bonded to the tooth surfaces.

The attachment of the materials used in dentistry to the oral tissue, and especially to hard tooth substance is, therefore, of the greatest significance in many dental procedures and is often the most important factor controlling clinical success. It is, however, a difficult problem to solve and, although considerable progress has been made in recent years with the development of substances that chemically bond to enamel and dentine, and of methods for pretreatment of tooth surfaces to enhance this bonding, there is still much to be learnt.

Since adhesion is so important in many aspects of dentistry, the basic concepts of the science of adhesion and surface interactions will be introduced in this chapter and the applications of adhesives in dentistry in general will be discussed. The status of adhesion in the various dental disciplines will be considered later in the relevant chapters.

### Definitions

Semantically there is some confusion over the word adhesion. The scientifically correct definition of adhesion is the attraction exhibited between the molecules of different materials at their interface. This is in contrast to cohesion, which is the attraction exerted between similar molecules within one substance. This definition of adhesion implies attraction at the molecular or submicroscopic level and must, therefore, involve valence forces.

Such a definition, however, is not entirely suitable when considering the technology of joining surfaces, because good bonding may be achieved in the absence of, or with minimal assistance from, such molecular attraction. Instead, adhesion may be defined as the state in which two surfaces are held together by interfacial forces, which may consist of forces of molecular

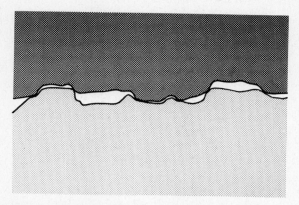

**Fig. 2.1** Adhesion achieved by micromechanical interlocking.

attraction or mechanical forces. The significance of this, as illustrated in Figure 2.1, is that the adhesion may be achieved by the interlocking of one surface with another on a microscopic scale, without the necessity for inter-molecular bonds. Furthermore, it is difficult to visualize, with the inherent microscopic roughness of virtually all surfaces, adhesion being achieved by molecular attraction without any assistance from mechanical interactions. It must, of course, be emphasized that it is microscopic mechanical inter-locking that is involved here rather than macroscopic mechanical retention.

It is this broad definition that must be used in dentistry, for microscopic mechanical interlocking plays a vital part in dental adhesion phenomena.

Sometimes the terms 'specific adhesion' and 'true adhesion' are used in this context, both referring to the molecular-attraction-based adhesion, to distinguish it from the mechanical interlocking. 'Specific adhesion' is the correct term to use for this, 'true adhesion' having no scientific meaning.

Most commonly, the joining of two substances by an adhesion phenomenon is achieved through the use of an adhesive, which is a substance capable of holding other materials together by surface attachment. That is, it will form an adhesive bond to the surfaces of two substances and thus hold them together. The surfaces to be joined and to which the adhesive is applied, are called the adherends or, more simply, the substrates.

Clearly, and as we shall see below, one of the important properties of an adhesive is its ability to be applied to the substance as a fluid, so that it covers the surface completely and readily, and then sets to give a mechanically sound interface. This is the basic reason why adhesives are almost universally required for joining two surfaces, as the substrates themselves rarely have this ability. It is of great importance to note, however, that this property is inherent and indeed desirable in many classes of dental restorative material, so that such materials may have adhesive properties themselves.

This concept has, in fact, led to a further confusion of terminology related to the use of restorative materials, with terms such as cement, luting agent, adhesive, and even lining and varnish being used with fairly arbitrary distinction. The term 'cement' has been used to describe simple filling materials without adhesive properties, such as silicate cement; for cavity linings which also have little or no direct affinity for tooth substances, such as zinc phosphate cement; for dental adhesives that can bond restoratives to enamel and dentine, as with the zinc polycarboxylate cement; and as filling materials that also display adhesion to tooth substances, the glass-ionomer cements providing the best example. Moreover, one type of material may be used on different occasions for quite different purposes, such as a filling or an adhesive.

In a non-dental context, a cement is a structural material consisting of a mixture of silicates and aluminates which, when mixed with water, slowly hardens. The similarity between such a material and the dental silicate cement is presumably how the latter obtained its name, a name which has been extended to other materials performing the same function. In its most common application, that is, bonding a restoration to a tooth, a dental cement functions in a complex manner. This may involve specific and mechanical adhesion and, in some circumstances, gross mechanical retention. The contribution from specific adhesion is often negligible, with the maximum contribution coming from mechanical adhesion. The term luting agent has been used to describe cements used in this way.

It is clear, therefore, that it is impossible to define these various types of dental material unequivocally as cements, luting agents, adhesives and so on. The procedure adopted in this book is that materials will be given their conventional name, and described in detail in the chapter that covers their most important clinical use, in which it will be made clear whether they are acting as an adhesive or not.

## THE NATURE OF ADHESION

As noted above, there are two basic types of adhesive mechanism; mechanical adhesion and specific adhesion, which involves molecular attraction. These categories may be subdivided further, as indicated in Table 2.1.

**Table 2.1** Categories of adhesion

| | |
|---|---|
| Mechanical adhesion | Micromechanical retention due to surface irregularities |
| | Retention due to dimensional changes |
| Specific adhesion | Primary valence forces |
| |    ionic |
| |    covalent |
| |    metallic |
| | Secondary valence forces |
| |    Keesom and Debye forces |
| |    London dispersion forces |
| |    hydrogen bonding |

## Mechanical adhesion

However smooth a surface may appear to the naked eye, on the atomic scale it will be relatively rough. This can lead to a degree of mechanical interlocking between two surfaces at their interface, giving some adhesion, as already illustrated in Figure 2.1. This type of adhesion can be enhanced by appropriate treatments to the surfaces to give greater irregularities, and by use of an adhesive which is sufficiently fluid to penetrate these irregularities and which, on setting, becomes constrained within them. Tooth surfaces may be pretreated by techniques, such as acid-etching of enamel, to promote adhesion.

The following points may be noted about the adhesion produced by microscopic retention.

**a** A very strong bond may be formed, even in the absence of strong molecular attraction.

**b** The bond will be especially strong under shear stress.

**c** The ultimate strength of such a bond is likely to depend on the cohesive strength of the adhesive; in other words, the adhesive (or possibly the substrate) may fail mechanically before the interface is disrupted.

**d** By adapting adhesive and substrate closely, forces of molecular attraction are enhanced.

The dimensional change produced by a change in temperature, state, or structure, may also be used to hold materials together. For example, differences in coefficients of thermal expansion can be employed to give a shrink fitting of one tube over another. Of greater relevance is the fact that most transformations of state or chemical reactions in the solid state are accompanied by a dimensional change, which may be utilized to produce an adhesive joint.

In dentistry, for the purposes of filling a cavity for example, it is expansion that is required, as illustrated in Figure 2.2. It is unfortunate that many changes of state or structure in dental materials are associated with a net

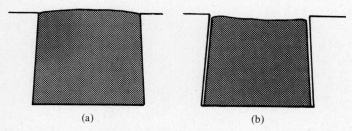

(a)                              (b)

**Fig. 2.2** Dimensional changes in a filling material: (a) expansion, indicating close adaptation to the cavity wall; (b) contraction, with a gap at the margin.

shrinkage. All polymerization and cross-linking processes exhibit a shrinkage since they establish stronger bonds between molecules. Similarly, the silicate cement filling material shrinks slightly on setting. All direct liquid to solid transformations (i.e. freezing) in metals are accompanied by a contraction, a point of some significance in the casting of metal dental appliances. Fortunately, a number of reactions in metals may produce an expansion. As will be discussed in detail in Chapter 4, the setting reaction of dental amalgam is associated with a complex series of dimensional changes and the net result may be either an expansion or contraction. This depends on variables such as the nature of the amalgam, alloy–mercury ratio, and the method of mixing. It is important to manipulate the amalgam in such a way as to produce a small overall expansion if close adaptation to the cavity wall is to be obtained.

## Specific adhesion

There are two broad categories of specific adhesion, involving primary and secondary valence forces. Sometimes the term 'chemical bond' is used for the primary valence bond and 'physical bond' for the secondary valence bond, although there is no justification for this and the terminology should be avoided. However, the terms 'chemical adhesion' and 'specific adhesion' are often correctly used synonymously.

### PRIMARY VALENCE BONDS

Primary valence bonds are those that hold atoms together to form molecules or macromolecular structures, i.e. ionic, covalent, and metallic bonds. These have been described in the previous chapter. They are exceptionally strong bonds and give rise to very strong joints. Soldering and welding, for example, are processes that allow metallic bonds to form across the interface.

In general adhesive technology, such bonds are not normally used. In dentistry, some adhesives are able to function through the formation of primary bonds with the various constituents of enamel and dentine and these are discussed later.

### SECONDARY VALENCE BONDS

These are far more important in most adhesive systems. Collectively known as Van der Waals forces, these are the inter-molecular forces of attraction that give cohesion to a structure. It has been shown in Chapter 1 that these forces are generally much weaker than primary valence bonds and that their strength determines the state of matter under given conditions.

There are several different types of secondary valence force, but all arise from interactions between molecules which are electrostatically unbalanced. Consider a simple molecule formed by the covalent bonding of two like atoms, such as two oxygen atoms or two chlorine atoms, for example (Fig. 2.3a). Since the atoms are alike, the shared electrons are equally distributed between

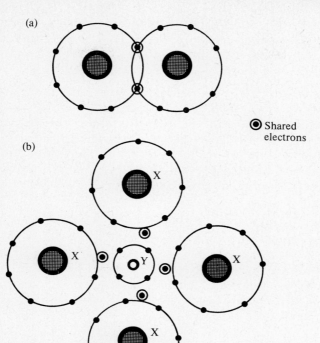

(a)

(b)

⊙ Shared
electrons

**Fig. 2.3** (a) Covalent bond between two similar atoms, showing equal sharing of the electrons; (b) covalently bound molecule of atoms X and Y, showing a displacement of the shared electrons towards the more electronegative X atom.

the two atoms. This equality of sharing gives a balanced molecule, which can be described as non-polar.

In a covalently bound molecule, however, where the constituent atoms have different degrees of electronegativity, as in Figure 2.3b, if the atoms X are more electronegative than those of Y, then the shared electrons are displaced towards X. Thus the X atoms have a net effective negative charge and the Y atoms a net effective positive charge, giving an electrostatic imbalance. Such a molecule is said to be polar and the pair of opposite charges in the molecule constitutes a dipole. Covalent molecules which contain atoms that are grossly dissimilar are usually polar, good examples being carbon tetrachloride, $CCl_4$, where there are four large chlorine atoms constituting the X of Figure 2.3b and one small carbon atom (Y), and methylene iodide, $CH_2I_2$. Of great interest is the fact that large organic molecules are frequently polar, polymers often containing polar groups which can be very useful for bonding purposes.

The forces of attraction involving polar molecules are the result of electrostatic attraction between dipoles. The different types of Van der Waals forces arise from the different types of dipole interaction and include the following.

**1** *Keesom and Debye forces.* Keesom forces arise from the direct interaction of permanent dipoles in neighbouring molecules of two or more polar compounds (Fig. 2.4a), where the dipoles orientate themselves to minimize internal energy and hence maximize the attraction. Debye forces, on the other hand, may exist between polar and non-polar molecules, the dipole moment of the former inducing a dipole in the latter by virtue of its electrostatic field. There is then attraction between the polar molecules and the induced dipoles (Fig. 2.4b).

**2** *London dispersion forces.* Electrons are in perpetual motion, which is essentially random within well-defined limits. This motion gives random instantaneous displacements of the electrons from the theoretical positions at which they give non-polarity, such that there is always an instantaneous dipole set up in any molecule, even a non-polar molecule. These instantaneous dipoles will be established in different molecules across an interface and each

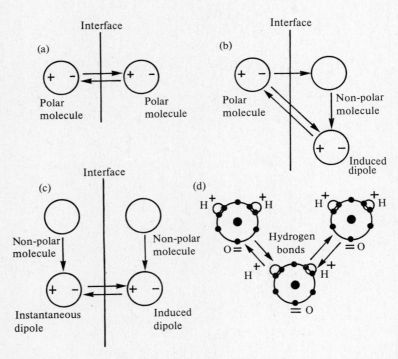

**Fig. 2.4** Secondary valence bonds. (a) Keesom forces; (b) Debye forces; (c) London dispersion forces; (d) hydrogen bonding in the water molecule.

will, additionally, tend to induce a corresponding dipole in the other. There is, therefore, a force of attraction between the instantaneous and induced dipoles (Fig. 2.4c) and this is called the London dispersion force. It is very important for the following reasons:

**a** it is not dependent on permanent dipoles in polar molecules but exists at any interface, and

**b** it is the strongest of the dipole interaction forces.

**3** *Hydrogen bonding.* This constitutes a special case of dipole–dipole interaction being a bond specifically involving hydrogen. It is the force of attraction that exists between two molecules each consisting of a highly electronegative atom or group, such as oxygen or fluorine and one or more hydrogen atoms. These two molecules are often, but not necessarily, of the same type, as with the case of water (Fig. 2.4d). Hence the water molecule is polar since the electrons are closer to the electronegative oxygen atom. This is, therefore, effectively negatively charged and each hydrogen atom effectively positively charged. This gives a dipole–dipole interaction between the hydrogen and oxygen atoms of neighbouring molecules, which is the hydrogen bond. This is a strong bond and is responsible for the relative stability of water when compared with similarly covalently-bound substances of equivalent molecular weight, such as hydrogen sulphide, $H_2S$, and ammonia, $NH_3$, which both exist as gases at room temperature.

Hydrogen bonds may also be formed when there are highly polar groups, such as the hydroxyl (—OH) and carboxyl (—COOH) groups on polymeric structures, and these play a significant role in many adhesive systems.

## CRITERIA FOR ACHIEVING ADHESION

Apart from the ability to participate in one or more of the above adhesive mechanisms, there are two characteristics a material must possess if it is to function efficiently as an adhesive.

**a** It must readily and completely cover, or 'wet' the substrate surface.

**b** It must undergo a liquid to solid transformation with minimal dimensional change.

In addition, the substrate must be clean so that the adhesive can gain intimate access to its surface.

### Wetting

Wetting is the ability to cover the substrate completely so that the maximum benefit is obtained from the forces of either mechanical or chemical adhesion. This ability is governed by both the driving force which is tending to produce the spreading of the adhesive over the substrate, and the resistance to the spreading, which is controlled by the viscosity of the adhesive, the surface irregularities of the substrate and the presence of contaminants.

The most important factor is the driving force behind the tendency to spread and this is controlled by the relationship between the surface energies of the liquid adhesive and solid substrate.

### SURFACE ENERGIES AND CONTACT ANGLES

In an ideal homogeneous solid or liquid, each molecule in the interior is completely surrounded by neighbouring molecules and, on balance, is attracted to molecules equally on all sides (Fig. 2.5a) giving a state of equilibrium. Near the surface, however, there is an imbalance of inter-molecular forces, with a net inward attraction towards the greater number of molecules (Fig. 2.5b). This inward force gives rise to the surface energy

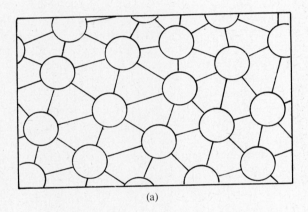

(a)

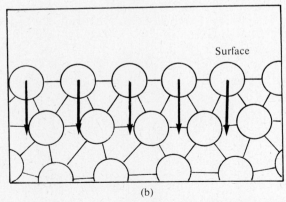

Surface

(b)

**Fig. 2.5** (a) Molecules in the interior of a solid or liquid, attracted equally to molecules on all sides; (b) molecules near the surface, with a net inward force of attraction, giving rise to the surface energy.

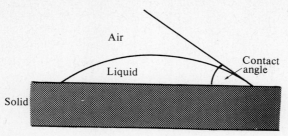

**Fig. 2.6** The contact angle at a liquid–solid interface.

of the material; in liquids this apparent inward force is called the surface tension. The surface tension of liquids and the surface energy of solids, being dependent on the molecular structure, are characteristic of a material under controlled conditions.

When a liquid and solid meet, the angle formed by the intersection of their respective interfaces with air (Fig. 2.6) is known as the contact angle, and is dependent on the surface tension of the liquid and the surface energy of the solid. A low contact angle implies that the liquid spreads over the solid surface, giving good wetting, whilst a high contact angle suggests that the liquid will form droplets on the surface rather than spread, giving poor wettability. Since any system will tend to adopt the lowest energy configuration possible (as discussed in Chapter 1) a solid with a high surface energy will encourage the spreading of a lower surface energy substrate over its own surface, giving rise to adsorption phenomena. Equally a low surface tension liquid will tend to spread out as much as possible in contrast to a high surface tension liquid which will minimize its surface area/volume ratio by forming spherical droplets. Hence, in general, low surface tension liquids will tend to spread over, or wet high surface energy solids.

This comparison is most meaningfully viewed in terms of the critical surface tension for the solid. If a number of liquids of a homologous series of known but different surface tensions are placed on a solid, each will yield its own contact angle. If a plot is made of the cosines of these angles as a function of the liquid surface tension, a straight line is produced (Fig. 2.7) in the so-called Zisman plot. The lower the surface tension, the lower the contact angle and the higher the cosine. Extrapolation to the contact angle of 0° (i.e. a cosine of 1) gives the critical surface tension of the solid, representing the surface tension of that liquid which will give complete wetting. Any liquid of surface tension greater than this gives incomplete wetting.

A crude criterion for wetting in an adhesive situation is, therefore, that the surface tension of the adhesive should be equal to or less than the critical surface tension of the substrate material. Thus domestic and industrial adhesives, such as epoxy resins, have low surface tensions $(3–3.5 \times 10^{-2}$ N/m) whilst those materials that are difficult to bond to anything, such as

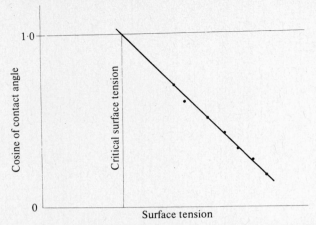

**Fig. 2.7** Graph of the cosine of the contact angle plotted against the surface tension of liquids placed on a solid surface. The surface tension at cosine = 1 is the critical surface tension of the solid.

polyethylene and PTFE (Teflon) have exceptionally low critical surface tensions ($1 \cdot 85 \times 10^{-2}$ N/m for PTFE).

In practice, the situation is slightly different, for it is found that optimum adhesion is achieved when the adhesive surface tension equals the critical surface tension of the substrate. All surfaces are microscopically rough and, indeed, this roughness may promote adhesion, as discussed earlier. However, an adhesive must be able to flow into the crevices and capillaries that constitute the rough surface. In order to do this, it must have a reasonably high surface tension since, as illustrated in Figure 2.8, the height to which a fluid rises in a capillary is directly proportional to its surface tension. Thus the best results should be achieved when the surface tension is high enough to encourage the adhesive to flow into the surface irregularities, but not higher than the critical surface tension of the substrate.

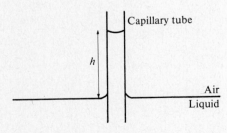

**Fig. 2.8** Rise of a liquid in a capillary. The height *h* if proportional to the surface tension.

Furthermore, the adhesive and substrate should be matched as closely as possible regarding the inter-molecular forces at their interface, to reduce the effective interfacial energy. Adhesives derived from polar substances, for example, are best suited to polar substrates.

SURFACE ROUGHNESS

As outlined above, surface roughness tends to favour greater adhesion, the intentional abrasion of surfaces prior to joining being a common procedure. The effect largely arises from an increased contribution from mechanical adhesion but the physical presence of solid projections into the adhesive, increasing its effective shear strength, and the increase in the potential surface area of contact over which specific adhesion can operate are also beneficial factors.

VISCOSITY

In some systems, although the surface energy considerations may suggest that an adhesive should wet a substrate, it may be prevented from doing so if it has a high viscosity. Viscosity is a measure of the consistency of a fluid, or its ability to flow. A thick 'viscous' fluid has a high viscosity while a freely flowing liquid such as water has a low viscosity. This property is not so important on very smooth surfaces but is of some significance when a rougher substrate is involved, when irregularities may hinder the fluid flow.

## Liquid–solid transformations

Although ideally an adhesive must initially have a low viscosity to facilitate complete wetting of the substrate, this viscosity must rapidly increase once bonding has taken place so that the shear strength of the adhesive reaches a suitable value. That is, the adhesive must undergo a liquid to solid transformation. Moreover, for a durable bond to form, this transformation must be accompanied by little or no dimensional change and, ideally, must result in a reasonably elastic solid.

There are a number of ways in which a liquid–solid transformation can be achieved, the most important of which are

**a** cooling of a liquid to below its melting-point,

**b** the rapid evaporation of a volatile solvent from a solution of the adhesive,

**c** polymerization of a monomer.

Soldering and the use of hot melt polymer adhesives are good examples of the first method, which are inappropriate for use in the oral environment because of the temperatures involved. Similarly, problems of solvent evaporation, including the toxicity of volatile solvents and the large contraction that must accompany the evaporation, make the second possibility impractical in structural dental adhesives. Polymerization is, therefore, the only viable alternative in adhesive dentistry.

Numerous adhesive systems provide perfectly satisfactory polymerization and cross-linking processes for this liquid–solid transformation, generally called the curing process. Their use in dentistry is limited by:

**a** the toxicity of the monomers used; many adhesive monomers and catalysts are too irritant for intra-oral use;

**b** the heat of polymerization, since reactions are usually exothermic and can give an appreciable temperature rise;

**c** the shrinkage associated with the curing. This is extremely important, and potentially arises from:

> **i** evaporation of by-products of the polymerization reaction, in the case of condensation polymers where water, alcohols, or similar substances are produced;
> **ii** formation of the primary bonds of adhesion, where inter-atomic distances are considerably reduced from those involved with Van der Waals bonds to those of covalent bonds.

The details of polymerization shrinkage with reference to dental polymers have been discussed in Chapter 1. In the context of adhesive polymers it is important to note that the effect of shrinkage is to induce internal forces. These tend to pull the adhesive away from the adherend, considerably reducing the contribution from mechanical adhesion and even disrupting the adhesive bond altogether. Obviously the greater the magnitude of the forces set up by the shrinkage, the greater this tendency and since the magnitude will be controlled, in part, by the volume of the adhesive, thin layers are far more efficient than thick layers. This is an important practical point, for it means that there is no advantage in using an excess of adhesive. It is also useful if the adhesive is reasonably elastic, for it may then be able to accommodate more shrinkage without inducing excessive stresses.

## ADHESION TO HARD TOOTH SUBSTANCES

The fact that good dental adhesives have not followed very readily from the development of general industrial adhesives is due partly to the constraints imposed on the adhesive by the need to function in an intra-oral environment, including the limitations of toxicity, moisture, and temperature, and partly by the nature of the substrates. It may be required to produce adhesion to enamel, as in techniques of orthodontics and preventive dentistry, or to dentine, or to both, as in restorative techniques. Since enamel and dentine differ in both composition and structure, it is necessary to discuss these aspects before describing methods of adhesion to them.

## ENAMEL

About 95 per cent of enamel consists of inorganic phases of the apatite structure. This is largely calcium hydroxyapatite $Ca_{10}(PO_4)_6(OH)_2$ but there will be varying amounts of fluorapatite and other structures. Only about 1 per cent of the enamel is organic. The remaining 4 per cent is water, a little of which is bound, but the majority is free and easily replaced. Thus, with enamel, specific adhesion has to be aimed solely at the inorganic phase. Care must also be taken to ensure that the loosely bound water does not adversely interfere with the establishment of adhesive bonds or their maintenance.

Structurally enamel is quite complex. The basic units are prisms, approximately $6\mu m$ in diameter, which extend through the thickness of the enamel, but with considerable microstructural variations. Within the prisms are small crystallites of the apatite, which are associated with the organic matrix. The boundaries between the prisms represent areas where the crystallite orientation changes (Fig. 2.9a), in a similar manner to the way grain boundaries represent the zone of crystal orientation mismatch in metals.

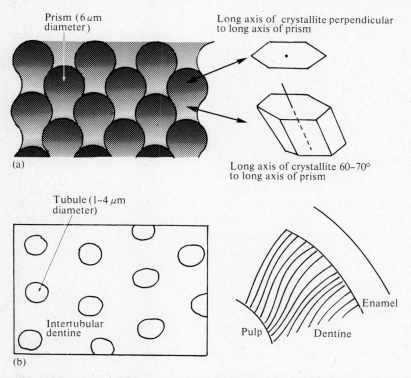

**Fig. 2.9** (a) Structure of enamel, showing section perpendicular to long axis of the prisms and the relationship between the crystallite orientation and positions within the prisms; (b) structure of dentine showing (left) a transverse and (right) a longitudinal section.

The reduced crystallite packing density in these areas means that there may be a greater concentration of organic phase and bound water associated with them. This prismatic structure is by no means consistent and uniform, numerous types of irregularity being observed. When considering mechanical retention of an adhesive to enamel, the exact structure of the enamel at the surface, including the orientation of the prisms, is of great importance, especially when the enamel surface is to be pretreated to encourage mechanical adhesion. This is discussed in more detail below.

One final point concerning enamel is that the prolonged contact with the oral environment leads to reactions with saliva and other substances resulting in a surface deposit on the enamel, which is structurally and compositionally very different from enamel. This must be regarded as a contaminant as far as adhesion is concerned and must be removed.

DENTINE

Dentine has a higher proportion of organic phase and water than does enamel. The organic content is given as between 20 and 30 per cent, this largely consisting of collagen but with a minor proportion of non-collagenous substances. Water, again mainly unbound, accounts for between 13 and 20 per cent leaving 50–67 per cent for the inorganic phase. Again this exists as calcium hydroxyapatite with variable amounts of other ions, such as fluoride ions, present. Account has to be taken of the organic phase when considering adhesion, as any adhesive which will bond only to the apatite, displaying no affinity for collagen, will give less than optimal results. Most dental adhesives, which do rely to a greater extent on specific adhesion to the mineral phase, give greater bond strengths to enamel than to dentine.

Dentine has a tubular structure (Fig. 2.9b). The tubules themselves are typically 1–4 $\mu$m in diameter and contain the protoplasmic extensions of the odontoblasts which line the pulpal aspect of the dentine. The apatite crystals in the intertubular dentine are much smaller than those in enamel and more randomly dispersed in the larger volume of organic matrix. Again the microstructure is complex and variable. Each tubule is curved and there are lateral extensions between them. The degree of calcification varies, with both hypo- and hyper-calcified areas present. All these factors have to be taken into account when considering adhesion to dentine, bearing in mind that a failure to produce adhesion over the whole of a surface will result in a considerably inferior bond.

It is also important to note that the presence of cellular components in the dentine, and its proximity to the pulp, place further limitations on the chemistry of the adhesive systems to be used.

## Materials for bonding to enamel and dentine

Many dental restorative materials, such as lining and anterior filling materials will, if allowed to set in contact with hard tooth substances, exhibit some bonding to them. That is, after setting, a finite force is necessary to separate the material from the tooth. Into this category come direct filling acrylic resin and composites based on the BIS-GMA resin (Chapter 5), and the zinc phosphate and zinc oxide/eugenol lining materials (Chapter 3). The nature of the adhesion achieved in these situations is not fully understood although there is unlikely to be any significant contribution from specific adhesion. Mechanical adhesion is probably responsible for this bond which is therefore attributable to the surface microstructure of the enamel or dentine. Usually in these systems a short period of immersion in water reduces the bond strength to zero, the water readily competing with the restorative material for the substrate surface.

Thus the use of these materials on untreated enamel or dentine does not usually give permanent, structurally useful bonds. Enamel is usually pretreated in some way to enhance mechanical adhesion of restorative materials, as discussed later.

Specific adhesion to enamel and dentine has, however, been achieved with certain types of materials which contain carboxyl (—COOH) groups. Two such materials of practical importance are the polycarboxylate cements, used widely as a dental cement and discussed in detail in Chapter 3, and the glass ionomer cements, used as filling and cementing materials and discussed in Chapter 5. Both these materials are based on the reaction between a solid (zinc oxide and calcium aluminosilicate respectively) and an aqueous polyacrylic acid solution. Their adhesion to tooth substances is particularly aided by their ability to wet the tooth surface and it is here that the benefit of matching polar adhesive to polar substrates is appreciated. When the cement is still reasonably fluid, there are many free —COOH groups which promote wetting of the polar tooth surface because of the tendency to form hydrogen bonds, which link polymer molecules to the substrate (Fig. 2.10a).

Once the substrate has been wetted and as the cements set, stronger forces of attraction take over from the hydrogen bond so that good adhesion is established between these polyacrylic acid based cements and a wide variety of materials. The initial adhesion takes place via the long-range dipole interactions discussed above. However, as the setting of the cement proceeds, the hydrogen atoms in the polyacid are gradually replaced by the cations from the ion-leachable powder, or possibly from the substrate, so that strong ionic bonds are formed in place of the weaker dipole interactions (Fig. 2.10b).

There are a number of features of this sequence that are clinically important. First, the fact that good wetting is dependent on the presence of free —COOH groups implies that the cement must be applied to the substrate at a very early stage during its setting. As the setting reaction proceeds, the number of such free groups is considerably reduced because of their reaction with the cation, so that if the cement is applied a little late, optimum wetting will not be achieved. Secondly, a pretreatment of the surface that cleans it thoroughly, especially removing proteinaceous debris, may be advantageous in allowing wetting to occur more rapidly. For example, a citric acid treatment has been recommended prior to the use of the glass ionomer cements.

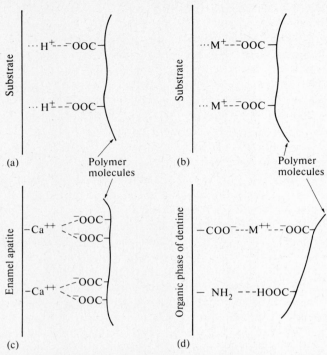

**Fig. 2.10** Specific adhesion of polyacrylic acid based materials to tooth substances. (a) Hydrogen bonds linking polymer to substrate; (b) replacement of hydrogen bonds by ionic bonds; (c) ionic bridge to enamel apatite; (d) bonding to amino acid and carboxyl groups in organic phase of dentine.

Thirdly, adhesion to the substrate is strongly dependent on the availability of suitable cations at the interface for promotion of the ionic bonding. Fortunately enamel is particularly good in this respect, the calcium ions of the apatite providing the ionic bridge (Fig. 2.10c). The smaller amount of apatite in dentine means that the adhesive bond to dentine is weaker than that to enamel. However, it is possible to achieve bonding to the organic phase of dentine via the pendant amino acid ($-NH_2$) and $-COOH$ groups and the cations supplied by the ion leachable glass (Fig. 2.10d).

Fourthly, these cements may adhere to a variety of substrates if these have polar surfaces. For example, adhesion to oxides may be achieved by the electrostatic attraction between cations, and both the negatively charged $-COO^-$ groups in the cement and the negatively charged oxygen layer of the substrate. Examples of bond strengths achieved between a glass ionomer cement and various substrates are given in Table 2.2. It is important to note that it is only polar surfaces to which it can adhere, in the case of metals implying a reactive metal yielding an oxide surface. Noble metals which do not passivate (as discussed in Chapter 1) cannot participate in this adhesive mechanism, and neither can unreactive porcelain. This is discussed further in Chapter 9.

A further important point to bear in mind is that the most significant difference between these cements and those that do not display specific adhesive properties is the presence of a polymeric hydrogen ion—donating liquid, rather than a monomeric acid such as phosphoric acid or eugenol. With the phosphate bonded cements, for example, the important metal–oxygen–phosphorus links are fully saturated and not available for adhesive bonding in the way that the numerous pendant —COOH groups are available in the polyacid.

**Table 2.2** Bond strength between glass ionomer cement and various substrates

| Substrate | Bond strength $(N/mm^2)$ |
| --- | --- |
| Enamel | 4·0 |
| Dentine | 2·9 |
| Stainless steel | 6·8 |
| Platinum | 0 |
| Gold | 0 |
| Porcelain | 0 |
| Platinum/tin oxide | 3·8 |

## Pretreatment of tooth surfaces

Several different techniques have been developed for the enhancement of adhesion to tooth surfaces. These may be grouped as follows:

**a** Cleansing treatments, to improve wetting.

**b** Calcifying treatments, to modify the tooth surface chemistry and enhance any bond formation that relies on calcium.

**c** Etching treatments, to improve mechanical adhesion.

**d** Application of coupling agents, to promote specific adhesion.

CLEANSING TREATMENTS

Any tooth surface is likely to be contaminated. This is true either for an enamel tooth surface or the wall of a cavity in dentine. Debris on the surface will hinder wetting by an adhesive and cleansing of the surface may be desirable prior to its application. As outlined in the section above, citric acid has been recommended for use prior to application of the glass ionomer cement. A 50 per cent solution has been found best, being applied for about 30 seconds and removed with an oil-free air/water spray. The bond strength achieved to both enamel and dentine is nearly twice that achieved when either of the alternative cleansing solutions, 20 vol. hydrogen peroxide or phosphoric acid are used.

CALCIFYING FLUIDS

Since the greatest degree of adhesion to tooth surfaces is achieved with enamel, where large amounts of calcium based mineral phase are present, attempts have been made to develop techniques for increasing the calcium content of the dentine surface. The basic method is to mineralize the dentine by exposure to some calcium-bearing fluid prior to use of the adhesive material. A number of different calcifying fluids have been investigated and typically contain an appropriate calcium compound such as Brushite (calcium hydrogen phosphate dihydrate) in a buffer solution (for example, phosphate buffer) containing a significant level of fluoride ions.

From such solutions, crystalline hydroxyapatite may be precipitated on to the dentine surface, apparently coherently with the original apatite of the dentine. Only a small layer of such a precipitate is necessary, since adhesive forces are very short range; indeed, a layer of molecular dimensions is sufficient. Widespread use of these calcifying fluids is awaiting the development of systems which can precipitate the mineral phase in a clinically acceptable time instead of the rather lengthy times necessary at the moment.

ACID-ETCHING

It has been recognized for some time that certain acids can etch the surface of enamel, etching being the slow dissolution of a solid by a fluid. In view of the heterogeneous structure of enamel, this clearly has great potential for facilitating mechanical adhesion, if the etching treatment can yield a microscopically rough surface. The first acid to be used was 85 per cent phosphoric acid, which is widely used to pretreat metal surfaces prior to their coating by paints and resins. Although many other acids have been investigated for this purpose, phosphoric acid remains as the most clinically acceptable etching medium, most frequently now as a 50 per cent solution. It produces a better compromise of enhanced adhesion, clinically acceptable application time, and lack of irritancy than any of the alternatives.

The acid causes dissolution of the enamel surface at a rate dependent on the microstructure. Generally the prism cores are dissolved faster than the inter-prismatic areas, giving the overall effect of a pitted surface. The variations in the enamel structure mean that this situation may be reversed in some areas, with depressions forming in the inter-prismatic areas, the prism core standing proud. Occasionally both core and peripheral areas dissolve at the same rate. Pits of other shapes may also be produced. These varying responses are due to the local differences in enamel constitution and orientation and possibly variations in the availability of the acid at the surface.

The significance of this etched structure is that the adhesive can penetrate the etched pits, as illustrated in Figure 2.11, considerably enhancing the effect of mechanical adhesion. The parts of the adhesive that penetrate the pits are called tags, and these typically extend $25\mu m$ into the enamel. Further beneficial effects of acid treatment are a general cleansing of the enamel

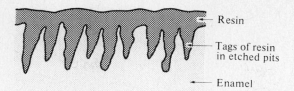

**Fig. 2.11** Penetration of etched enamel surface by adhesive.

surface, in a similar manner to that discussed above in the case of citric acid, and the provision of a potentially much greater surface area of contact over which the forces of specific adhesion may operate.

COUPLING AGENTS

Coupling agents are, in effect, adhesives that work in a special way. As illustrated in Figure 2.12, they have extremely reactive molecules that are polyfunctional, that is, different parts of the molecule are able to react in different ways at the same time. They may, therefore, be used to adhere to a substrate, by specific adhesion, via one of the functional groups in the molecule, leaving another type of functional group available for forming an adhesive bond to another substance. A very good example of a coupling agent is the silane that is used to promote adhesion between a resin and a filler in a composite as discussed in Chapter 1. In the context of adhesive dentistry it is possible to increase the adhesion of some resins to enamel by the use of coupling agents. For example, a molecule that has a functional group that is able to chelate with the calcium of the apatite phase of enamel and one functional group that could participate in a polymerization reaction in a self-curing resin will promote adhesion between the resin and the enamel.

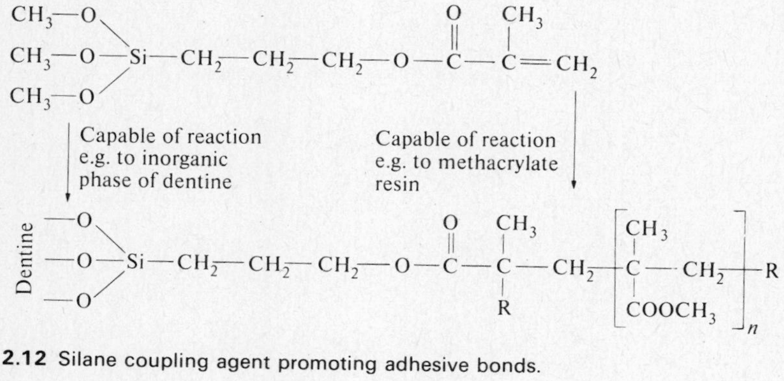

$$CH_3-O$$
$$CH_3-O-Si-CH_2-CH_2-CH_2-O-\overset{\overset{O}{\|}}{C}-\overset{\overset{CH_3}{|}}{C}=CH_2$$
$$CH_3-O$$

Capable of reaction e.g. to inorganic phase of dentine

Capable of reaction e.g. to methacrylate resin

$$Dentine \begin{cases} -O \\ -O-Si-CH_2-CH_2-CH_2-O-\overset{\overset{O}{\|}}{C}-\overset{\overset{CH_3}{|}}{\underset{R}{C}}-CH_2 \\ -O \end{cases} \left[ \overset{\overset{CH_3}{|}}{\underset{COOCH_3}{C}}-CH_2 \right]_n R$$

**Fig. 2.12** Silane coupling agent promoting adhesive bonds.

### Adhesives in clinical practice

As outlined in the opening paragraph of this chapter, much work still remains to be done in the field of adhesive dentistry. However, a number of clinical treatments rely on adhesion between dental materials and hard tooth substance for their success. These include the following:

**a** repair of fractured incisors with composite resins;

**b** fissure sealing;

**c** restoration of cervical erosion cavities;

**d** direct bonding of orthodontic appliances;

**e** cementation of inlays, crowns, and bridges.

In addition, adhesion is a highly desirable property in direct cavity filling.

These situations are discussed in detail in the appropriate chapters. It is important to remember, however, that techniques of adhesive dentistry at the present time are largely confined either to acid-etch treatments or the use of polyacrylic acid-based cements.

# 3

# Lining materials and cements

There is a risk of pulpal irritation with many restorative materials if they are applied directly to the exposed dentine in a prepared cavity. This irritation may be thermal, from temperature extremes transmitted by a metal filling or from the heat evolved during the exothermic polymerization of some of the resin-based restoratives. Chemical irritation from these and other filling materials may also cause pulpal damage. Less of a problem is trauma from pressure during the condensation of dental amalgam and electrical irritation from small currents produced by galvanic action when dissimilar metal restorations are placed in close proximity. To minimize the pulpal reaction associated with irritation from these sources the majority of prepared cavities are lined with a protective material (Fig. 3.1). Lining materials are also used to reconstruct, to a certain extent, the internal form of deep cavities, allowing the clinician to reproduce more closely the classical cavity design. It is claimed that certain linings have a therapeutic effect on the inflamed dental pulp, having an antibacterial and anti-inflamatory action. Others appear to stimulate the production of secondary dentine when used in a similar situation. This group of 'therapeutic' lining materials have been employed as pulp capping agents, covering the exposed dental pulp, in an attempt to maintain its vitality.

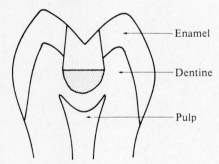

Enamel

Dentine

Pulp

**Fig. 3.1** Lining (shaded) placed beneath filling to protect the underlying pulp.

All the lining materials protect the pulp from some or all of the influences mentioned above but there are some, such as zinc phosphate cement, which, while giving very adequate protection from all varieties of irritation, are themselves chemically irritant. The ideal lining material should be non-irritant to the tissues.

After mixing, the material should set hard in the cavity in a time that allows adequate manipulation, but permits rapid increase in strength in order that the placement of the filling can follow without delay. Considerable compressive strength is necessary to allow the forceful condensation of amalgam. Lining materials should ideally adhere to dental tissues and, if used to cement restorations, to the restorative materials concerned. For this latter function, the cement should be insoluble in oral fluids, as a small section will always be available to the oral environment at the margins of the restoration. Dimensional stability is desirable but not as critical as with filling materials. Linings must be compatible with the restorative materials they contact, disrupting neither their setting reactions nor final properties. To minimize the transmission of thermal stimuli they should have a low thermal conductivity. In addition the attributes of cheapness and a long shelf-life are, of course, desirable, but sometimes unattainable.

Many lining materials are used in modified forms and using modified techniques to cement inlays, crowns, and bridges. Here, adhesion and solubility become factors of greater importance. Some lining materials, such as zinc oxide/eugenol, are used as temporary dressings although there are other products specifically designed for the purpose. The conflicting requirements for a material to be used for a dressing are that while good strength and adhesion are necessary it must be easily and cleanly removed when required.

Most of the cements discussed in this chapter are based on those materials, described in Chapter 1, which are the product of an acid–base interaction between an acidic liquid and a basic (or amphoteric) solid. Zinc oxide/eugenol; zinc oxide/eugenol and ortho-ethoxybenzoic acid; zinc oxide/phosphoric acid; zinc oxide/polyacrylic acid; and aluminosilicate glass/polyacrylic acid cements all fall into this category. In addition to these there are a smaller number of miscellaneous materials which do not readily fall into any category.

## Zinc oxide/eugenol cement

The hardened mass resulting from the reaction between zinc oxide and eugenol has many applications in dentistry. These include lining cavities, cementing restorations and taking impressions. Rarely, however, are the reagents used in pure form and additives to the powder and liquid alter the rate of reaction and the properties of the set material.

### CONSTITUENTS

Zinc oxide is the principal constituent of the powder although magnesium oxide may also be present in small quantities and reacts with eugenol in a similar way. Various fillers, such as white rosin, are used to improve the final strength and reduce brittleness, and may form up to 28 per cent of the powder. Colophony resins, for example abietic acid, are among the accelerators used and they also lead to the production of a smoother, more cohesive mix. The rate of reaction is usually increased by the addition of zinc salts such as the acetate, stearate, succinate, or propionate in concentrations of up to 1 per cent.

The liquid is mainly eugenol (Fig. 3.2), but another oil such as olive oil or cotton seed oil is usually added in a concentration of about 15 per cent to mask the taste of the eugenol and modify the viscosity. Accelerators may be present in the liquid to increase the rate of reaction, acetic acid being commonly used.

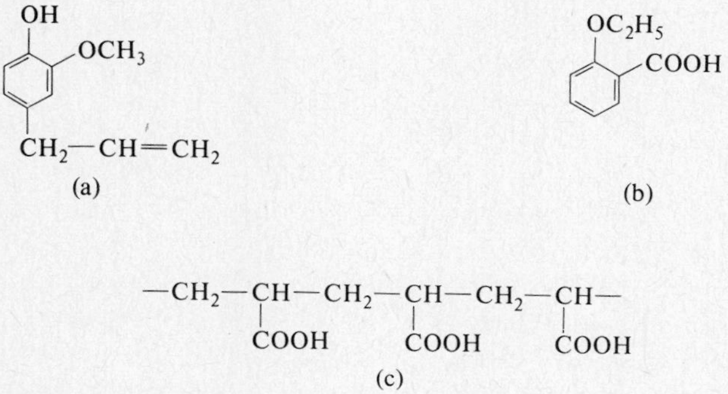

Fig. 3.2 Structure of (a) eugenol; (b) o-ethoxybenzoic acid; (c) polyacrylic acid.

SETTING REACTION

The zinc oxide powder initially absorbs some eugenol, but this is largely confined to the superficial layer of the powder particles, where a reaction takes place between the two. The product is amorphous zinc eugenolate, which binds the central, unreacted portions of the powder particles together. A trace of water is necessary to start the reaction which probably leads initially to the formation of zinc hydroxide which subsequently reacts with eugenol. Water is a by-product and when the setting reaction has commenced it is self-perpetuating.

In the presence of excessive zinc acetate (over 5 per cent) the zinc eugenolate formed is crystalline and stronger than the amorphous form. However, the setting reaction is too rapid for clinical use and advantage cannot be taken of this property.

RATE OF REACTION

The complete reaction between zinc oxide and eugenol takes place in about 12 hours, far too slowly for clinical convenience. The main factor that increases and controls the setting rate of the commercially produced cement is the presence of accelerators included by the manufacturer. However, other factors play a part. If the particle size in a given mass of powder is relatively small, a larger surface area of zinc oxide is available for reaction and this leads to more rapid utilization of eugenol. The rate of reaction is therefore increased. An increase in temperature also increases the rate of reaction, as does the presence of moisture (the addition of water, however, is not an acceptable way of modifying the reaction rate). Inclusion of a greater amount of powder in a given volume of liquid (a high powder/liquid ratio) leads to more rapid absorption of eugenol by zinc oxide and hence to more rapid reaction. The reactivity of zinc oxide is partly dependent upon the way in which it is manufactured; if it is prepared by the oxidation of the metal it is less reactive than when it is produced by heating the carbonate or hydroxide. In practice the cement powder generally contains a mixture of zinc oxide prepared by both methods.

PROPERTIES

Set zinc oxide/eugenol cement has a pH of 6·6–8·0 and is not irritant to the pulp when placed in deep cavities. Reports of the effect of the cement on the exposed pulp differ. While zinc oxide/eugenol has been used as a pulp capping material, it is generally agreed that eugenol is mildly irritant. The cement has an obtundent effect on tissues, reducing pain when it is present. Advantage has been taken of this property, not only in the lining material, but also in periodontal and extraction wound dressings, as indicated in Chapter 14. Free eugenol, always present in the set cement, is responsible for this effect. It also has an antibacterial action which reduces pulpal irritation from this source.

**Table 3.1** Strength of lining materials and cements

|  | Compressive strength $(MN/m^2)$ | Tensile strength $(MN/m^2)$ |
|---|---|---|
| Zinc oxide/eugenol | 14 | 1·4 |
| Zinc oxide/eugenol plus polymers | 42 | 3·0 |
| EBA | 62 | 4·2 |
| Zinc phosphate | 100 | 5 |
| Zinc polycarboxylate | 90 | 14 |

Zinc oxide/eugenol is a relatively weak material with a compressive strength of 15–40 $MN/m^2$ (Table 3.1). The most rapid increase in strength occurs in the first 15 minutes after mixing. While offering good insulation by virtue of its low thermal conductivity and protection of the pulp from electrical and chemical irritation, its low strength does not insure against transmission of pressure during the condensation of amalgam. Indeed, many clinicians consider that, in the basic form described, it is not strong enough to withstand these pressures and should therefore be covered with a stronger material such as zinc phosphate cement. Other operators limit its use to simple, single surface restorations, where adequate support can be achieved on all sides from the cavity walls. In these circumstances it is essential that a very thick mix is used to give maximum strength and rapid setting. The use of zinc oxide/eugenol as a lining material is further limited by its lack of compatibility with tooth-coloured filling materials. Resin-based materials are plasticized by the oils present and these also interfere with the setting of silicate cement and lead to its discoloration.

As a cement, zinc oxide/eugenol relies on mechanical adhesion as little or no specific adhesion operates in the absence of any suitable functional groups on the molecule of eugenol (Fig. 3.2). The tensile strength of the basic material is low at $0{\cdot}12{-}0{\cdot}4$ MN/m$^2$ (Table 3.1), although this and the compressive strength are improved in modified forms. The effectiveness of the latter varieties as cements is correspondingly greater. The main failing of zinc oxide/eugenol as a longer term cement is its high solubility. As it dissolves, eugenol is released and the cement disintegrates. As a consequence zinc oxide/eugenol is rarely used as a permanent cement, but is ideal for the placement of temporary restorations. The solubility of the final material is reduced by increasing the powder/liquid ratio.

Zinc oxide/eugenol is a widely used material for dressing prepared cavities. Its ease of application and removal, and its obtundent effect, are clearly advantageous. As there is virtually no contraction on setting, the marginal seal is superior to other materials, including zinc phosphate cement. This good seal may be a significant factor in reducing pulpal irritation as the ingress of fluid contaminated with bacteria is minimized. However, its solubility and disintegration lead to poor abrasion resistance which limits the life of the dressing. For the periods of time usually involved, zinc oxide/eugenol is a durable and satisfactory dressing material.

## Modified zinc oxide/eugenol cements

Additions to the powder and liquid serve to improve the physical properties of set zinc oxide/eugenol cement. Polystyrene or methyl methacrylate polymer dissolved in the liquid to a concentration of about 10 per cent, or the addition to the powder of 10 per cent hydrogenated rosin, a natural resin, increases both the compressive and tensile strength of the final material (Table 3.1). The increase in strength is thought to be due to the dispersion of the added materials in the matrix, binding the unreacted zinc oxide particles, with the production of a composite.

Because of their improved strength, modified zinc oxide/eugenol cements may be used satisfactorily as lining materials in larger, more complex cavities, being able to withstand the pressure of amalgam condensation. As they are non-irritant to the pulp they may be applied directly in deep cavities, obviating the need for a sub-lining.

ETHOXYBENZOIC ACID CEMENTS

Ethoxybenzoic acid (EBA) cement is a modification of zinc oxide/eugenol cement. Zinc oxide comprises 60–74 per cent of the powder, fused quartz or alumina 20–34 per cent, and hydrogenated rosin about 6 per cent. The last constituent reduces the brittleness of the set cement while the quartz or alumina acts as a filler allowing the final matrix to behave as a composite. Alumina is the more commonly used filler as quartz particles impart a gritty texture to the cement which is undesirable in a material used to cement inlays, crowns, and bridges.

The liquid is 37·5 per cent eugenol and 62·5 per cent o-ethoxybenzoic acid by volume. EBA, the structure of which is shown in Figure 3.2, is also a chelating agent and encourages the formation of a crystalline matrix which has greater strength. The improvement in compressive and tensile strengths is shown in Table 3.1. The physical properties of the cement approach those of phosphate cement, but EBA cements are less irritating to the pulp and can be applied to deep cavities without a sub-lining.

EBA cements are used as lining materials and to cement restorations to prepared teeth on a temporary and permanent basis. There is little or no specific adhesion of EBA cements to tooth substance or restorative materials and the material adheres mechanically at a microscopic level. Despite their superior properties, EBA cements are not as satisfactory as zinc oxide/eugenol for dressings, some products disintegrating and wearing rapidly in the mouth. The solubility of the formulation described is low. However, if EBA cement does not contain alumina and hydrogenated rosin the solubility is markedly increased.

## Zinc phosphate cement

Zinc phosphate cement is a material widely used as a lining and as a cement for indirect restorations. It is presented as a powder and a liquid which, when mixed, set to a hard mass.

CONSTITUENTS

The powder is fundamentally zinc oxide, although magnesium oxide is usually present up to 10 per cent. Other oxides, often those of bismuth and silicon, are present in small proportions to improve the quality of the set material and to produce a variety of shades. Fluorides have been added to some preparations with a view to reducing the solubility of adjacent enamel and thus the incidence of recurrent caries around cemented restorations. The components of the powder are mixed in the appropriate proportions and heated to a temperature between 1000 and 1400 °C. The resultant mass is ground to a powder of controlled particle size.

The liquid is an aqueous solution of o-phosphoric acid, the concentration of which varies from one product to another, but is usually between 30 and 40 per cent. The solution is buffered by the addition of metal oxides and hydroxides. Zinc and magnesium oxides and aluminium hydroxide are used for this purpose and form phosphates in the liquid.

SETTING REACTION

The setting reaction may be considered in two stages. First the superficial layer of the zinc oxide powder particles is dissolved by the acid with the formation of acid zinc phosphate which, in the second phase of setting, forms hydrated zinc phosphate. This substance is virtually insoluble and crystallizes to form a phosphate matrix that binds together the central unreacted portions of the zinc oxide powder particles. The reaction is exothermic and results in contraction. Magnesium oxide reacts in a similar way to zinc oxide.

RATE OF REACTION

Clinically it is important that the rate of reaction is within well-controlled limits. This is determined largely by the manufacturer but, as will be seen later, the clinician is able to modify the rate to a limited extent while maintaining the properties of the material.

The reactivity of zinc and magnesium oxide is determined by the sintering temperature used during manufacture. This is normally between 1000 and 1400 °C and the higher the temperature used, the less reactive the oxides become. The exact composition of the powder also influences the reaction rate; for example, bismuth trioxide is thought to slow the setting reaction in some preparations. Particle size affects the rate of reaction. Smaller particles, by offering a greater surface area for a given mass of material, lead to a more rapid reaction while the converse is true of larger particles.

The reactivity of the liquid may be modified by the manufacturer and, inadvertently, by the clinician. By adding oxides the manufacturer buffers the solution and at the same time reduces the reactivity, as phosphates are produced. Water content is a critical factor carefully controlled during manufacture and care must be taken clinically if alterations, detrimental to the rate of reaction and final set, are not to be introduced. o-Phosphoric acid is the most stable form of phosphoric acid, and therefore the least reactive. The water content determines the degree of dissociation of this acid into its more reactive forms. An increase in the water content allows more dissociation, greater reactivity, and consequently an increase in the rate of the setting reaction. Loss of water from the liquid has the opposite effect.

From the foregoing it will be appreciated that care should be taken to ensure that water loss from, or gain by, the liquid is minimized. Most dispensing bottles are designed to minimize evaporation by incorporating a nozzle. An eyedropper for dispensing would leave the contents of the bottle open to the air to a greater extent each time it was used. The nozzle should be covered while not in use. Loss of water by evaporation slows the setting reaction and may be evidenced, in extreme cases, by clouding of the liquid as crystallization occurs. Bottles are designed to carry about 20 per cent more liquid than required to react with the corresponding bottle of powder. While this does not reduce the amount of evaporation that takes place it minimizes the effect on the concentration of the residual solution. When all the powder has been used, the remaining liquid, which is the most severely affected, should be discarded. In a humid atmosphere, water will be taken up by the liquid with a consequential increase in the rate of setting. Water should never be added during mixing as a means of modifying the rate of reaction as this will produce deleterious effects on the physical properties of the set material.

Within certain limits, the clinician is able to modify the rate of setting by his manipulation of the material. An increase in the temperature increases the rate of reaction, and reduced temperature slows the rate. It is this latter effect that is useful, giving a longer working time and allowing the clinician to incorporate as much powder as possible in the time available for mixing. As will be seen, this leads to improved physical properties in the set material. The simplest way of achieving a reduction in the temperature of the reagents is by cooling the glass mixing slab, most frequently by immersion in cold water. Two dangers in this technique become apparent, both involving the contamination of the mix with water. If the slab is not thoroughly dried before the reagents are dispensed they will become contaminated directly, and if it has been cooled below the dew-point, condensation may produce a similar result. In both events the rate of reaction is increased, the opposite result from that intended, and the set material displays inferior physical properties.

The more powder that is incorporated into a given amount of liquid, the faster will be the rate of reaction. In this situation the increased surface area of powder available to the liquid leads to more rapid formation of a saturated solution of hydrated zinc phosphate, which, as a result, crystallizes earlier. The more rapid reaction is also accompanied by a more rapid evolution of exothermic heat which is less readily dispersed. The consequent rise in temperature may also contribute to an increased reaction rate.

By introducing the powder into the liquid slowly the rate of reaction may be reduced. This is enhanced by spreading the mix over a wide area on the glass slab, which should be bulky, in order to disperse the heat of reaction more efficiently. In practice the powder is added to the liquid in increments. Early increments do not lead to the rapid formation of crystalline hydrated zinc phosphate as saturation is not achieved and the reactivity of the remaining liquid is further reduced. Increments should be added at intervals so that as much powder as possible is included, generally over a period of 1·5 minutes. The total amount of powder that can be added will be determined by the desired viscosity of the final mix, and this will vary depending on the clinical use.

The setting time must be between certain limits for clinical convenience as this determines the working time of the material. If the rate of reaction is too rapid, continued spatulation breaks up the crystalline matrix as it forms, leading to a weakened mix lacking cohesion. On the other hand, an extended setting time delays the sequence of treatment. After a mixing time of 1·0–1·5 minutes the material should set in 5·0–9·0 minutes, depending on the manipulation variables described and the particular clinical task being undertaken.

PULPAL REACTION

Freshly mixed, setting zinc phosphate cement, by virtue of its low pH, induces an inflammatory response in the pulp when placed over exposed dentine, particularly when the preparation is deep. The pH of freshly mixed cement may be as low as 1·6, but will vary depending on the initial powder/ liquid ratio. As the material sets the pH increases and approaches neutrality in 1–2 days, but the differential between initially thick and thin mixes is maintained, even when the material is set.

It is generally recommended that deep cavities should be sub-lined with a less irritant material, such as calcium hydroxide or zinc oxide/eugenol, before the placement of a zinc phosphate cement lining (Fig. 3.3). While the depth of a cavity may be a fundamental consideration in the selection of a lining material, the nature of the tissue to be covered should not be over-looked. Dentine is a mineralized tissue traversed by tubules containing odontoblast processes which provide continuity of the pulp with the pre-pared cavity. It seems reasonable that a shallow cavity in relatively sound tissue in a young patient will present dentine far more prone to the trans-mission of harmful stimuli to the pulp than a deep, long-standing cavity in an older person. Here the dentine is often sclerosed and accompanied by considerable deposits of secondary dentine. A certain amount of clinical judgement must therefore temper the choice of material based on a con-sideration of cavity depth alone.

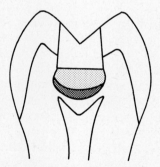

**Fig. 3.3** Sub-lining placed beneath lining in deep cavity.

Over-drying of the dentine prior to the direct application of zinc phosphate cement has been criticized, as desiccated dentinal tubules allow deeper pene-tration of free acid with a possible increase in pulpal irritation. While pulpal irritation is the biggest single disadvantage of zinc phosphate cement, this problem should not be overemphasized as it is only a temporary one, lasting until the cement has set. For many years crowns have been cemented, using zinc phosphate cement, on preparations that have exposed coronal dentinal tubules. Although a number of patients complain of pain during, and for a short time after, cementation only a few have long-term problems associated with the procedure.

STRENGTH

Compared with other lining materials zinc phosphate is strong. Its final strength, however, depends on manipulation variables under the control of the clinician. In general, the more powder incorporated into the liquid, the stronger will be the final material, and this amount can be increased by cooling the mixing slab and introducing the powder slowly. There is, however, an upper limit beyond which the addition of more powder does not contribute towards an increase in strength. Indeed, if too much powder is incorporated inadequate wetting of the particles leads to a dry, crumbly mix with poor physical properties.

Quoted values for the strength of lining materials may be misleading and often refer to an 'average' mix; considerable variation occurs (Table 3.1). Most of the strength (about 70 per cent) is achieved in the first hour after mixing and the maximum strength occurs in 24 hours. Magnesium oxide is thought to contribute towards an increased compressive strength.

The strength of zinc phosphate cement is closely related to its solubility. In general, a mix that produces a strong set results in a less soluble cement. If, however, the material is undergoing dissolution the strength is markedly reduced.

SOLUBILITY

Set zinc phosphate cement is virtually insoluble in water but dissolves to a greater extent in dilute organic acids. The site at which the cement may be exposed and available to the oral fluids is around the margins of inlays and crowns. Dental plaque in the vicinity of these margins, in particular the gingival margin, produces an acidic environment which may lead to the more rapid dissolution of the cement. The deficiency that results between the tooth and its restoration leads to greater plaque accumulation and, with progressive loss of cement, caries is more likely.

In water the phosphate matrix is dissolved extremely slowly, but it is thought that dilute acids dissolve the unreacted zinc oxide. The solubility can be minimized, however, by incorporating as much powder as possible during mixing, a procedure that also improves the strength. The water content of the liquid, as explained earlier, is carefully controlled by the manufacturer in order to determine the rate of reaction and final physical characteristics. Deviation from the formulation by loss or gain of water is accompanied by increased solubility (Fig. 3.4).

Contamination of zinc phosphate cement with moisture during mixing and in the early stages of setting must be avoided or constituents will be leached out and the final set will possess inferior physical properties and be more soluble. Tooth preparations should, therefore, be isolated from moisture

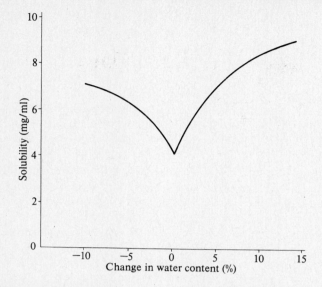

**Fig. 3.4** Effect of deviation from optimal water content of liquid on solubility of set cement.

prior to the application of the cement and during the initial set. The solubility gradually decreases over the first 24 hours, as the cement hardens, and protection of an exposed cement lute with varnish during this early period is beneficial. After 7 days the solubility of the cement in water is 0·1–0·2 per cent.

DIMENSIONAL CHANGE

Zinc phosphate cement contracts to a small extent on setting. Under water this is only 0·05–0·1 per cent but in air is somewhat greater at almost 0·3 per cent. Most of the contraction occurs in the first 2 hours. However, the set cement should not be allowed to dry out as shrinkage will be followed by crazing, disintegration, and increased solubility.

Contraction on setting, even at the upper limit of the range quoted, is not of clinical significance when the cement is used as a lining, as such contraction will tend to be directed towards the cavity surfaces. Moreover, when used to cement restorations in place the layer of material is so thin that, in absolute terms, the contraction is negligible. However, if zinc phosphate were used as a temporary dressing, in an inlay cavity for example, the amount of contraction would prejudice the marginal seal and allow leakage of fluid between the tooth and the dressing. Although, in the short term, caries would not occur, pulpal irritation would be increased. Zinc phosphate cement is not, therefore, usually considered suitable as a temporary filling material especially as it is chemically irritant and difficult to remove from the cavity.

ZINC PHOSPHATE AS A LINING

Zinc phosphate cement offers good protection to the pulp from thermal, electrical, and pressure stimuli. Although it provides protection from chemical irritation produced by certain restorative materials, it may damage the pulp directly as a result of its initially low pH. In deep cavities, and where the dentine is relatively sound, a sub-lining should be used. One benefit of the low pH of the setting cement is that it has an antibacterial effect. The fewer viable micro-organisms remaining on the cavity floor, the less will be the pulpal irritation.

By varying the powder/liquid ratio the operator may alter the viscosity and handling properties of the cement. However, where possible the maximum amount of powder should be included to gain maximum strength. The relatively high strength of phosphate cement allows the material to withstand the high compressive forces applied during the condensation of amalgam. This is particularly important when a restoration is being placed in a tooth with a pulp exposure, as pressure transmitted through the lining would be an additional traumatic burden for the tissue to overcome. A degree of structural alteration of the cavity form may be achieved with the cement by virtue of its strength, for example, the reconstruction of the pulpal and axial walls in a deep proximo-occlusal cavity.

Ideally, an adequately thick mix of zinc phosphate cement should have a similar consistency to thick putty and be sticky in texture. Some variation in consistency is acceptable to accommodate operator preference. Stickiness may lead to difficulty in separating the material from metal instruments and a thin film of alcohol on the latter is helpful as a separating medium. Zinc phosphate is compatible with all restorative materials, neither interfering with their setting reactions nor their final properties.

ZINC PHOSPHATE AS A CEMENT

Zinc phosphate has been used to cement inlays, crowns, and bridges to prepared teeth for many years. It is important that the mix has a low viscosity to ensure that excess cement escapes easily as the restoration is seated. Theoretically the final thickness of the cement lute is governed by the particle size, the smaller the size the closer the fit. However, a reduction in particle size increases the rate of the setting reaction and compensatory changes must be made, generally in the composition of the liquid, to maintain an adequate working time. It is, of course, desirable that a material used to cement restorations has a long working time. This allows the operator time to apply the mixed cement to the restorations and seat them carefully in the teeth. In practice a compromise is achieved by the manufacturers, and a cement film thickness of 15–40 $\mu$m is usually possible with most proprietary brands. As described earlier the working time may be extended by the slow addition of the powder into a mix spread over an extensive area of a cooled mixing slab. In this way it is possible to incorporate more powder to produce a stronger, less soluble cement.

It is unfortunate that the thinner mix used for cementation purposes has a lower pH, and is therefore more irritant to the pulp. However, in most preparations, even on non-carious teeth, this does not appear to create a clinical problem. Only a small proportion of patients complain of transient pain or discomfort from the tooth as the restoration is cemented.

Zinc phosphate offers little or no chemical or specific adhesion, the adhesive effect being mechanical. For the most part this is achieved at a microscopical level by the intrusion of the cement into minute irregularities on the prepared tooth surface and on the fitting surface of the restoration. In view of this mechanism the fitting surfaces of restorations should not be polished. Occasionally this effect may be augmented by the cement engaging gross mechanical undercuts in the tooth, but these are not a usual feature of crown and bridge preparations. Forces applied to the cement that may lead to its failure are complex and difficult to analyse. It is generally agreed that shearing forces are the most damaging and it is probable that these lead to the failure of the cement. The thicker the cement lute, the more effective these forces are, another indication for minimizing the amount of cement between the restoration and the tooth. The thinner the cement lute, the better retention will be, partly for the reason given above and partly because fewer voids will be incorporated during the placement of the restoration. Forces tending to displace restorations from parallel-sided crown and inlay preparations induce a shear stress rather than a tensile stress in the cement lute. In view of the very low tensile strength of zinc phosphate cement (5 $MN/m^2$), this is fortunate.

### Copper phosphate cements

These cements are esentially similar to zinc phosphate cements but a portion of the powder is replaced with a copper compound. Most frequently this is cupric oxide, which gives the powder a black colour. Other compounds, such as cuprous oxide, iodide, and silicate, have also been used and they impart characteristic colours. The cupric oxide usually added makes up 2–25 per cent of the powder. A similar liquid to that used in zinc phosphate cement is used but the acidity is normally lower and may be less than pH 1. Formation of hydrated crystalline phosphates occurs during setting to form a matrix that binds unreacted powder particles.

PROPERTIES

Copper compounds were originally added to this group of materials to enhance their antibacterial properties, the higher the proportion in the powder, the greater being the effect. Unfortunately this improvement is accompanied by an increase in solubility and therefore decreased efficiency of the material as a cement. Substances such as mercuric salts, including phenyl mercuric nitrate, have also been added for their antibacterial action, but their liberation is again dependent on the dissolution of the cement.

Like zinc phosphate cements, copper cements are acidic and among the most irritant of restorative materials. The pH of the liquid is exceedingly low and neutrality is never reached, the pH of the set material being about 5·3. This, and the dark colour, make copper phosphate cement unsuitable as a lining material, despite its strength which is similar to that of zinc phosphate.

### APPLICATIONS

Copper phosphate cements have been used as fissure sealants and as semi-permanent restorations in primary teeth, especially where it has not been possible to remove all the caries. However, such restorations are unsightly and dissolve fairly rapidly. As some varieties of copper cement set fairly well in the presence of saliva, they have been used in the cementation of cap splints in maxillo-facial surgery, and this is perhaps the commonest application at the present time.

## Zinc polycarboxylate cement

This more recently developed material also has a powder/liquid presentation. It is the first lining material and cement to display substantial specific adhesion to tooth substance.

### CONSTITUENTS

The powder is predominantly zinc oxide with small amounts of magnesium oxide. Other metal oxides are sometimes included to modify the setting reaction and one product contains stannous fluoride in an attempt to reduce caries in the adjacent dental hard tissues. Alumina is included to 43 per cent in another preparation and may operate to produce a composite matrix in the same way as in EBA cements.

The liquid is an aqueous solution of polyacrylic acid (Fig. 3.2) which may be presented with different viscosities, a low viscosity being used for the cementation of restorations while the higher viscosity is used for linings. The viscosity is generally controlled by varying the molecular weight of the acid but similar effects may be produced by altering its concentration. A representative example is a 40 per cent solution of acid, the low viscosity liquid containing acid of molecular weight 22 000, and the high viscosity having a molecular weight of about 50 000.

### SETTING REACTION

Polyacrylic acid is a chelating agent and binds metallic ions. During the setting reaction of the cement, the superficial layer of the zinc oxide particles is attacked and zinc ions are chelated by the carboxyl groups on the acid chains (Fig. 3.5a). It is possible that polyacrylate chains are cross linked by

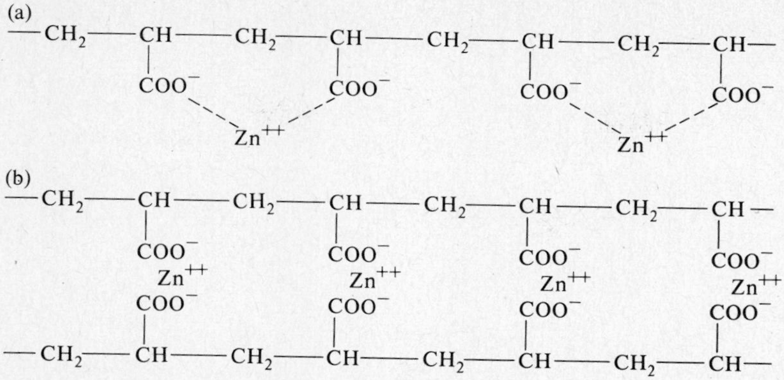

(a)

(b)

**Fig. 3.5** (a) Chelation of zinc ions by polyacrylic acid; (b) salt bridge formation in the setting of zinc polycarboxylate cement.

a similar mechanism involving the formation of salt bridges (Fig. 3.5b). The result of the reaction is a cored structure in which unreacted powder particles are bound by a matrix of zinc polyacrylate.

RATE OF REACTION

The setting reaction proceeds rapidly but may be slowed by cooling the mixing slab or incorporating less powder in the mix. As a paper mixing pad is often supplied, and as a reduction in the powder/liquid ratio reduces the strength of the final set, it is generally left to the clinician to incorporate the optimal amount of powder into the liquid in the shortest possible time. This is facilitated by the relatively high viscosity of the liquid. A powder/liquid ratio of about 1·5:1·0, by weight, is representative and mixing should be complete in 30–40 seconds to give adequate working time. Some manufacturers provide a measure for the powder that dispenses an amount for inclusion into a single drop of liquid. While measurement of the powder by volume is not accurate, the error introduced is probably small compared to that resulting from other clinical variables. The surface of the resultant creamy mix should be shiny when the material is used. If it is matt and tends to form 'cobwebs' when touched with an instrument, setting is too far advanced and the mix should be discarded. Slight loss of water from the liquid has a considerable deleterious effect on the strength of the final cement and the liquid should, therefore, be dispensed immediately before use and not left exposed on the mixing pad for any longer than is necessary.

PULPAL REACTION

Although the pH of the liquid is 1·0–1·7, and that of the freshly mixed cement is 3·0–4·0, pulpal reaction appears slight. This may be due, in part, to the high molecular weight of the acid which impedes its penetration of the dentinal tubules. The tendency of polyacrylic acid to form complexes with protein may also contribute to its slow progress through dentine. After 24 hours the pH of the cement is 5·0–6·0. While the pulpal response is slight compared to that induced by zinc phosphate cement, it is wise to place a sub-lining in very deep cavities, where microscopic pulp exposures may be present, prior to the placement of a zinc polycarboxylate cement lining. One product contains 15–18 per cent polyacrylic acid in the powder which allows a less concentrated solution to be used in the liquid, giving a correspondingly higher pH of 4·2–4·5.

### STRENGTH

The compressive strength of zinc polycarboxylate cement is comparable with that of zinc phosphate cement (about 90 MN/m$^2$), while the tensile strength is higher at 14 MN/m$^2$ compared to 5 MN/m$^2$ for zinc phosphate (Table 3.1). The final strength is dependent on the powder/liquid ratio, the more powder incorporated the greater the strength. The concentration and molecular weight of the polyacrylic acid solution in the liquid also plays a part. Thus the low viscosity liquid used to prepare a mix for cementation purposes produces a weaker set than the more viscous liquid used for linings.

### SOLUBILITY

Zinc polycarboxylate cement tends to absorb water and is slightly more soluble than zinc phosphate cement. This is a limitation when it is used to cement restorations as marginal dissolution of the cement may lead to recurrent caries. However, some presentations are more satisfactory in this respect, having solubilities similar to that of zinc phosphate cement. As with the latter material, zinc polycarboxylate is more soluble in dilute organic acids, such as those produced by dental plaque, than in water.

### ADHESION

Zinc polycarboxylate cement displays specific adhesion to tooth substance, in particular enamel (Chapter 2). It is thought that the initial stage in the process is the wetting of the tooth surface, which is favoured by the tendency of the carboxyl groups on the polyacid chain to form hydrogen bonds with the substrate surface. These bonds, however, are progressively replaced by ionic bonds between calcium ions in the tooth and the carboxyl groups following the displacement of hydrogen (Fig. 3.6). The capacity of the carboxyl groups to undergo hydrogen bonding may also play a part in the formation of complexes with the organic constituents of the tooth. However, the superior adhesion of the cement to enamel suggests that the principal reaction is with the inorganic phase, as this constitutes a higher proportion of enamel than dentine. The adhesion of zinc polycarboxylate cement to a smooth surface is superior to that achieved with a rough one, in contrast to zinc phosphate cement. Although polycarboxylate cements are hydrophilic, the

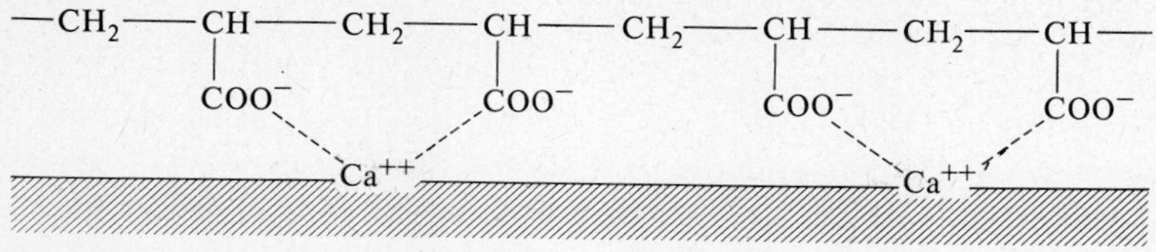

$$-CH_2 \quad CH \quad CH_2 \quad CH \quad CH_2 \quad CH \quad CH_2 \quad CH-$$

$$COO^- \qquad COO^- \qquad COO^- \qquad COO^-$$

$$Ca^{++} \qquad\qquad\qquad Ca^{++}$$

**Fig. 3.6** Adhesion between polycarboxylate cement and inorganic tooth substance.

cavity surface must be clean and dry if adhesion is to be optimal. The presence of saliva markedly reduces the adhesion between the cement and the tooth.

Experiments have shown that pretreatment of clean dentine surfaces with buffered saturated solutions of Brushite (calcium hydrogen phosphate dihydrate) leaves a thin layer of precipitated calcium hydroxyapatite. This increases the bond strength between dentine and polycarboxylate cement to the order of that between the cement and enamel. In the future this may form part of the technique for handling polycarboxylate and glass ionomer cements (Chapter 5). Under ideal circumstances any failure of the union between the tooth and polycarboxylate cement would be cohesive within the cement, the bond between the two remaining intact.

APPLICATIONS

By using the appropriate liquid, zinc polycarboxylate cement may be used as a cavity lining or a cement for the placement of indirect restorations. In the former role the strength is sufficient to allow condensation of amalgam and its effect on the pulp is mild enough to obviate the need for a sub-lining in many instances. The thermal conductivity of the cement is low, offering good protection against thermal stimuli transmitted by metallic restorations.

Polycarboxylate cement undergoes an initially slow rise in viscosity which allows adequate time to apply it to the fitting surfaces of restorations and seat them in the prepared teeth. This latter procedure is aided by the high degree of flow exhibited by the material. These properties, in combination, enable a relatively high powder/liquid ratio to be used for cementation mixes, giving greater strength and reduced solubility.

The specific adhesion between polycarboxylate cements and tooth substance has obvious advantages when they are used as cementing media. Adhesion is enhanced by good wetting of the substrate surface (Chapter 2) and hydrogen bonding by carboxyl side groups facilitates this in poly-carboxylate cement. However, the effect of this mechanism diminishes as the cement sets and early application to the tooth is essential if maximum adhesion is to be achieved. Unfortunately the adhesion to gold and porcelain is poor, and when a restoration is displaced it is usually at the interface between the cement and the restorative material. This problem may be overcome in the future by coating the fitting surface of restorations with a layer of a material bearing functional groups to induce specific adhesion. Adhesion of polycarboxylate cement to stainless steel is greater and this has application in orthodontic practice. There may be a place for zinc poly-carboxylate in the cementation of stainless steel brackets to the enamel surface in fixed appliance therapy; however, so far clinical results have been variable. The adhesion of cement to stainless steel instruments should be avoided by using a separating medium, such as alcohol or dry cement powder. Instruments should be cleaned thoroughly immediately after use.

### Glass ionomer cement

This adhesive restorative material is described in detail in Chapter 5. While it was originally designed as a tooth-coloured filling material, it has been modified to allow its use as a lining, cement, and fissure sealant.

The powder of the modified product is still an aluminosilicate glass but the particle size has been reduced to an average diameter of 15 $\mu$m. This not only allows closer adaptation of a restoration to the tooth preparation when the material is used as a cement, but also facilitates mixing. Proportioning of the powder and liquid is achieved using measures, and twice as much powder is used in a mix for a lining as in a mix for cementation purposes. Specific adhesion occurs to both enamel and dentine and also to polar surfaces, such as the oxide layer on the inner aspect of bonded porcelain crowns (Chapter 9). A system therefore exists that offers specific adhesion to both restoration and tooth. It is recommended that a varnish is applied around the margins of restorations cemented with this material, as soon as the excess has been removed, in order to protect the cement lute from the oral environment during setting and for some hours afterwards. It is thought that this enhances the durability of the adhesive bond to tooth substance. As a lining material, glass ionomer cement can be used in all but the deepest cavities without a sub-lining, as the pulpal reaction appears slight.

It is too early to assess glass ionomer cements in the proposed clinical roles. However, the adhesion to tooth substance and its mild effect on the pulp have clear advantages. It is also possible to enhance the adhesion to dentine by pretreatment of the tooth surface with Brushite solution, just as with polycarboxylate cement.

## PULP CAPPING AGENTS

There are occasions when a vital dental pulp is exposed during cavity preparation. Contamination of the exposure with saliva generally occurs and is superimposed, in most instances, upon established bacterial invasion from the carious process itself. In a proportion of these cases it is possible to maintain the vitality of the pulp by covering the exposure with a suitable material before restoring the tooth by a conventional technique (Fig. 3.7). Clearly a material used in this way must not be markedly irritant, and ideally it should stimulate the formation of a calcific barrier, preferably of ordered secondary dentine, to wall off the pulp from the prepared cavity. In order

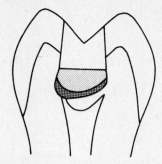

**Fig. 3.7** Exposed pulp covered with pulp capping material that also acts as sub-lining.

to minimize pulpal infection and inflammation an antibacterial action is advantageous. The material used functions as a lining or sub-lining and should not have to be removed subsequently, which would, in effect, re-expose the pulp. This allows the immediate, and hopefully permanent, placement of a restoration in the tooth.

### Calcium hydroxide

Calcium hydroxide has been used in a wide variety of preparations for pulp capping and sub-lining deep cavities. In the latter situation the remaining dentine in the floor of the cavity may be extremely thin and there is always the possibility that microscopic exposures are present but clinically undetectable.

PRESENTATION

Although calcium hydroxide may be applied in aqueous suspension, this is not an easy procedure and the resultant dried material is easily broken up and may be dislodged during the placement of the lining. Therefore, most popular presentations have a vehicle that makes the material easier to handle and gives a set with greater cohesion. The most common presentations are two-paste systems in which a setting reaction occurs in the vehicle that results in binding of the calcium hydroxide. The latter generally plays no part in the reaction. Various vehicles are used, some based on the solution of a polymer in a volatile organic solvent, others on an aqueous suspension of methyl cellulose.

PROPERTIES

Calcium hydroxide induces mineralization in the adjacent pulp, but the mechanism by which this occurs is not clear. It is known, however, that the calcium incorporated into the mineral bridge is of systemic origin and does not come from the pulp cap.

The pH of calcium hydroxide preparations is 11–12 and this produces a degree of tissue irritation leading to a band of necrotic and inflamed tissue between it and the healthy pulp. The basicity of calcium hydroxide is considered to be responsible for its demonstrable antibacterial action. Not all preparations, however, are equally effective in this respect. Some vehicles do not allow the egress of calcium hydroxide from the set mass and these have a correspondingly reduced antibacterial potential. The basicity also helps to neutralize acidic lining materials, such as zinc phosphate cement, that are placed over calcium hydroxide, reducing possible pulpal irritation from this source.

Most preparations of the two-paste type set more rapidly if temperature and humidity are increased. While the setting time on the mixing pad may be some minutes, the materials harden rapidly when applied to the tooth surface. Placement of the lining or filling may therefore be carried out with little delay. Care must be taken to avoid contaminating the mix on the pad and the applicator should, therefore, be wiped clean after each application to the cavity before more material is taken from the pad.

Calcium hydroxide is widely used as a pulp capping agent and as a sub-lining in deep cavities. It is also used extensively as a lining for tooth-coloured filling materials. However, the vehicle should not contain solvents, such as chloroform, that plasticize the resin used in some of these restorative materials. While two-paste systems produce a more cohesive result than simple suspensions, they are weak and unable to withstand the pressure of amalgam condensation. A newer product attempts to overcome this problem by using a vehicle that results in a set of higher compressive strength.

### Therapeutic pulp capping materials

Pulp exposure is always accompanied by bacterial contamination which leads to inflammation of the pulp. If untreated, fluid exudate from pulpal blood-vessels leads to an increase in pressure within the pulp chamber which, in turn, causes stasis of the blood-flow. It is the cessation of circulation that leads to pulp death.

Certain pulp capping materials include drugs in an attempt to prevent this sequence of events. One such product contains the antibiotic demethylchlor-tetracycline, to eliminate infection and an anti-inflammatory steroid, triamcinalone, to reduce exudation within the pulp. The preparation is presented in two forms, a paste and a cement. The paste, made up of calcium chloride, zinc oxide, anhydrous sodium sulphite, polyethylene glycol, and distilled water, in addition to the drugs, is used to cover the pulp exposure at the time of cavity preparation and the tooth is dressed. After 3–5 days, if the tooth is symptomless and has retained its vitality, the dressing is removed and the paste is replaced with the cement which carries the same drugs in lower concentrations. The cement is essentially a modified zinc oxide/eugenol preparation, and the powder, which includes the drugs, contains zinc oxide, Canada balsam, resin, and calcium hydroxide. The liquid consists of eugenol and rectified turpentine. Although the cement sets hard, unlike the paste, it is not sufficiently strong to allow the condensation of amalgam and must be covered with a stronger lining.

There has been a move away from the use of materials containing steroids because they may allow an infection to proceed unchecked because of the absence of an adequate inflammatory response. The true situation may, therefore, be masked. It is also undesirable to have to re-expose the pulp in a two-stage technique where further contamination may take place and further trauma is inevitable. The maintenance of pulp vitality is less effective with these materials, and the formation of a calcific barrier across the exposure rarely occurs.

## Cavity varnishes

Cavity varnishes generally consist of a natural resin, such as gum copal or rosin, in a volatile organic solvent. Many such solvents have been used, including ether, chloroform, acetone, benzene, and alcohol. More recently synthetic compounds such as polystyrene have been used in solvents and the resultant varnish is more effective in preventing the penetration of acid.

Applied to cavity walls, varnishes reduce the penetration of fluid between the tooth and the subsequently placed restoration. This is particularly so with recently placed amalgam fillings. The permeation of acid into dentine from cements, particularly zinc phosphate and silicate cements, is markedly reduced by the presence of varnish on the cavity floor, but as the layer is usually thin (from 3–20 $\mu$m per application), thermal protection is inadequate unless several layers are built up. Resistance to acid penetration is further increased by the inclusion of calcium hydroxide and zinc oxide, but their addition increases the solubility and, as the resultant varnish is coloured, there may be aesthetic consequences if the cavity margin is involved. The solubility of the basic varnish is very low and it appears to remain at the margin where it is exposed, provided it is in thin section. In general two, and sometimes three, layers are required to ensure a continuous film over the cavity surface, each layer being allowed to dry before the application of the next. As the presence of silicate cement adjacent to the enamel wall has an anticariogenic effect (Chapter 5) it is recommended that varnish should not be applied to the enamel walls of cavities to be restored with silicate cement.

In view of the small film thickness involved, cavity varnishes may be valuable to cover the dentine in shallow cavities to be restored with silicate cement without prejudicing the anticariogenic effect. In the management of deep cavities, especially if there is a pulp exposure present, it may be desirable to use a sub-lining of, for example, calcium hydroxide. In such cases the cavity varnish should be applied after this, but before the main lining. Certain cavity varnishes are not compatible with some resin-based restorative materials. In such circumstances the solvent in the varnish may interfere with the polymerization of the filling, leaving it soft, but it is more likely that free resin monomer will dissolve the varnish layer. As acrylic resin is no longer widely used as a filling material this problem is of reduced significance. Manufacturers of some composite restorative materials recommend the use of a varnish with their product.

Cavity varnishes have been widely used to protect the surface of freshly placed silicate fillings, preventing their early contamination with saliva and the loss of volatile constituents. A similar application now occurs with glass ionomer cement (Chapter 5) where improved adhesion follows the use of a varnish after the placement of the filling.

## TEMPORARY DRESSINGS

Following the preparation of gold inlay cavities it is necessary to restore the teeth temporarily while the permanent restorations are being made. Here the dressing maintains the relationship between the treated tooth and those adjacent and opposed to it, as well as protecting the exposed dentine and underlying pulp. There are other situations where it may not be possible to place a permanent restoration following cavity preparation and where temporary dressings are used until the tooth is restored permanently. Other forms of treatment may be phased over several visits, for example root-canal therapy, and temporary fillings are used during the intervening periods.

While a temporary dressing should be strong enough to withstand masticatory forces for a limited period, it should be possible to remove it easily and cleanly. Marginal leakage should not occur if pulpal irritation, consequent upon the ingress of fluid between the dressing and the tooth, is to be minimized. The material used should not, therefore, contract on setting. Ideally the coefficient of thermal expansion should be similar to that of tooth substance to eliminate marginal percolation for the same reason. Clearly a dressing material should be non-irritant to the pulp and have a low thermal conductivity, so that separate linings should not be necessary prior to their placement, even in deep cavities.

Several lining materials and cements are used as dressings and this, together with their merits and limitations, has been indicated in the relevant sections. Other preparations, however, have been used in this role, some specifically designed for the purpose.

### Gutta percha

Gutta percha has several applications in dentistry and is described as a root filling material in Chapter 12. A mixture of gutta percha with zinc oxide as a filler and waxes as plasticizers is still occasionally used as a temporary filling material. It is presented as small sticks which are softened by heat before insertion into the cavity. The temperature involved, however, is sufficiently high to cause pulpal damage and in certain circumstances, the pressure required to introduce it into the cavity may also bring about pulpal irritation. Marginal leakage is a major disadvantage and this may, in part, be due to the poor adaptation of the temporary filling to the cavity wall which often occurs. By applying a solvent, such as oil of cajuput, to the surface of the dressing the marginal seal may be improved. It is now widely recognized that the disadvantages outlined are sufficient to make gutta percha unsuitable as a temporary filling material, although it has another use in the application of a hot stimulus to the tooth during pulp vitality testing.

## Temporary filling putties

There are a number of products in the form of a putty or viscous paste which harden after insertion into the cavity. It appears that the presence of saliva brings about the transition from putty to solid. These presentations are most frequently based on zinc oxide/eugenol but have other constituents, some of which are probably concerned with keeping the putty free from moisture to prevent setting until the time of use. One such product contains potassium alum, aluminium phosphate and sulphate, calcium sulphate, paraffin, and menthol in addition to zinc oxide and eugenol, while another contains calcium hydroxide. These materials are quick and convenient to use and are easily removed from the cavity subsequently. Manufacturers suggest that the deeper part of a temporary dressing may be left as a lining for the permanent restoration. While this is technically feasible, it must be remembered that products containing eugenol may have a deleterious effect upon the setting and final properties of the tooth-coloured filling materials.

# 4
# Dental amalgam

An amalgam is an alloy of mercury with one or more other metals. Mercury is unique in that it is the only metal which is liquid and therefore able to react with other metals at room temperature. This particularly desirable property is put to great advantage in dentistry where restorative materials are required to set in a short period of time at mouth temperature, producing a strong solid.

Most of the dental amalgams in use today are specifically called silver amalgams since silver is the principal constituent of the alloy that reacts with the mercury. Other types have been used in the past, such as the copper amalgams, but these are no longer common.

In the silver amalgams, the mercury is mixed with an alloy that contains tin, copper, and possibly a few other metals in addition to the silver. This alloy is called the dental amalgam alloy. This terminology is not entirely logical for 'dental amalgam alloy' does not usually contain mercury and must not be confused with 'dental amalgam' which is the product of the reaction between the dental amalgam alloy and mercury.

Dental amalgams have been used for many years and since the beginning of the twentieth century have been the most popular of all filling materials. Many silver amalgams in use today are not vastly different from that developed by G. V. Black eighty years ago although there have been considerable refinements in their composition and method of presentation. In spite of the considerable advances in the composite filling materials discussed in the next chapter, amalgam remains the only available material that can withstand the high stresses applied to the posterior teeth and is, therefore, used for most Class I and II cavities and for many Class V cavities. Amalgam is, therefore, used in every situation where aesthetic appeal is not considered important (approximately 70–80 per cent of all fillings).

## Mercury used in dental amalgam

Mercury is a metal which freezes at $-39\ °C$. When used for the preparation of dental amalgam it must be very pure and, in fact, purity represents the only criterion upon which the metal is judged for this application. Contamination by traces of other metals can lead to changes in the properties of the amalgam and may also lead to changes in the effects of amalgam on the pulp since the contaminants themselves are often toxic.

Since it is the absolute concentration of trace elements that is important in defining the purity of mercury, the terms most frequently used, such as double distilled, redistilled, and triple distilled have no legal or scientific standing. The purity can, in fact, be checked easily by visual examination for even slight traces of contaminants such as 0·001 per cent of copper, zinc, lead, tin, bismuth, arsenic, antimony, or cadmium transform the normal, highly reflective surface of pure mercury to a dull surface. Two metals which do not do this are silver and gold, which can be present in amounts up to 0·1 per cent without causing any detectable change. The concentration of these elements can be determined by volatilizing the mercury and analysing the residue.

Standard specifications for dental mercury, such as those of the American Dental Association or the British Standards Institute require there be a bright mirror-like finish (i.e. contaminants to be less than 0·001 per cent of those base metals identified above) and less than 0·02 per cent of total non-volatile residues.

## COMPOSITION OF DENTAL AMALGAM ALLOYS

The conventional dental amalgam alloys supplied by different manufacturers have slightly varying compositions but generally fall within the compositional range given in Table 4.1. The A.D.A. specification (No. 1) allows a minimum of 65 per cent silver and maxima of 29, 6, 2, and 3 per cent for tin, copper, zinc, and mercury respectively. These figures are based to a large extent on the composition requirements to give adequate tarnish resistance.

**Table 4.1** Normal composition range of dental amalgam alloy

|     | %     |
| --- | ----- |
| Ag  | 67–74 |
| Sn  | 25–28 |
| Cu  | 0–6   |
| Zn  | 0–2   |
| Hg  | 0–3   |

The high-copper, dispersion-type amalgam alloys have a different composition and structure, some of the tin being replaced by copper. A typical composition is given in Table 4.2. This type of alloy has been developed in an attempt to eliminate some of the undesirable properties that are due to the higher tin content. It is likely that other modifications to the composition will be introduced in the near future to further this aim.

**Table 4.2** Typical composition of high-copper, dispersion-type amalgam

|     | %   |
| --- | --- |
| Ag  | 70  |
| Sn  | 16  |
| Cu  | 13  |
| Zn  | 1   |

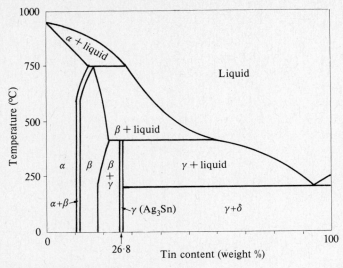

**Fig. 4.1** Silver–tin phase diagram.

## The silver–tin alloy system

The phase diagram for the silver–tin system is shown in Figure 4.1. Of greatest significance in relation to dental amalgam alloy is the $\gamma$ (gamma) phase, which is an intermetallic compound corresponding to the atomic formula $Ag_3Sn$. This is stable up to 480 °C but, in the silver–tin system is found only over the range 25–27 per cent tin. The composition of the $Ag_3Sn$ phase by weight is 26·85 per cent tin; 73·15 per cent silver. It is most important that the conventional type of dental amalgam alloy contains as much of this phase as possible, as it is the $Ag_3Sn$ phase that controls the reaction with the mercury and gives the desirable properties to the resulting amalgam. If any other phase is present it will be the $\beta$ phase, which is slightly richer in silver than $Ag_3Sn$. The presence of the $\beta$ phase tends to increase the rate of reaction with mercury, as discussed later.

In practice, small amounts of copper and zinc will be present in the alloy, altering slightly the compositional limits on the phase diagram. The copper tends to replace the silver, yeilding a $Cu_3Sn$ or $Cu_6Sn_5$ phase in addition to the $Ag_3Sn$.

### INDIVIDUAL ELEMENTS IN CONVENTIONAL DENTAL AMALGAM ALLOY

*Silver.* Silver is the major element present in the $Ag_3Sn$ phase and, therefore, contributes significantly to the reaction with mercury. Silver contents towards the higher end of the range generally result in a slightly larger expansion on setting and a better resistance to tarnish in the resulting amalgam.

*Tin.* The tin is present to control the reaction between the silver and mercury. Without tin the reaction would be too fast and the setting expansion would be clinically unacceptable. The tin reduces both the rate of reaction and the expansion to optimal values. It is important that the tin content is kept within well-defined limits as excessive tin may result in a very undesirable setting contraction, inferior mechanical properties, and reduced tarnish resistance.

*Copper.* Copper has played a significant role in dental amalgam metallurgy for a long time. 'Copper amalgams' are still available as alternatives to silver amalgams but rarely used since the reaction between copper and mercury does not take place unless they are heated. A small amount of copper, typically 3 per cent, is used in many types of silver amalgam, however, where it can modify the amalgamation process. In particular, it increases the hardness and strength of the amalgam. A far more dramatic effect is found when copper is present in larger amounts in the so called dispersion-type or high-copper amalgams that are discussed below.

*Zinc.* Zinc itself, in small quantities, does not influence the setting reaction or the properties of amalgam. It is added to the alloy as a scavanger or deoxidizer, thus aiding the manufacture of the alloy. When the various elements are fused together, zinc preferentially reacts with the oxygen, and any impurities present, preventing the oxidation of the more important elements and thus preserving their optimal concentrations.

*Mercury.* In some formulations a small amount of mercury is added to the alloy, usually just sufficient to cover the surface of the alloy particles. This gives a more rapid reaction and is referred to as pre-amalgamation.

### Dispersion-type amalgams

The silver–copper phase diagram is shown in Figure 4.2. This is a simple system, exhibiting a eutectic structure (Chapter 1) at a composition of approximately 71 per cent silver, 29 per cent copper. This eutectic is used in the preparation of the dispersion-type amalgams. Generally the manufacturer mixes a very fine dispersion of this eutectic, with a particle size of the order of 1 $\mu$m, with the conventional $Ag_3Sn$ phase in proportions of about 1 part Ag–Cu to 2 parts $Ag_3Sn$ to form the alloy powder. The proportions vary from one product to another.

## MANUFACTURE OF DENTAL AMALGAM ALLOYS

There are two basic methods of preparing the conventional dental amalgam alloy, which yield products of different physical form. These are the lathe-cut alloys and the spherical particle alloys. The dispersion-type amalgam alloys are prepared by a combination of these two methods.

### Lathe-cut alloy

For many years only lathe-cut alloys were available and most of the

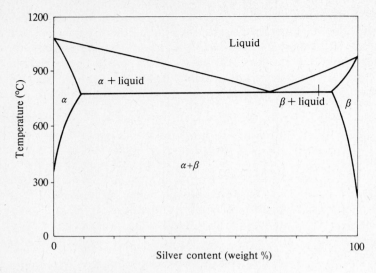

**Fig. 4.2** Silver–copper phase diagram.

characteristics of amalgam were determined using this type of material. The particles are produced mechanically from a cast ingot of the amalgam alloy. The various constituent metals are melted together and cast into a suitable shape. The speed of cooling from the high temperature is very important for it controls the structure of the alloy. As discussed in Chapter 1, a phase diagram may indicate that a certain phase will be stable at room temperature, but rapid cooling may prevent atoms from occupying sites in the lattice of that phase by allowing insufficient time for diffusion at the appropriate temperature. In the case of the silver–tin system, rapid cooling of an alloy of composition corresponding to the $\gamma$ phase may yield a $\gamma + \beta$ structure because of this effect (Fig. 4.3a). Since the $\beta$ phase should be kept to a

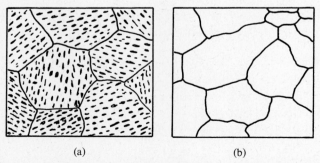

(a)                          (b)

**Fig. 4.3** (a) $\gamma + \beta$ structure in amalgam alloy produced by rapid cooling; (b) $\gamma$ structure resulting from homogenizing anneal.

minimum, it is desirable that the equilibrium condition of maximum $\gamma$ content should be allowed to develop (Fig. 4.3b). This may be achieved by slow cooling, but it is more practical and common for the alloy to be rapidly cooled and then reheated to about 400–450 °C for a suitable time, say 12–24 hours, for this equilibrium structure to be achieved. This operation is referred to as an homogenizing anneal.

The ingot is then placed in a lathe and cut with a suitable tool to produce filings, which are themselves comminuted, or broken down, in a ball-mill or similar equipment. The final particle size is important since it influences the setting reaction and handling qualities of the amalgam. This size may differ from one manufacturer to another and indeed, many manufacturers supply amalgams of different particle size. It is now generally agreed that a small particle size is desirable, and the adjectives 'fine-cut' and 'micro-cut' are frequently used to describe the products. Although distinction between such grades is arbitrary, fine-cut alloys typically have a mean particle size of about 35 $\mu$m while that of the micro-cut alloys is nearer 25 $\mu$m. Naturally there will be a distribution about the mean although it is important that careful sieving and grading is performed to ensure a controlled range of particle size. A sample of a lathe-cut alloy is shown in Figure 4.4.

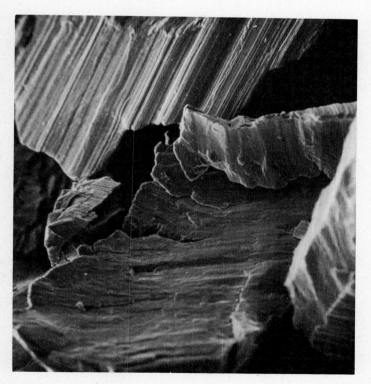

**Fig. 4.4** Sample of lathe-cut alloy as observed in a scanning electron microscope.

The mechanical method of producing these particles results in high residual stresses, representing a high internal energy of the particles. These stresses would normally be relieved spontaneously but over a long period of time, this being achieved by the gradual readjustment of the atoms, as in a normal annealing process. However, the reactivity of the particles will depend, to some extent, on their internal energy so that the relief of the internal stresses would result in a reduction in reactivity, thereby giving a variable product. This situation may be aggravated by a tendency for the particles to oxidize slowly over a period of time. To overcome this problem, the alloy particles are given an anneal, during which the residual stresses are considerably reduced, so that the product will suffer little or no change during storage. This process is called ageing and involves heating the particles to between 60 and 100 °C, often using boiling water, for up to 6 hours.

### Spherical particle alloy

The production of spherical particle alloy is considerably easier than that of the lathe-cut variety. Molten alloy is atomized in a stream of inert gas within a closed chamber. The atomization process results in the formation

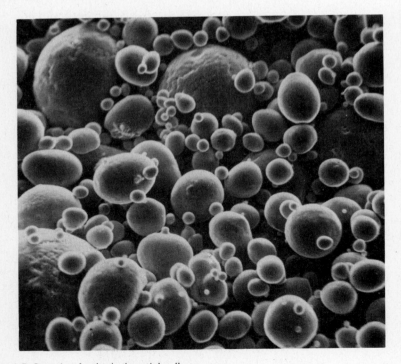

**Fig. 4.5** Sample of spherical particle alloy.

of large numbers of minute droplets which rapidly solidify as they lose heat. A range of particle sizes is produced and in this case, to optimize their packing within the amalgam during mixing and condensation, a wide range is incorporated. Typically the diameters will range from 5 to 40 or 50 $\mu$m, as illustrated in Figure 4.5.

The microstructure of each individual particle is essentially the same as that of a large cast ingot, consisting of $\gamma$ and $\beta$ phases. The particles may be given an homogenizing anneal to remove this cored structure but manufacturers differ in the heat treatments given.

### Dispersion-type amalgam alloy

As noted above, the dispersion amalgam alloys contain larger amounts of copper than do the conventional alloys. The method of incorporating the copper into the structure may vary from one product to another, but the most widely established method utilizes the silver–copper eutectic. This eutectic is prepared in spherical particle form and is mixed with particles of $Ag_3Sn$, which may be spherical or lathe-cut, an example being shown in Figure 4.6.

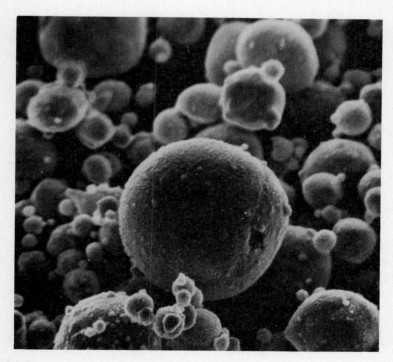

**Fig. 4.6** Sample of high-copper, dispersion-type amalgam.

## THE MANIPULATION OF AMALGAM

Apart from the finishing procedures, which are dealt with later, there are three important steps involved in the manipulation of the amalgam which influence the reaction between the alloy and the mercury. These are (a) the proportioning of alloy and mercury, (b) the mixing, or trituration, and (c) the packing of the amalgam into the cavity, known as condensation.

### Proportioning

Here it is necessary to consider the relative proportions of the alloy and mercury, the methods by which they are dispensed and the total volume of the mix.

#### MERCURY/ALLOY RATIO

When mixing mercury and amalgam alloy together there must be sufficient mercury available to wet all the particles so that the reaction can proceed uniformly throughout the mass. This places a lower limit on the mercury/alloy ratio. On the other hand, as discussed more fully later, the presence of excess mercury in the final amalgam has a very deleterious effect on the properties, placing an upper limit on this ratio.

In practice, the desirable ratio varies a little from one amalgam to another, but it is generally agreed that the finished restoration should contain less than 50 per cent total mercury. It is this final mercury content that is important and it is of no great significance if there is more mercury present in the initial mix as long as the excess is removed during condensation. For a long time it was customary to use proportions of 5:7 or 5:8, alloy to mercury, and at these values a very convenient plastic mass was produced. However, the optimum ratio has changed with the method of mixing and it is widely held that equal volumes of mercury and alloy give a good usable product with most varieties of amalgam.

The amount of mercury recommended for spherical particle alloy is often slightly less than for lathe-cut alloy, due to the smaller surface area/volume ratio of the former, which requires less mercury to give complete wetting of particle surfaces. Dispersion-type amalgams usually use equal volumes of mercury and alloy.

#### METHOD OF PROPORTIONING

Several techniques are available for dispensing the mercury and amalgam alloy in the correct proportions for mixing. The alloy may be dispensed by manual weighing or by automatic weight or volume dispensers. The mercury may also be dispensed by either volume or weight. However, these methods have been largely superseded by the use of preweighed alloy tablets or pre-proportioned capsules containing both alloy and mercury.

Although quite accurate ratios of mercury to alloy can be achieved by the weight or volume dispensing methods, both methods do have disadvantages. For example, volume dispensing of the powder can give variable weights depending on the particle size, and the distribution and density of packing. Also the powder tends to cling to the wall of some dispensers. Any method of pouring mercury from one container to another may increase mercury contamination in the surgery and involves the danger of spillage.

Most manufacturers now supply their amalgam products either in the form of preweighed tablets of alloy to be used with a good mercury dispenser, or in proportioned capsules. In these capsules, there are two compartments separated by a very thin membrane (Fig. 4.7). The mercury is contained in one compartment and the alloy in the other, the relative amounts being determined by the manufacturer. The membrane is ruptured mechanically immediately before mixing is performed by the mechanical methods discussed below. These disposable capsules are usually more expensive but they do have the advantage of convenience. There is also the further theoretical advantage of consistency as the responsibility for correct proportioning has been transferred to the manufacturer.

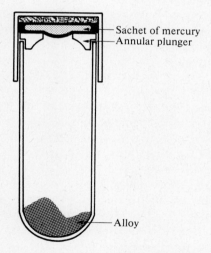

Sachet of mercury
Annular plunger

Alloy

**Fig. 4.7** Section through capsule containing preproportioned amalgam alloy and mercury.

SIZE OF MIX

This depends, to some extent, on the size of the restoration and the method used for trituration. With preproportioned capsules, the amount is already determined and is typically 400–600 mg of alloy per capsule. Although large cavities will require larger amounts of amalgam, it is usual practice to make up 2 or even 3 smaller mixes as required, rather than one large mix.

## Trituration

It is essential that the mercury thoroughly wets the alloy particles in order to ensure that the two components are adequately mixed. This process of mixing is called trituration and it may be achieved either by hand or, more commonly, by mechanical amalgamators.

### HAND MIXING

Although at one time the only method available for mixing, this is now rarely used, being suitable only for individually dispensed alloy and mercury. Mixing is achieved with a pestle and mortar, both made of glass, with ground surfaces. Trituration is complete when a smooth homogenous mass is produced, the time taken depending on the force used and the speed of mixing. Typically a 25–45 second period is sufficient.

### MECHANICAL AMALGAMATORS

Hand mixing is neither a convenient operation nor one which is likely to give consistent results, since it is difficult to judge the important variables of force and speed. Mechanical amalgamators are superior in both respects and are almost universally used. It is likely, however, that the properties of an amalgam will be the same when mixed carefully by either technique.

The exact procedure used with mechanical amalgamators depends on the method of proportioning. If tablets of alloy and dispensed mercury are used, these are placed in a capsule with a small metal or plastic pestle, and the capsule placed in the amalgamator, where it is vibrated at high speed. With preproportioned mercury and alloy, the membrane is first ruptured and then the capsule is simply placed in the amalgamator and again vibrated.

The time to complete trituration depends on the characteristics of the machine. The efficiency of the trituration is basically controlled by the amount of energy supplied, which in turn is dependent on the speed and force of the mixing, just as it is when mixing by hand. Typically a vibratory frequency of 2000–4000 cycles per minute is used with a total amplitude of 50 mm. It does seem, however, that the more rapidly the energy is applied, the better the amalgamation, so that high-speed amalgamators are preferred.

It is important to note that the amount of trituration is extremely important in developing an amalgam of optimal properties, and the effect on these properties of under- and over-trituration will be discussed later. Generally an under-triturated amalgam will be difficult to manipulate and may crumble, since not all the alloy particles will be wetted by the mercury. By contrast, in an over-triturated amalgam, too much interaction will have taken place and it may be too plastic to manipulate.

Since different amalgam preparations appear to require slightly different trituration times, and since different amalgamators have different characteristics, it is important to follow the manufacturer's instructions concerning the time setting to use with any particular machine.

## Condensation

The amalgam is placed in the cavity after trituration. Then, using suitable instruments, force is applied to the amalgam in order to

**a** adapt it to the cavity walls;

**b** remove excess mercury; and

**c** enhance packing of the amalgam particles and reduce the risk of void formation.

This process is called condensation. It is obviously desirable for the amalgam to be packed well into the cavity, but the removal of excess mercury is equally important since, as mentioned above, free mercury has a significant deleterious effect on the properties of the restoration.

The following factors related to condensation influence the quality of the restoration:

**a** the time between trituration and condensation;

**b** the method of condensation used;

**c** the size and shape of the condenser;

**d** the force of condensation; and

**e** the size of the increments of amalgam used.

### TIME BETWEEN TRITURATION AND CONDENSATION

The amalgam should be condensed in the cavity as soon as possible after trituration. If there is any appreciable delay, the strength of the restoration will be reduced and the dimensional change associated with the setting will be altered. This is because the setting reaction will have started before condensation takes place, making it far more difficult to remove excess mercury. This again points to the need to avoid large mixes so that all the amalgam may be condensed in the cavity in a suitably short time. Generally 3–4 minutes is regarded as the maximum time between trituration and condensation.

### METHOD OF CONDENSATION

Condensation may be performed either with hand instruments or with mechanical condensers. A variety of instruments is available for hand condensation, and their design is described below. Mechanical condensers are usually attached to a handpiece and their design allows either a tapping action or vibratory movement on the amalgam. It is also possible to use ultrasonic condensers. Once again the mechanical method does not intrinsically produce a better amalgam than the hand method, if both are used correctly. Mechanical methods may, however, give more reproducible results and may reduce operator fatigue, although it is important to remember that a certain amount of force has to be applied by the operator of a mechanical condenser to make full use of the tapping or vibratory action.

SIZE AND SHAPE OF CONDENSERS

Hand instruments have a variety of tip shapes and sizes. They may have an oval, crescent, trapezoidal, triangular, or circular shape and vary in size up to about 3 mm diameter in the case of the latter. The tip itself may have a smooth or serrated surface, the instrument almost invariably being made of stainless steel. The type used is often a matter of operator preference, but the size and shape are largely governed by the shape of the cavity and the stage of the process. With the placement of the first increment in a small cavity, it is often desirable to exert a large force over a small area in a particular direction, in which case a 1 to 1·5 mm tip of a shape appropriate to the cavity is used. As more amalgam is placed in the cavity, the size of the tip represents a compromise between the need to have a small tip to give maximum pressure and a large tip to cover a wide area and prevent the tip from penetrating into the amalgam. A 1·5 to 2 mm tip is commonly used. For the final increment a large tip, 2–3 mm in diameter, is often used to facilitate contouring and preserve the surface finish. It is noticeable that the spherical particle amalgam requires less pressure for condensation, and so a tip larger than that used for lathe-cut amalgam is often employed.

FORCE OF CONDENSATION

Figures are often quoted for the optimal force of condensation. In clinical practice these figures are of no great value as there is no way for the operator to assess the force he is applying. It is important, however, to use a large force if good adaption and good properties are to ensue. It should be noted that less force of condensation is required in spherical amalgams.

SIZE OF INCREMENTS

Amalgam is placed in cavities in a series of increments. It is generally desirable that these increments are small enough to allow for sufficient condensation in each part of the restoration. This is particularly important if it is not possible to use a high condensation pressure. If large increments are used, it is difficult to remove all the excess mercury and, since the packing will be less efficient, voids may form, leading to a reduction in strength. Any mercury-rich material that is brought to the surface should be removed to prevent its entrapment. However, the surface must not be too dry as it would then fail to bond to the next increment. In effect, a compromise has to be reached. It is usual to overpack a cavity with amalgam so that the mercury-rich superficial layer that arises during condensation can be removed during contouring, increasing the amount of mercury that is eliminated.

## MERCURY–AMALGAM ALLOY REACTION

The reaction that occurs between mercury and the silver–tin alloy is complex and incompletely understood. However, the reaction can be quite adequately represented by the equation

$$Ag_3Sn + Hg \longrightarrow Ag_3Sn + Ag_2\,Hg_3 \text{ (or } Ag_5\,Hg_8) + Sn_6\,Hg$$
$$\text{(or } Sn_7\,Hg \text{ or } Sn_8\,Hg).$$

The $Ag_3Sn$ phase is denoted by $\gamma$, and the reaction products are $\gamma_1$ and $\gamma_2$ respectively. $\gamma_1$ is a mercury–silver phase of body-centred cubic structure and composition approximating to $Ag_2\,Hg_3$ or $Ag_5\,Hg_8$. The $\gamma_2$ phase is a hexagonal tin-rich tin–mercury phase, the composition of which is quoted as between $Sn_6\,Hg$ and $Sn_8\,Hg$. In the set amalgam there is, in addition to these two reaction products, a substantial amount of unreacted $Ag_3Sn$. Thus, the reaction may be conveniently written

$$\gamma + Hg \longrightarrow \gamma + \gamma_1 + \gamma_2.$$

Since the $\gamma$, $\gamma_1$, and $\gamma_2$ phases are structurally and compositionally so different, the properties of the amalgam will largely depend on the relative proportions of each and their relationship to each other. It is essential that there is a large amount of unreacted $\gamma$ in the set amalgam, for this is the strongest phase. This is especially significant during the early stages of the setting reaction when $\gamma$ is effectively the only phase contributing to the strength. Typically about 30 per cent by volume of the set amalgam will be unreacted $\gamma$. The $\gamma_1$ phase is present in the greatest amount. It is reasonably strong and corrosion-resistant. On the other hand, the $\gamma_2$ phase, which contains about 80 per cent tin, is weak and far more susceptible to corrosion.

Amalgam can be regarded in much the same way as the cements discussed in the previous chapter, since the desirable structure of the set product, as illustrated in Figure 4.8, is a substantial core of unreacted alloy, held together

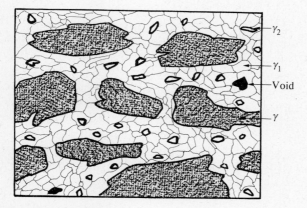

**Fig. 4.8** Microsctructure of set amalgam.

by a minimum of the reaction products consistent with complete wetting of the particles and integrity of the structure. In this case the core is $\gamma$ and the matrix is $\gamma_1$ and $\gamma_2$, with preferably a high $\gamma_1$ and low $\gamma_2$ content.

On mixing, the process commences by the wetting of the alloy particles by the mercury. There is some controversy concerning the next stage of the reaction, but it would appear likely that the twin processes of the mercury diffusing into the alloy particles and some $\gamma$-phase dissolving in liquid mercury take place simultaneously during both trituration and condensation phases, as illustrated in Figure 4.9. The $\gamma_1$ and $\gamma_2$ phases then start to crystallize in this zone between the mercury and the alloy particles where, in effect the $Ag_3Sn$ is in solution in the mercury. The $\gamma_1$ phase tends to form a continuous network in this matrix, with the $\gamma_2$ phase forming in discrete areas. It is not known at exactly what stage this crystallization begins, although it is likely that the process has started by the end of trituration or during condensation.

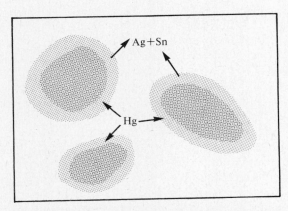

**Fig. 4.9** Diffusion of mercury into superficial layers of alloy particles and dissolution of surface $Ag_3Sn$ in mercury.

As noted above, the reaction does not go to completion, the final amalgam restoration containing a considerable proportion of unreacted $\gamma$. There are two basic reasons for this. First, as the $\gamma_1$ and $\gamma_2$ phases crystallize, some of the crystals that are formed will coat the $\gamma$ particles. This slows down the reaction by separating the particles and causing the reaction to be controlled by diffusion through the solid phases. Secondly, although the reaction is dependent on the alloy–mercury ratio used, the amount of mercury available for reaction is reduced during condensation, so that the source of mercury indicated in Figure 4.9 is depleted. Thus, less mercury is available, whilst at the same time it becomes more difficult for it to gain access to the unreacted $\gamma$.

The exact extent of the reaction depends on both the characteristics of the alloy used and the clinical variables associated with its manipulation, since they will control the ability of the $\gamma_1$ and $\gamma_2$ phases to separate the reactants. These factors include the alloy–mercury ratio, the alloy particle size, the trituration time, the time between trituration and condensation, and the condensation pressure. For example, any $\gamma_1$ and $\gamma_2$ phases that form at a very early stage in the process and coat the alloy particles, may have an immediate effect on the reaction by causing it to become partially diffusion-controlled at this point. A large particle size, giving a small surface area/particle volume ratio will tend to have this effect. However, if trituration is prolonged, this structure will be broken up, exposing fresh $\gamma$ to the mercury, with the original $\gamma_1$ and $\gamma_2$ no longer preventing the mercury from reacting with the remaining $\gamma$ particles.

### SETTING REACTION OF HIGH COPPER AMALGAMS

The setting reaction in dispersed-phase, high-copper type amalgams is somewhat different. Although the $Ag_3Sn$ particles of the alloy react with the mercury in the same way, the tin that is in solution in the mercury as a result of the dissolution of the surface of the $Ag_3Sn$ particles reacts with the silver–copper eutectic rather than the mercury. In effect the tin displaces some of the silver from the eutectic, forming a copper–tin compound, approximating to $Cu_6Sn_5$.

## PROPERTIES OF AMALGAM

### Dimensional changes on setting

An undesirable feature of a direct restorative material is contraction on setting, since, in the absence of adhesion, this could cause the restoration to shrink away from the cavity walls and lead to a greater susceptibility to recurrent caries, as discussed in the next chapter. It is also undesirable for there to be any large-scale expansion leading to excessive stresses in both the restoration itself and the surrounding tooth.

Theoretically, therefore, a restorative material should either exhibit no dimensional change at all on setting, or should have a slight expansion. In practice, however, it has been difficult to show whether an amalgam exhibiting a slight expansion is any better than one exhibiting a slight contraction, provided excesses of either are avoided. Thus the A.D.A. specification for amalgam now quotes a range of dimensional change of $+20$ $\mu m/cm$ to $-20$ $\mu m/cm$ as acceptable.

The classical behaviour of a setting amalgam is shown in Figure 4.10. There is a short phase of contraction, followed by a longer and more significant period of expansion, reaching a peak and leading to a small final contraction, levelling off typically between 5 and 10 $\mu m/cm$ net expansion.

Not all amalgams display this behaviour, however, and indeed the curves for any one amalgam formulation may vary substantially with clinical factors such as trituration time, condensation pressure and, in the case of mechanical trituration, with the type of amalgamator used. The dimensional change is so variable, in fact, that it is difficult to achieve consistent results with a material, and it is possible to have either a net contraction or net expansion with the same material under different circumstances.

The curve shown in Figure 4.10 is explained in the following way. A slight initial contraction is the result of the diffusion of the mercury into the alloy and the solution of the latter in the mercury. In practice this contraction is often minimal and short-lived, and is quickly followed by expansion. This expansion is attributed to the crystallization of the new $\gamma_1$ and $\gamma_2$ phases and their effective outward growth. The observed expansion at this time must be considered as the net result of the expansion due to this effect and an opposing tendency to contract because of the further mercury diffusion and alloy solution. In this classical situation, the apparent expansion due to the outward growth of $\gamma_1$ and $\gamma_2$ phases is greater, and so a net expansion is observed. Towards the end of the reaction, the contraction may, in fact, become dominant as the final traces of mercury diffuse into the solid-state reaction products.

Among the important variables affecting the dimensional changes are the composition of the alloy, the mercury/alloy ratio, the alloy particle size, the trituration time, and the pressure of condensation. The effect of these material and clinical variables is to alter the balance between the tendencies to give

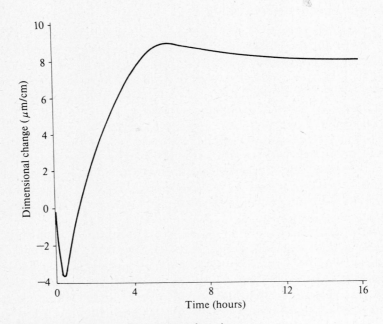

**Fig. 4.10** Dimensional changes on setting of amalgam.

contraction and expansion and to vary the rate of the reaction and hence the relationship between the various stages in the setting reaction and the stages of clinical manipulation.

## ALLOY COMPOSITION

As discussed previously, greater silver content of the conventional alloy results in greater expansion of the amalgam, whilst conversely an increase in the tin content tends to give greater contraction. A net contraction may result from an alloy containing more than 29 per cent tin.

## ALLOY PARTICLE SIZE

For a given weight of alloy, as the alloy particle size decreases, the total alloy surface area increases. This greater surface area presented to the mercury results in a more rapid diffusion of the mercury into the particles during trituration, giving a more pronounced initial contraction and a greater contribution to the tendency to contract during the middle stages. This effect is enhanced by the relationship between the time taken to form $\gamma_1$ and $\gamma_2$ in a fine particle size alloy, and the length of trituration time as discussed below. Thus, a very fine particle size results in a reduced overall expansion of the amalgam.

## MERCURY/ALLOY RATIO

The more mercury present the greater the extent of the reaction, and hence the greater the amount of $\gamma_1$ and $\gamma_2$ phases produced. Thus, the expansion associated with the formation of these new phases dominates, giving an increased net amount of setting expansion with high mercury/alloy ratios. This emphasizes the significance of the trend towards lower mercury/alloy ratios, since the expansion observed with a very high ratio can be excessive. It also demonstrates the importance of the removal of excess mercury during the condensation process.

## TRITURATION

The trituration time is perhaps the most important variable. In general, the longer the trituration time the less the expansion, as illustrated in Figure 4.11. Curve 1 represents the behaviour of an amalgam given a normal trituration time. If the trituration time is shortened, very little diffusion of the mercury into the alloy takes place, resulting in little tendency to contract and a greater net expansion (curve 2). If the trituration time is lengthened, two factors come into play. First, the continuous mechanical attrition results in the breakdown of the particles and the removal of newly formed $\gamma_1$ and $\gamma_2$ phases from the particle surfaces, giving a greater tendency for mercury diffusion into the alloy and a greater contraction. Secondly, there is a tendency for more $\gamma_1$ and $\gamma_2$ to be formed during the trituration stage, as distinct from after the trituration stage when the amalgam has been placed in the cavity.

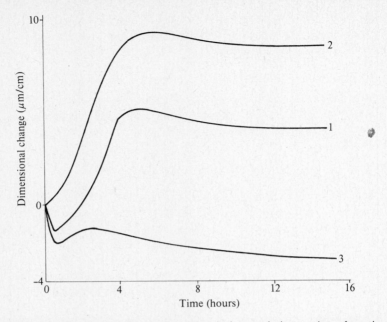

**Fig. 4.11** Effect of trituration time on dimensional change during setting of amalgam. Curve 1: normal time, Curve 2: short time, Curve 3: long time.

Any $\gamma_1$ and $\gamma_2$ formed before placement in the cavity cannot, of course, contribute to any observed expansion in the cavity, so there is a net loss of apparent expansion in an over-triturated amalgam. Thus, these two effects combine to give dimensional change behaviour similar to that of curve 3.

This explanation can be used to amplify the reasons outlined above for the effect of alloy particle size, for an alloy with a small particle size will be effectively over-triturated in comparison with a large-particle-size alloy for a given trituration time. That is, part of the $\gamma_1$ and $\gamma_2$ formed with the fine particle size is produced too early and does not contribute to any apparent expansion in the cavity.

CONDENSATION

If an amalgam is left after trituration, without being condensed, a large initial contraction will be observed as a result of the undisturbed diffusion of mercury into the alloy. However, without condensation, excess mercury is not removed, so that far more $\gamma_1$ and $\gamma_2$ are ultimately produced, giving a very substantial and continued expansion. With condensation, the excess mercury is removed and the amount of expansion limited. In practice, little difference is observed between amalgams condensed with different but clinically acceptable pressures.

Occasionally an expansion considerably greater than the 10 $\mu$m/cm range discussed above may be observed. This may happen 4–5 days after setting and occurs only in amalgams that are made from alloys containing zinc and which become contaminated with water (or saliva) during trituration or condensation. The problem arises because the available zinc in the alloy may react with water in this situation to yield hydrogen gas

$$H_2O + Zn \longrightarrow H_2 \text{ (gas)} + ZnO.$$

This hydrogen collects in the form of bubbles and the resulting pressure causes the amalgam to flow outwards, hence giving an apparent expansion.

This delayed expansion is sufficiently great to cause clinically significant problems with the restoration and must be avoided. This can be done by either preventing the contamination or by using a zinc-free amalgam. It should be possible in all but a few difficult cases to avoid moisture contamination, and this is the best method of prevention. Zinc-free alloys are available, and indeed there is little need for zinc in spherical particle alloys since its scavenging action is not required in the inert atmospheres used for atomization. However, great care should still be taken to avoid contamination even with zinc-free alloys since, although there may be no delayed expansion, other properties, especially the corrosion-resistance, are affected.

## Mechanical properties

A major cause of failure in amalgam restorations is fracture. Restorations may be subjected to high forces such that compressive, shear, and especially tensile stresses developed within the amalgam may exceed the ultimate strength of the material. Of particular importance are three aspects of the mechanical properties, the ultimate strength of the set amalgam, the rate at which this strength is obtained, and the susceptibility of the amalgam to creep or flow.

Since dental amalgam has a multiphase structure, its strength will depend on the properties of the individual phases and their relationship to one another. Typical figures for the tensile strengths of the individual phases and a set amalgam are as follows,

| | |
|---|---|
| $\gamma$ (Ag$_3$Sn) | 170 MN/m$^2$ |
| $\gamma_1$ (Ag$_2$ Hg$_3$) | 30 MN/m$^2$ |
| $\gamma_2$ (Sn$_7$ Hg) | 20 MN/m$^2$ |
| Dental amalgam | 60 MN/m$^2$ |

Clearly the unreacted $\gamma$ phase is significantly stronger than either of the two reaction products. This underlines the importance of using amalgams and clinical techniques which result in the greatest proportion of retained $\gamma$. The tensile strength of the set dental amalgam lies between that of the $\gamma$ phase and the $\gamma_1$ and $\gamma_2$ phases. As an amalgam fractures, cracks usually propagate through the weak $\gamma_1$ and $\gamma_2$ phases, avoiding the much stronger and harder $\gamma$ particles.

Dental amalgam is a brittle material, fracturing with little evidence of plastic deformation. As with most brittle materials, the tensile strength of an amalgam is much lower than the compressive strength, with typical figures of 60 MN/m$^2$ and 300 MN/m$^2$ respectively. This compressive strength is quite satisfactory, but it is the low tensile strength that is largely responsible for fractures in amalgam.

Several factors control the strength of amalgam, including the mercury/ alloy ratio, the alloy composition, the particle shape and size, porosity, and the clinical variables of trituration and condensation techniques.

*Mercury/alloy ratio.* The effect of the mercury content on the properties of an amalgam is clearly demonstrated by its effect on the mechanical properties. If too little mercury is used, the alloy particles are not completely wetted so that in parts of the restoration the alloy will not react with mercury, leaving increased local porosity and a lack of continuity and giving a weaker amalgam. On the other hand, an excess of mercury results in the formation of a large amount of weak reaction products. This is clearly seen in Figure 4.12 which shows the fall in compressive strength that accompanies an increase in residual mercury content.

*Alloy composition.* Provided the composition of the amalgam alloy is within the limits discussed earlier, the actual composition does not have a very

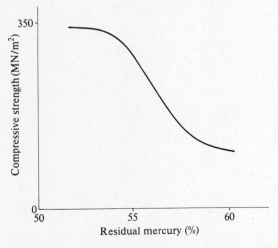

**Fig. 4.12** Relationship between compressive strength of amalgam and residual mercury content.

significant effect on the strength of the set amalgam. Most of the commercially available lathe-cut and spherical-particle alloy amalgams give 24 hour compressive strengths between 280 and 350 $MN/m^2$, the variation being largely due to factors other than composition.

While it is claimed that the high-copper, dispersion-type amalgams are much stronger than the conventional composition alloys, it is uncertain whether they will prove to give any exceptional improvement in clinical performance in this respect. The real advantage, as discussed below, is in the improvement of corrosion-resistance.

*Particle size and shape.* Although spherical particle alloy amalgams give a faster rate of gain of strength, the mechanical properties of the set amalgam are little different from those of the lathe-cut. Whatever the nature of the particles, it is clear that superior strengths are produced with small particle sizes, emphasizing the trend towards fine or microfine particles. As noted earlier, the best results with a spherical particle amalgam are obtained when there is a range of sizes, typically 5–40 $\mu$m, to give efficiency of packing of the particles, reducing the volume of the weaker matrix between them.

*Porosity.* Even a small amount of porosity in an amalgam will significantly affect the strength, and the influence of voids on the properties of brittle materials has already been discussed in Chapter 1. Cracks propagating through the $\gamma_1$ and $\gamma_2$ matrix can often be seen to pass through the voids, which clearly offer little resistance. The amount of porosity is minimized by correct trituration and, more importantly, by good condensation technique. In this context it must be noted that retaining pins in the amalgam reduce the strength in a similar manner to porosity, crack propagation being aided by their presence.

## RATE OF GAIN OF STRENGTH

It is frequently suggested that many fractures of amalgam restorations are initiated during the first few hours after condensation, small cracks formed during this time opening up to produce fractures at a later stage. It is naturally difficult to prove this, but certainly amalgam gains strength quite slowly. Figure 4.13 illustrates the rate of gain of strength of a lathe-cut alloy, only 15–20 per cent of the final strength being attained after one hour. The strength in the very early stages is controlled by the characteristics of the alloy particles and the relatively fluid nature of the matrix. Clearly the highest early strengths are obtained with amalgam alloy particles of high strength and in systems which retain a large proportion of unreacted $\gamma$ phase. This early rate of gain of strength will also be influenced by clinical variables.

One of the main differences between lathe-cut and spherical-particle alloys is the appreciably faster rate of gain of strength observed with the latter. A two-hour compressive strength of the spherical-particle alloy may be 70–90 per cent of the 24-hour strength, while the equivalent value for a lathe-cut

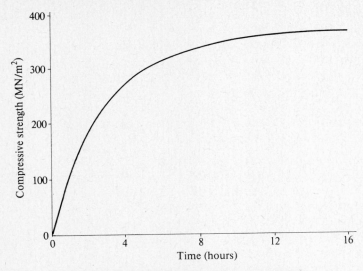

**Fig. 4.13** Rate of gain of strength during setting of lathe-cut amalgam.

alloy may be between 40 and 70 per cent. It must be remembered, however, that the final strength will be similar in these two cases.

CREEP OR FLOW OF AMALGAM

The phenomenon of 'creep' was introduced briefly in Chapter 1 where it was defined as the time-dependent deformation of a material under a constant stress. Creep behaviour is not normally observed in metals at room or mouth temperatures, which are low in comparison to the melting-point. However, the melting-point of dental amalgam is relatively low, so creep is theoretically possible. The significance of creep is that an amalgam restoration may change its shape over a long period of time under the influence of occlusal stresses, a phenomenon which most often results in the flattening of occlusal surfaces and the distortion of proximal boxes, leading to overhanging margins. Although these stresses may be insufficient to cause mechanical fracture, the changes in the restoration, especially at the margins, may eventually contribute to marginal failure.

In the context of dental amalgam, the terms 'creep' and 'flow' are sometimes used interchangeably. While creep is a well-defined metallurgical term, flow is not so precise. Quite frequently it is used to denote the creep behaviour that is observed in an amalgam that has not fully hardened. Indeed, in the A.D. A. specification for dental amalgam the flow test specifically relates to an amalgam specimen three hours old. In this test, a cylindrical, three-hour specimen is subjected to a constant axial compressive stress of 10 MN/m$^2$ at 37 °C for 21 hours, and the reduction in length recorded.

Naturally the amount of flow or creep observed at this time will be much greater than in the fully set material.

Generally the same factors that control the strength of amalgam control the creep behaviour. In particular, excess residual mercury and porosity both increase the creep rate. It is difficult to estimate the clinical significance of creep, but it does seem likely that modern alloy selection and good condensation techniques give amalgams which creep very little in practice. However, should an amalgam of a higher creep rate be produced it is more likely to suffer marginal breakdown and result in a poorer clinical performance.

## Tarnish and corrosion of amalgam

Although dental amalgam is a relatively corrosion-resistant alloy, the oral environment is quite corrosive and so some corrosion is observed in amalgam restorations. This is particularly significant when it occurs at the margins, for it is a major contributing factor in producing marginal breakdown and ditching, as will be discussed later.

It is necessary here to distinguish between the two phenomena of tarnish and corrosion in relation to amalgam. As outlined in Chapter 1, tarnish essentially involves a deposition of substances onto the surface of a metal, causing that metal to loose its lustre, but without significantly affecting the underlying structure of the metal. Amalgam restorations frequently tarnish in the mouth, with sulphides, especially tin sulphides, forming on the surface. Although this tarnish radically alters the appearance of the restoration, it may in fact be beneficial, as the surface deposits may passivate the restoration and reduce the corrosion rate.

Corrosion is a process in which the metal reacts with the environment and so affects the structural integrity of the metal. It is, therefore, of far greater significance than tarnish.

### CORROSION MECHANISMS IN AMALGAM

There is still much speculation about the corrosion mechanisms in amalgam. At least two factors seem to be important, both related to the previously described galvanic and concentration cell corrosion mechanisms. The presence of three chemically-distinct phases in the conventional composition amalgams leads to the formation of a multitude of microgalvanic cells on the surface of a restoration, as depicted in Figure 4.14. Of particular importance is the fact that the $Sn_7 Hg$ $(\gamma_2)$ phase is significantly more electronegative than either the $\gamma$ or $\gamma_1$ phases. Thus, the $\gamma_2$ phase in isolation would corrode in oral fluids more rapidly than either of the other two, but, more significantly, when present in a multiphase $\gamma$, $\gamma_1$, and $\gamma_2$ structure, the $\gamma_2$ areas become anodic in these microgalvanic cells and dissolve at a relatively fast rate. Thus, the corrosion of amalgam is largely controlled by the presence and distribution of the more reactive $\gamma_2$ phase.

Concentration cell corrosion arises when there are variations in the

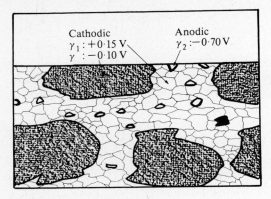

**Fig. 4.14** Microgalvanic cells on amalgam surface.

composition of the corrosive environment over the metal surface. Especially important is the oxygen content of the fluid within crevices. The oxygen is slowly utilized by the corrosion process and, if further oxygen is unable to diffuse to that area, the crevice becomes relatively depleted of oxygen. Thus the crevice becomes anodic with respect to the remainder of the surface and hence corrodes at an accelerated rate. This is important, for it explains corrosion in areas of porosity, at the margins of a restoration, and in areas where the $\gamma_2$ has dissolved.

The presence of plaque or other deposits on the surface of the restoration may also influence corrosion by the same concentration cell mechanism. It has been postulated, for example, that with a non-uniform distribution of plaque on the surface, corrosion is initiated underneath the areas of plaque, since these become depleted in oxygen and therefore anodic. This explains the more rapid corrosion of inaccessible areas, such as proximal surfaces, where plaque removal by the patient is difficult.

### SIGNIFICANCE OF CORROSION AND THE EFFECT OF CLINICAL VARIABLES

The reactions that take place during amalgam corrosion are complex, but the major reactions may be summarized as follows:

Tin–mercury phase + oral fluids (oxygen, chloride, etc.) $\longrightarrow$
tin salts (tin oxides, chlorides, etc.) + mercury.

Certainly it is tin oxides and tin oxychlorides that predominate in corrosion products found on the surface, the most significant feature of this process being the release of mercury. This free mercury is able to diffuse into the remaining $\gamma$ phase areas where it can react to produce even more $\gamma_1$ and $\gamma_2$. The result is a further expansion of the amalgam and the replacement of the strong and corrosion-resistant $\gamma$ by more of the weak and corrosion-susceptible $\gamma_2$ phase. As the reaction proceeds so the amalgam is weakened and eventually may break down, especially at the margins, contributing to the ditching effect.

It is clearly important to adopt techniques that are going to result in minimal amounts of $\gamma_2$ formation. This is largely associated with the mercury content so that good condensation technique is especially important. In view of the comments on concentration cell corrosion associated with surface pits and plaque, it is also desirable to produce as smooth a surface as possible to avoid such surface irregularities and minimize food and plaque accumulation. Finishing techniques are discussed below.

CORROSION IN DISPERSED PHASE AMALGAMS

Since the corrosion of amalgam is predominantly associated with the $\gamma_2$ phase, any method of reducing the amount of this phase should produce superior corrosion-resistance. This is, in fact, the situation with the high-copper, dispersion-type amalgams. Here the tin forms a tin–copper phase in preference to the $\gamma_2$ phase. The virtual absence of $\gamma_2$ in these amalgams has led to superior results in respect of corrosion and marginal breakdown.

## Toxicity and biocompatibility of mercury and amalgam

It is well known that mercury is a toxic element. For example, exposure to organo–mercury compounds and inhalation of mercury vapour both have significant physiological or pathological effects. For this reason there has been extensive discussion, over many years, of the possibility of toxic effects arising from the use of mercury in amalgams. This problem can be divided into two aspects, concerning first the effects on dental personnel of mercury vapour in surgeries and secondly the effects of amalgam restorations on the patients.

In the first case there is considerable evidence to show that mercury vapour may accumulate in a surgery as a direct consequence of the repeated use of mercury in the preparation of amalgams. Naturally the level of mercury contamination will vary with the methods employed. For example, the use of preproportioned capsules containing both the alloy and the mercury results in considerably less mercury vapour release than the older methods of dispensing mercury and hand trituration. On the other hand, the modern ultrasonic condensation technique increases mercury vapour levels.

The exact effect of this mercury contamination on the dental personnel is unclear. It appears, however, that poor mercury hygiene in the surgery does result in contamination of personnel, with high levels of mercury on the skin, hair, and fingernails, and that systemic toxicity may arise. A little care in the use of mercury and amalgams, especially by using good ventilation, should result in the contamination being reduced to tolerable levels. For example, waste amalgam should be stored under water, and handling of amalgam should be kept to a minimum.

In contrast, there seem to be few documented cases of adverse effects arising in patients with amalgam restorations. On very rare occasions a patient may be sensitive to mercury, but the amount of mercury vapour taken up by a patient in a course of treatment is too small to produce any toxic effects. Metallic mercury is very poorly absorbed by the gastro-intestinal tract so that the release of mercury-containing compounds from the surface of restoration is very unlikely to result in raised mercury levels in the body. Furthermore, the mercury cannot be converted into the harmful organo-mercury compounds. It is known that elements from amalgam could diffuse into the dentine from a restoration, and may conceivably reach the pulp. It is not known whether this affects the pulp in any significant way, but the use of lining materials should minimize this risk.

## CAVITIES FOR AMALGAM

Amalgam, being a brittle material, is not suitable for use in thin section. For restorations which will have to withstand the forces of occlusion and articulation, the amalgam must be used in reasonable bulk; and those restorations that are deep and narrow are mechanically more favourable than those that are shallow and broad. Generally at least 2 mm of amalgam must be used in occlusal situations, especially when a large proximal box is involved.

The greatest risk of fracture occurs marginally where the anatomy of the tooth and the design of the cavity may lead to a tapered feather edge of amalgam. Ideally the cavo-surface angle should be about 90°, which allows the amalgam to abut against the tooth in considerable bulk. Figure 4.15 shows a situation where this has not been achieved and where marginal breakdown is likely to occur, giving a ditched amalgam. There are several situations that may bring about marginal ditching, including fracture of weakened enamel, delayed expansion, and the retention of lining material at the margin of the cavity, which is subsequently lost by dissolution. The accumulation of plaque in the ditch defects may lead to recurrent caries and aggravates marginal corrosion, as explained earlier. Corrosion at these sites also contributes further to the formation of marginal defects.

The coefficient of thermal expansion of amalgam is about 25 ppm (more than twice that of tooth substance) and some marginal percolation on thermal

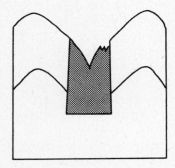

**Fig. 4.15** Tapered feather edge of amalgam restoration, leading to marginal breakdown.

cycling must occur (Chapter 5). Marginal leakage is greatest in the newly placed amalgam, and this reduces with time. It has been widely suggested that corrosion products deposited at the interface between the restoration and tooth are responsible for this reduction.

Temperature changes applied to amalgam are transmitted rapidly through restorations as the thermal conductivity of the material is high. It is necessary therefore, in all cavities except those of minimal depth, to place a lining. It is important in this situation to select a material that has sufficient strength to withstand the forces of condensation, which, as mentioned earlier, are considerable. Zinc phosphate, zinc polycarboxylate, and reinforced zinc oxide/eugenol products are suitable for this purpose.

As amalgam does not display adhesion to tooth tissue it must be retained in the cavity by mechanical means. This is usually achieved by preparing an undercut cavity which will allow the set amalgam filling to be retained. Obviously retentive features must prevent the loss of the filling in every possible direction. Where a cavity is so large that this is no longer possible, for instance when cusps have been completely removed, additional aids to retention are necessary. Most frequently these take the form of metal pins placed strategically into the dentine to about half their length, the amalgam being condensed around them. As each pin produces a focus through which the amalgam may fracture, as few pins as possible are used. The introduction of simple and effective systems of pin retention has greatly added to the versatility of amalgam as a restorative material. It must be appreciated, however, that the pins do not strengthen the amalgam; indeed they actually reduce the strength. Their importance lies solely in the improved retention. Fresh amalgam does not display adhesion to set amalgam, and patches or additions to restorations must be prepared in such a way that they themselves are retained by adequate mechanical means.

## FINISHING AMALGAM RESTORATIONS

After the amalgam has been condensed into the prepared cavity it is carved with a sharp instrument to conform to the contour of the tooth. It is particularly important to contour the filling to accommodate occlusion with the opposing teeth without interference. If this is not achieved, small cracks may develop in the first few hours, which later lead to gross fracture, as explained earlier. With slower setting amalgam it is wise to allow one or two minutes before commencing carving, so that sufficient strength has been gained to offer some resistance to the carving instrument.

The surface of a carved amalgam is rough and will allow plaque to accumulate fairly readily. As dental plaque may play an important part in the corrosion mechanism it is generally thought to be beneficial if an amalgam is smoothed and polished. Polishing procedures leave the surface amalgam more homogeneous, and this will also help reduce corrosion. Finally, in large restorations a smooth surface improves patient comfort—

although it is true to say that this is a retrospective discovery on the part of the patient.

While most of the finishing techniques available should be carried out at least 24 hours after the placement of the restoration, burnishing is applied shortly after carving at the original visit. For many years burnishing was thought to be a detrimental process, as the application of pressure over the surface tends to concentrate mercury in the surface layer, so reducing resistance to corrosion. Certainly the surface of a burnished amalgam is smoother than that of an untreated one. It is now generally agreed that light burnishing around the margins improves the adaptation of the amalgam to the cavity walls and reduces early marginal leakage. While burnishing may be a compromise, it is felt that marginal corrosion is not increased to an appreciable degree.

The smoothest finish may be produced on an amalgam by using a series of abrasives at a subsequent appointment. Operators have their own preferred sequence, but the use of fine-bladed finishing burs followed by the application of a dentifrice with a brush or cup is typical. While the high lustre produced in this way is soon lost, the surface remains smooth and resists corrosion more favourably.

# 5
# Tooth-coloured filling materials

While a carefully placed amalgam restoration can give clinically satisfactory results in posterior teeth, it would be totally inadequate aesthetically for anterior teeth. Neither the original metallic lustre nor the tarnished surface that may ensue are acceptable for a restoration which is easily visible. There is, therefore, a need for tooth-coloured filling materials in these situations.

Although generally it may be said that the requirements for a tooth-coloured filling material are just the same as those for a posterior filling material, with the added demand for an aesthetically pleasing appearance, it is instructive to review these requirements at this point so that the properties of the available materials may be discussed and compared.

## REQUIREMENTS OF TOOTH-COLOURED FILLING MATERIALS
These may be grouped as follows.

### CLINICAL HANDLING

As with many dental materials, the use of a direct anterior filling material must be based on a setting reaction that allows a small volume of the material to be mixed and placed in the cavity, where it then sets in a conveniently short time. Adequate properties should then be achieved within a few hours. Of importance, therefore, are:

**a** the ease with which the material may be prepared for use;

**b** a suitable working time;

**c** a viscosity compatible with insertion and adaptation to the cavity;

**d** a setting reaction that is readily activated and that can continue to completion if necessary, under the conditions within the mouth, not being adversely affected by these ambient conditions;

**e** a conveniently short setting time;

**f** a long shelf-life where there is no danger of the setting reaction taking place prematurely or of components evaporating to the detriment of the properties.

### DIMENSIONAL STABILITY ON SETTING

One of the most critical features of the setting of a filling material is the dimensional change that may accompany the reaction. As discussed earlier in relation to amalgam, the clinical significance of minor dimensional changes is not clear, but ideally there should be no contraction on setting nor should there be any excessive expansion. Both of these produce marginal catches and stagnation areas, which may lead to marginal leakage, a common cause of clinical failure. None of the materials used for anterior restorations show any expansion, but all exhibit some degree of contraction.

AESTHETICS

Of relevance here are both the initial aesthetic appearance and the possible changes in appearance that can take place over a period of time. It is important to note that it is not just the surface colour that contributes to the aesthetics of a restoration. Both enamel and dentine are translucent, allowing part of any incident light to be absorbed and part to be transmitted, as discussed in Chapter 1. This means that the overall appearance of a tooth is a property of the bulk of the tooth and not just its surface. Ideally, therefore, a restoration that is to simulate the appearance of a tooth should have the same optical properties, including:

**a** colour and shade;

**b** translucency (measured by the amount of light absorbed);

**c** refractive index.

Whatever the bulk properties of the restorative material, the appearance will be modified if there are significant irregularities of the surface. Irregularities, if large enough, can scatter light, making the restoration appear dull. Thus, it is desirable to achieve a good surface finish on the restoration, a requirement which poses significant problems in practice. Also in this context, it is important that the setting reaction should not result in porosity, which can radically alter the surface finish.

Reactions between restorative materials and the oral environment are discussed later. One effect of such reactions, however, is an alteration to the appearance of the restoration, usually to its detriment. Long-term changes may be due to:

**a** chemical reactions between components of a filling material and the oral fluids (for example, impurities in cements can react with sulphides in the saliva to form coloured sulphides);

**b** solution or erosion of the filling material leading to greater light-scattering at the surface and reduced translucency;

**c** accumulation of plaque or food debris on rough surfaces;

**d** diffusion of fluids into a restoration leading to staining;

**e** dehydration of a restoration;

**f** slow but continuous chemical changes in the material which lead to changes in optical properties.

MECHANICAL PROPERTIES

Restorations in anterior teeth are not generally subjected to the same stresses as those in cavities involving the occlusal surfaces of posterior teeth, but nevertheless they must have adequate mechanical properties. It is difficult to quantify the strength requirements of these filling materials, but most in current use have compressive strengths in the region of 200–300 MN/m², and this would appear adequate. It is additionally desirable for the material to have good abrasion-resistance to avoid loss of anatomical form due to wear.

In recent years, because of the improvements in the mechanical properties of tooth-coloured filling materials, attempts have been made to use these materials as alternatives to amalgam for cavities in posterior teeth, partly for aesthetic reasons and partly in anticipation of further problems associated with mercury toxicology. Under these conditions, the strength and abrasion-resistance become far more critical, and different minimum performances are required. A compressive strength of at least 300 MN/m² and a tensile strength of 50 MN/m² or more would be required in addition to higher abrasion-resistance.

PHYSICAL PROPERTIES

In addition to the optical properties already reviewed above, certain physical properties are important, particularly the thermal properties, where it is necessary to consider both conduction and expansion.

*Thermal conductivity.* Ideally a restorative material should be a poor conductor of heat, so that excesses of temperature in the mouth are not transmitted to the pulp. In practice this is easily overcome in most clinical situations, where a lining should effectively limit heat transmission even when a highly conductive metallic restoration is used. In the context of anterior restorations, where the use of metals is clearly incompatible with the requirements of aesthetics, the alternatives of ceramics, polymers, and composites are all good insulators.

*Thermal expansion.* This is more significant as it can influence the phenomenon of marginal leakage. As fluids of different temperatures are taken into the mouth, it is possible for the temperature of the teeth to fluctuate from about 4 °C to perhaps 50 °C in the case of hot drinks. Even if these temperatures are only attained transiently in the tooth substance, the tooth will expand and contract accordingly.

If a tooth contains a restoration, that restoration will expand and contract itself. However, the amount of expansion and contraction will depend on its coefficient of expansion and, in any combined system of tooth and restoration, in the absence of adhesion between the two, each part will expand and contract independently according to its own expansion coefficient. If there is a considerable difference in these coefficients then there will be differential dimensional changes. In particular, if the restoration has a much higher coefficient than the surrounding tooth it will contract more on cooling, causing a gap to form between the filling and the tooth. Oral fluids may then penetrate this gap intermittently in a process called marginal percolation. This may result in either solution of the restoration at the margins or secondary caries around the margins. The coefficient of expansion of dentine is $8.3 \times 10^{-6}/°C$ and that of enamel is $11.4 \times 10^{-6}/°C$. Not surprisingly, ceramic structures have coefficients approximating to these figures but polymers often give values much higher.

COMPATIBILITY WITH ORAL TISSUES AND FLUIDS

The effect of interactions between anterior restorative materials and fluids and tissues of the oral environment can be divided into adverse effects on restorations, adverse effects on oral tissues, beneficial effects on oral tissues, and adhesion.

**a** *Adverse effects on restorative materials.* There are two possible problems here. First, oral fluids may tend to dissolve the material, and it is therefore most desirable for the solubility to be effectively zero. One of the more important factors is that the oral fluids are quite variable. Saliva is a complex substance of constantly varying composition. Moreover, the fluid in contact with a restoration may be influenced by plaque, and here in particular the pH is lowered. It is important, therefore, that the material is resistant to solution in oral fluids of variable composition and in a variety of conditions, including a range of pH which may reach as low as 4·0. It is further desirable that the resistance to solution is not too critically affected by variations in clinical manipulation.

Secondly, there may be a tendency for filling materials to absorb water from oral fluids. This may lead to internal structural changes, which can affect the mechanical properties, or swelling. The significance of swelling caused by water absorption is difficult to ascertain, for while an excess of swelling is undesirable as it could have a detrimental effect on the filling, a limited amount may be advantageous since it could compensate for the setting shrinkage. Typically a resin-based composite filling material will have a water absorption of 1–2 per cent and this may be considered acceptable.

**b** *Adverse effects on tissue.* It is conceivable that thermal trauma to tooth substance could occur with exothermic setting reactions in filling materials. Certainly some materials do set exothermically, but it is uncertain whether the temperature rise is sufficient to cause any harm.

Chemical effects of the setting reaction are more important. Acid–base setting reactions, such as those discussed in Chapter 3, may involve very low pH values and the diffusion of acid through the dentine to the pulp. Similarly the curing of polymerizing systems involves monomers and cross-linking agents, catalysts, and so on, which are toxic and could have damaging effects on the pulp.

While it is recognized that most filling materials do cause some pulpal irritation, the mechanisms are not known with any certainty. It is standard practice with many of these materials to use a lining in the cavity to minimize the pulpal irritation.

**c** *Beneficial effects on tissues.* This is solely concerned with the possible inhibition of secondary caries by the activity of the filling material and arises from the beneficial effect of fluoride contained within silicate cement, which is discussed below. Since these restorations are undoubtedly associated with a smaller incidence of recurrent caries, this must be considered an ideal requirement. However, great care has to be taken in this context, for if fluoride in a restoration is to have a beneficial effect, it has to be released into the surrounding tooth structure, which implies either diffusion or dissolution processes. Diffusion of fluoride is unlikely to be successful in the long term, while achieving fluoride release by increasing solubility is a self-defeating process.

**d** *Adhesion.* The problems of marginal leakage and secondary caries arising from setting shrinkage or differential expansion could be minimized if there was adhesion between the restoration and the tooth. As discussed in Chapter 2, adhesion to tooth substances is very difficult to achieve.

It must be realized that these requirements are rather general in nature, usually being difficult to quantify and often impossible to satisfy completely. In practice, however, adequate results are achieved without realizing these ideal requirements and present-day materials represent a compromise.

These materials are now discussed in detail. They fall into two categories, the acid–base cements, similar to those described in Chapter 3, which are used as lining materials, and the resin-based materials usually referred to as 'composites'. It will be appreciated that since the ideal restorative material does not exist, developments are continually being made and new products emerge frequently.

## Cements used as tooth-coloured filling materials

As described in Chapter 3, most dental cements are based on the reaction between an acidic liquid and a basic, or possibly amphoteric, oxide, which results in a large volume of unreacted powder held together by a matrix of some kind of salt gel. Usually the powder consists of either a simple oxide, a mixture of simple oxides, or a suitable ion-leachable glass, while the liquid is either phosphoric acid, eugenol, or a polyacid such as polyacrylic acid. Two such cements may be used as filling materials. Silicate cement, which has been in use since the beginning of this century, is based on the ion-leachable glass–phosphoric acid system while the much more recent glass-ionomer cement involves the glass–polyacrylic acid reaction.

## SILICATE CEMENT

Although called a cement, this is used solely as an anterior filling material. It appears to have been introduced into dentistry well before 1900 and the present-day formulation was in use by about 1910.

### Composition

As indicated above, silicate cement is produced by the reaction between an ion-leachable glass and phosphoric acid. Many different commercial preparations have been marketed over the years and their formulations have varied slightly. However, all are, or have been, presented as a powder and liquid combination, with fairly similar compositions.

*Powder.* The powder is prepared by the manufacturer, by fusing a mixture of silica ($SiO_2$) and alumina ($Al_2O_3$) in a fluoride-based flux, typically consisting of fluorite ($CaF_2$) and cryolite ($Na_3AlF_6$). The amount and nature of the fluxes present control fusion temperature, which will usually be in the region of 1200 to 1300 °C. Other materials may also be added to the mixture, including lime (CaO) and phosphates (for example, $Ca(H_2PO_4)_2 \cdot H_2O$).

After thorough mixing at the fusion temperature, the material is cooled very quickly. This shock-cooling causes the glassy structure to crack, which facilitates grinding of the material into a fine powder. This whole process is called fritting.

The proportions of the various constituents in the powder control its structure, the rate of reaction with the liquid, and the properties of the set cement. A typical cement powder could be prepared from materials in the proportions given in Table 5.1.

**Table 5.1** Composition of the powder of silicate cement

|  | % |
|---|---|
| $SiO_2$ | 38 |
| $Al_2O_3$ | 30 |
| $CaF_2$ | 4 |
| $Na_3AlF_6$ | 20 |
| $Ca_3(PO_4)_2$ | 8 |

The structure of the resulting powder is basically that of a continuous three-dimensional array of $SiO_4$ and $AlO_4$ tetrahedra, as illustrated in Figure 5.1, with small, dispersed spherical areas of a fluoride-rich phase. Since, in a representative cement, there are approximately equal numbers of silicon and aluminium atoms, there will be an equal number of $SiO_4$ and $AlO_4$ tetrahedra linked together to give what is essentially an alumino-silicate glass. Such a structure itself cannot be electrically neutral, because of the threefold

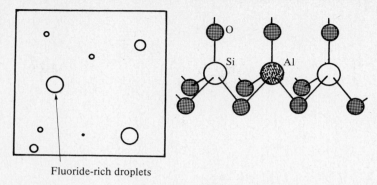

Fluoride-rich droplets

**Fig. 5.1** Microsctructure and molecular structure of an aluminosilicate powder used in silicate cement.

valency of aluminium in contrast to the fourfold valency of silicon. Each aluminium atom is, therefore, negatively charged. This is, however, balanced by the presence of positively charged calcium ($Ca^{2+}$) and sodium ($Na^+$) cations, supplied by the fluxes and present within the tetrahedra.

If the aluminium–silicon ratio differs from unity, the density of negative charges on the aluminosilicate network will vary and this will have a significant effect on the rate of reaction as discussed below.

A pure aluminosilicate glass would be quite translucent. The presence of the spherical, fluoride-rich areas in this aluminosilicate matrix, however, serves to opacify the material, giving the powder a characteristic opal appearance. Other metallic oxides may be present to produce a variety of shades.

*Liquid.* The liquid is an aqueous solution of phosphoric acid which also contains some metal ions as buffering agents. The ratio of phosphoric acid to water is important, although commercial preparations vary from 45 per cent acid up to 65 per cent acid. A concentration of phosphoric acid in the region of 50 per cent is most desirable. As noted in Chapter 3, the properties of phosphoric acid in relation to the reaction with a glass or oxide depend on its degree of dissociation, and this is of significance in the case of silicate cement. As the acid concentration increases, the rate of reaction decreases, and therefore excessively high acid concentrations give prolonged setting times. This is of importance not only in the selection of phosphoric acid concentration by the manufacturers, but also in the storage of the liquid in the surgery, for a loss of water from acid in an unstoppered bottle will give an artificially raised acid concentration.

The presence of metal ions in the liquid influences the setting reaction and also affects the properties of the set cement, especially the strength. Clearly the metals used must be moderately soluble in phosphoric acid and must be non-toxic. Any metal that is weakly basic, or possibly amphoteric, would be suitable from the point of view of forming a suitable glass. Such metals include aluminium, magnesium, beryllium, and zinc. Beryllium is a toxic metal and so aluminium and zinc are usually selected, and are typically present in proportions up to 2 per cent and 9 per cent respectively.

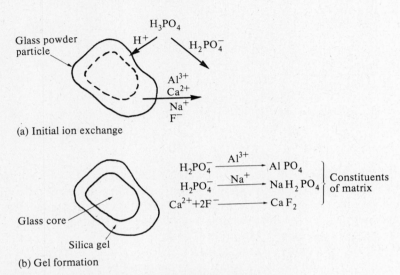

**Fig. 5.2** Stages in the setting reaction of silicate cement.

## Setting reaction

The setting reaction is that of an acid–base reaction between the phosphoric acid solution and the fluoride-containing aluminosilicate glass. The mechanism of this reaction is depicted in Figure 5.2. The stages in this process are as follows.

1  Hydrogen ions from the acid, in the form of hydrated protons ($H_3O^+$), penetrate the surface of the glass particles.
2  These attack the aluminosilicate structure, releasing $Al^{3+}$ cations and some of the $Ca^{2+}$, $Na^+$, and fluoride ($AlF_2^+$, $CaF^+$, etc.) ions.
3  The loss of aluminium ions from the aluminosilicate structure and their replacement by $H_3O^+$ ions results in the formation of a hydrated silica gel, referred to as a siliceous gel, on the surface of the particles.
4  The cores of the particles remain unattacked.
5  The ions released from the particles accumulate in the liquid phase, together with with $Al^{3+}$, $Zn^{2+}$ and phosphate ions already present.
6  As a result of the loss of $H_3O^+$ ions, the pH of the liquid increases. As this happens, and the concentration of $Al^{3+}$ ions increases, a gel starts to form in the liquid phase. This may be represented by a continuous replacement of the hydrogen ions by aluminium ions in the phosphate structure

$$H_3PO_4 \xrightarrow{Al^{3+}} Al(H_2PO_4)_3 \xrightarrow{Al^{3+}} Al_2(HPO_4)_3 \xrightarrow{Al^{3+}} AlPO_4.$$

The formation of this aluminophosphate structure is accompanied by a poly-merization process, giving a structure of the type illustrated in Figure 5.3. This results in the transformation of the liquid phase to an aluminophosphate gel. It is this gel formation that gives the initial set to the material.

7 Further hardening results from the continued polymerization of the gel phase as more $Al^{3+}$ ions are released and the pH continues to rise.

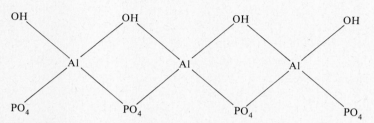

**Fig. 5.3** Molecular structure of the aluminophosphate matrix in the set silicate cement.

## Structure of set cement

The structure of the set cement is illustrated in Figure 5.4. As much as 80 per cent of the aluminosilicate glass remains unattacked and this constitutes the major phase of the set structure. These unreacted particles are covered with a siliceous gel and are bonded together by a matrix which is largely an aluminium phosphate hydrogel. This is essentially amorphous, or glass-like, which gives the cement characteristic brittle properties. There is some tendency for small crystalline areas to form, both of the aluminium phosphate itself (as $Al_2(PO_4)(OH)_3$) and as fluoride-containing areas (especially $CaF_2$).

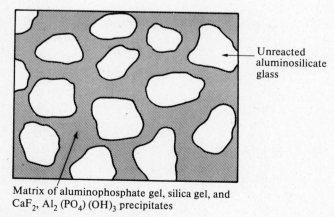

Unreacted aluminosilicate glass

Matrix of aluminophosphate gel, silica gel, and $CaF_2$, $Al_2(PO_4)(OH)_3$ precipitates

**Fig. 5.4** Microstructure of set silicate cement.

## Properties of silicate cement

The characteristics and properties of the silicate cement are discussed here in relation to the requirements of anterior filling materials outlined earlier in the chapter.

CLINICAL HANDLING

**1** *Mixing.* Mixing is easily achieved but it is important that it is done correctly as the technique used influences the setting reaction and the properties of the set cement. It may be performed by hand or alternatively by mechanical methods. The following factors are significant in hand mixing.

**a** The correct powder/liquid ratio must be used. This may vary from one commercial preparation to another but it is always stated clearly by the manufacturer. If the mix is too thick, there will be incomplete wetting of the particles, giving a crumbly substance. A low powder/liquid ratio (i.e. an excess of acid) will give a longer setting time because of the greater length of time needed to increase the pH in the liquid phase and initiate the alumino-phosphate gel formation. Properties such as the strength and solubility are also adversely affected.

**b** The temperature should be as low as conveniently possible, since the rate of the setting reaction increases significantly as the temperature rises. A low temperature is best achieved by using a thick glass slab which has been cooled with cold water.

**c** The reaction is also seriously affected by the presence of moisture. It is very important to dry the glass slab thoroughly after cooling and to avoid cooling below the dew-point when condensation would result in moisture collecting on the slab. It is preferable that mixing should be confined to a small area of the slab to prevent the hygroscopic powder from picking up too much moisture from the air.

**d** Since the cement is abrasive, soft metal spatulas should be avoided. Either agate (a hard ceramic), cobalt–chromium alloy, or plastic spatulas are suitable, but stainless steel is too soft and must not be used since small particles abraded from it are incorporated into the cement and cause it to discolour.

**e** Mixing should be achieved as quickly as possible, folding the powder rapidly into the liquid. It should preferably be complete within a minute.

*Mechanical mixing.* Some commercially available materials are presented in capsules with preproportioned powder and liquid separated by a seal. The seal is broken immediately before mechanical mixing, in much the same way as amalgam alloy and mercury are triturated in a capsule using an amal-gamator. This mixing is achieved far more rapidly than by hand. As with preproportioned amalgams, this method should eliminate dispensing errors and should minimize contamination. There is little evidence to show, however, that a cement prepared in this way has any superior properties to a hand-mixed cement, but it does appear that the process of mechanical mixing causes a rise in temperature which gives shorter working and setting times.

**2** *Working time.* It is essential that the silicate cement is placed in the cavity and contoured as soon as possible after mixing because, as far as possible, the setting reaction should take place in the cavity. Any manipulation of the cement after setting has started results in a disruption of the structure and a detrimental effect on the properties.

**3** *Consistency of the cement.* Provided the mixing has been performed correctly and without undue delay, the consistency of the cement is quite suitable for insertion. Ideally the cement should be inserted in one portion, as complete bonding may not occur between increments placed in the cavity. As soon as the material is in the cavity, a celluloid or cellulose acetate strip is placed over the restoration and held under pressure. It is important that the strip should not be moved until the initial set has occurred as otherwise the gel that is forming will fracture, weakening the cement.

**4** *Setting reaction.* Obviously with this system the setting reaction starts as soon as the powder and liquid are mixed and needs no further activation. As indicated above, the reaction is influenced both by the temperature and the presence of moisture. Protection from contamination by moisture is, perhaps, the most important factor. Water absorption effectively alters the ratio of phosphoric acid to water in the liquid, and this will affect the final properties. Also, as the setting reaction proceeds by the formation of the aluminophosphate gel, much of the aluminium and phosphate is soluble in the early stages, and should any excess moisture be present, they may dissolve and thus impair the ability to form a strong gel.

It is important, therefore, that not only should moisture contamination be avoided during mixing, but that the cement should be inserted into a dry cavity and that the restoration should be protected from saliva for a few hours after its placement. A rubber dam may be used to keep the operating area dry and it is usual to paint the surface of the restoration with a varnish immediately after the cellulose acetate strip has been removed to avoid subsequent contamination.

**5** *Setting time.* The initial set, indicating the point at which the liquid-to-gel transformation occurs, takes place within 3–6 minutes. The reaction, however, continues for a much longer time, and it may be several days before the pH of the cement stabilizes and the maximum strength is achieved. The setting time will depend on both the composition of the powder and liquid and the particle size of the powder, as determined by the manufacturer. Generally a longer setting time also results when the temperature is lowered, if water is lost from the phosphoric acid solution, if the mixing time is extended, or if a low powder/liquid ratio is used.

**6** *Shelf-life*. The powder has an unlimited shelf-life. However, problems may arise with the liquid during use, because of its hygroscopic nature. It is possible for the liquid to either lose or gain water from the atmosphere, depending on the relative humidity. For example, a 50 per cent phosphoric acid solution will tend to lose water if the relative humidity is less than 70 per cent and gain water if it is much greater than 70 per cent. In practice this means that the liquid will normally tend to lose water if left exposed. The loss can be quite significant if the bottle of liquid is left unstoppered for any length of time, but can also be appreciable during the lifetime of a bottle with normal use. Since the structure and properties of the cement depend on the $H_3PO_4:H_2O$ ratio such a loss can clearly influence the restoration. It is obviously important to replace the stopper on the bottle immediately after withdrawing the required liquid. Also, manufacturers normally supply an excess of liquid so that the residue can be discarded when all the powder has been used up. The formation of crystalline deposits in the liquid is indicative of an undesirable change in the acid concentration, and such liquid should not be used.

DIMENSIONAL STABILITY ON SETTING

The setting reaction of silicate cement is accompanied by a slight contraction. This, however, is not considered to be of any great clinical significance. Dimensional changes can also take place if either the cement is allowed to be contaminated by moisture soon after its insertion in the cavity, when it swells, or if it is allowed to dehydrate significantly at a later stage, when it shrinks. These effects are discussed in more detail later.

AESTHETICS

Silicate cement restorations probably have the best aesthetic properties of all filling materials. The colour and shade can be accurately controlled by the dentist by the selection of the appropriate powder from a wide range supplied by the manufacturer. The combination of a finely divided glass core bound by an amorphous gel matrix gives an ideal degree of translucency. The aluminosilicate glass itself has a refractive index of between 1·47 and 1·68 with that of the gel matrix being close to 1·45. These compare with figures of 1·56 and 1·62 for the refractive indices of dentine and enamel.

The best surface finish is obtained with the cellulose acetate matrix. If any further contouring and finishing has to be performed, it is very difficult to achieve as good a surface finish as that left by the matrix.

Reactions with the oral environment may lead to changes in the appearance of the restoration. These arise for numerous reasons, including:

**a** *Solution or erosion of the cement*. This is discussed in some detail below but has relevance here as it alters the appearance of the surface, especially decreasing the translucency.

**b** *Staining*. Solution of the cement is most significant in areas of plaque deposition and at the margins of the restoration. Sulphides appear to form in these areas leading to staining, especially noticeable as a black line around the margins.

**c** *Dehydration.* If the set restoration is allowed to become dry it will dehydrate at the surface. This causes the restoration to shrink slightly, thereby losing some of its translucency and hence taking on a chalky appearance, and it is likely to crumble. Although the cement will rehydrate on further exposure to water, it will not fully regain its original properties or appearance. Thus, care has to be taken to prevent the tooth drying out at subsequent procedures on that or adjacent teeth and silicate cements are contra-indicated in mouth-breathers.

**d** *Reactions involving contaminants.* Any contaminants present in the cement may react with the oral fluids at the restoration surface to produce coloured sulphides, which naturally affect the aesthetics. It is important that the manufacturer should avoid any such impurities. Discoloration may also arise if the cement is contaminated during mixing with, for example, oils or metal particles, or by reaction with medicaments taken by the patient, any preparation containing Hibitane being particularly effective in this respect. Toothpaste containing stannous fluoride may also cause discoloration.

MECHANICAL PROPERTIES

In comparison with other inorganic cements, silicate cement has a high compressive strength, typically of the order of 225 $MN/m^2$. In terms of restorative materials, however, this is not very high and is only just adequate for anterior fillings. Of greater significance is the fact that, as with all brittle materials, the cement is much weaker in tension, often giving a tensile strength no greater than 15 $MN/m^2$.

Greatest strengths are achieved when, for given powder and liquid compositions, the greatest powder/liquid ratio, compatible with complete wetting is used. The reason here is the same as that given to explain the effect of amalgam alloy/mercury ratio on the properties of amalgam, for the strength in both cases is dependent on large amounts of unreacted particles with just sufficient of the weaker matrix to bind these together.

As outlined above, care has to be taken during the clinical handling of the cement if the highest strength is to be realized. In particular, any procedure which involves disturbing the cement once it has started to set is likely to result in reduced strength.

It naturally takes some time for the maximum strength to develop. Most cements will have developed less than 50 per cent of the final strength by 30 minutes and only 60 per cent by three hours. Even at one week only 80 per cent of the maximum strength may have been attained.

The other mechanical property of relevance is the hardness, for this largely controls the abrasion-resistance. Again the hardness compares very favourably with other cements and is, in fact, very similar to that of dentine. However, it is appreciably less than enamel.

THERMAL PROPERTIES

The thermal conductivity of set silicate cement is about 0·8 W/mK, which compares very favourably with the values of 0·88 and 0·59 W/mK respectively for enamel and dentine. This is not too surprising in view of its ceramic structure.

For the same reason, the coefficient of thermal expansion of the cement, at $8 \times 10^{-6}/{}^{\circ}C$, is also similar to those of enamel ($11·4 \times 10^{-6}/{}^{\circ}C$) and dentine ($8·3 \times 10^{-6}/{}^{\circ}C$). This is, perhaps, one of the most important properties of silicate cement, for it means that the restorations should not be susceptible to percolation.

COMPATIBILITY WITH ORAL TISSUES AND FLUIDS

Some very significant characteristics of silicate cement, both desirable and undesirable, are associated with its reaction with oral tissues and fluids.

**a** *Solubility of the cement*. Silicate cements have a poor resistance to dissolution in oral fluids. The exact mechanism of this process is not entirely clear but it is largely associated with a susceptibility of the aluminium phosphate matrix to attack by acids. This matrix, and therefore the cement itself, is relatively insoluble within the range of pH 5·5 to 7·5 normally found in saliva, but as the pH is lowered below 5·5 the solubility increases, becoming very rapid should a pH of 4·0 be reached. This becomes important should plaque accumulate on the restoration, as the pH under plaque may be below 5·5 and even as low as 4·0. Plaque is particularly prevalent around the margins, especially the gingival margins, and the erosion is therefore most significant in those areas.

The solubility of the cement varies with the nature of the acidic environment. Citric acid in particular dissolves the aluminophosphate very readily, especially at pH 4·0, but also when present in a buffered near-neutral solution. Lactic acid and acetic acid also dissolve the cement but at much slower rates. This varying rate appears to depend on the solubility of the aluminium and phosphate complexes that form with the acids; citrates, for example, are particularly soluble. Although citric acid may be present in the mouth, it is the lactic acid produced within the plaque that is most prevalent and which appears to be mainly responsible for the erosion of silicate restorations.

This solubility also varies with time. The attack may be quite rapid initially as some soluble phosphate, sodium, and fluoride ions are released from the matrix. The erosion slows down, however, as the amount of phosphate that is released diminishes.

Clinical failure due to this solubility arises largely because of the extent of erosion that occurs at the margins in a self-perpetuating process. The attack is initially rapid because food debris and plaque tend to accumulate in these areas, but the erosion itself leads to a roughening of the surface, which encourages further plaque formation within that area and the creation of areas of very low pH. This may lead to aesthetically unacceptable staining and to eventual disintegration of the restoration at the margins.

Since it is the aluminophosphate matrix that is acid-soluble, best results are achieved with a maximum of unreacted core aluminosilicate glass and a minimum of this gel matrix. A high powder/liquid ratio is therefore indicated again.

**b** *Effect of silicate cement on enamel.* It will be noticed from the above explanation that fluoride ions predominate in the list of released species during cement erosion. This constant release of fluoride results in its transfer to, and accumulation in, the surrounding enamel. This has beneficial effects of increasing the resistance of this enamel to acid attack and inhibiting plaque formation, and because of this, silicate cement restorations appear to be associated with an anticariogenic or cariostatic effect. It is certainly well established that such restorations seldom fail through recurrent caries in the adjacent enamel, and that this fluoride release, along with the resistance to marginal leakage, must be largely responsible.

**c** *Effect of silicate cement on pulp and gingivae.* The pH of the liquid used for preparation of a silicate cement will be of the order of 1·0, or possibly less. After mixing, the pH rises slowly, reaching 3·0 at 10 minutes and 4·0 by 1 hour. After two days the pH has only reached 5·0 and never rises much above the 5·0–5·2 range. Since the tubular structure of dentine allows some fluid movement, and since pulp is seriously and irreversibly damaged by even transient exposures to low pH, it is not surprising that silicate cement restorations have a tendency to cause pulpal injury. It is, in fact, regarded as one of the most damaging of restorative materials. It is most important, therefore, to use a suitably protective lining, a calcium hydroxide-based material usually being preferred. It is important that silicate cement should not be placed in direct contact with a zinc oxide/eugenol material whilst the latter is setting, since unreacted eugenol may react with the silicate cement affecting the setting time and physical properties and leading to discoloration.

It is also possible for silicate cement to irritate the gingivae, a factor which is of particular importance in cavities which extend subgingivally. This largely arises because of the tendency for the restoration to erode at its margins, leaving a surface susceptible to food debris and plaque accumulation, which results in gingival inflammation.

**d** *Adhesion.* There is no adhesive bond formed between silicate cement and either dentine or enamel.

### Summary of clinical performance of silicate cement

A silicate cement mixed and placed with care can have a clinical life of many years. Such success is achieved because of the very favourable thermal expansion properties which lead to a resistance to marginal leakage, the lack of a significant dimensional change on setting, the anticariogenic effect of the released fluoride, and the excellent aesthetics.

The key to success, however, is good technique, since a poorly handled silicate cement may fail very early. The precipitating factor for failure is the poor resistance to solution in oral fluids which leads either to staining, or marginal breakdown, or both. Either of these failure mechanisms may, in fact, become manifest within a few months. Although good technique will minimize the risk of failure, some well-placed restorations may also erode at an early stage because of the presence of a low pH environment, so the life of a restoration is quite unpredictable.

## GLASS IONOMER CEMENT

This material has been discussed in Chapter 2, since it is an adhesive restorative material, and in Chapter 3, since it has potential as a cementing agent as well as a filling material. The material, which is widely referred to as ASPA cement, was developed in 1969 and introduced clinically a few years later, so that the amount of clinical experience has been rather limited and it is uncertain how successful it will prove as a material for anterior fillings.

### Composition

This cement is based on the reaction between an aluminosilicate glass and a polycarboxylic acid, such as polyacrylic acid: hence the name ASPA. Glass ionomer cement will clearly possess some characteristics of silicate cement (since they have the powdered aluminosilicate glass in common) and of zinc polycarboxylate cement (which has an essentially similar liquid).

*Powder.* The powder is prepared in much the same way as the powder in the silicate cement, that is, by fusion and shock cooling, but it has a slightly different composition, as indicated in Table 5.2.

**Table 5.2** Composition of the powder and liquid of glass ionomer cement

|  | % |
| --- | --- |
| POWDER | |
| $SiO_2$ | 29 |
| $Al_2O_3$ | 17 |
| $CaF_2$ | 34 |
| $Na_3AlF_6$ | 5 |
| $AlF_3$ | 5 |
| $AlPO_4$ | 10 |
| LIQUID | |
| Poly (-acrylic acid -itaconic acid) | 47·5 |
| Water | 47·5 |
| Tartaric acid | 5·0 |

The structure is again that of a continuous aluminosilicate phase containing a dispersion of fluoride-rich spherical droplets. The powder has a maximum particle size in the region of 45 $\mu$m.

*Liquid.* The liquid is an aqueous solution of polycarboxylic acids, the general structure of which has been discussed in Chapter 1. Polyacrylic acid is a widely used polycarboxylic acid but does not have entirely suitable viscosity and stability for this application. Instead an aqueous solution of a copolymer of acrylic acid and itaconic acid, with a small amount of tartaric acid to control the setting rate, is used in the proportions indicated in Table 5.2.

### Setting reaction

The setting reaction is similar in principle to that involved with silicate cement, but differs in detail (see Fig. 5.5). On mixing the glass powder with the acid, calcium and aluminium ions are displaced from the glass as $Ca^{2+}$ and $Al^{3+}$ along with the fluoride ion. The composition of the glass has been chosen to allow this process to occur quite rapidly and is frequently referred to as an ion-leachable glass because of this property. The calcium ions react rapidly in the liquid, forming salt bridges between the negatively charged carboxyl groups as shown. The polycarboxylate chains become cross-linked by this process, soon forming a gel which marks the initial set of the cement. The aluminium ions react more slowly, largely because they are trivalent and have more difficulty in forming the salt bridges, but they

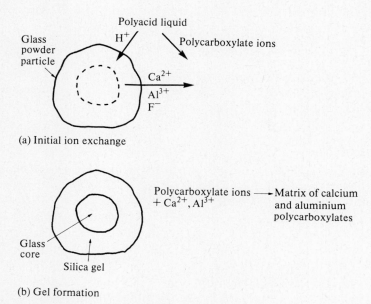

Fig. 5.5 Setting reaction of glass ionomer cement.

do slowly increase the degree of cross-linking, producing further hardening until the final set is achieved.

## Structure of the set cement

Again the most critical aspect of the reaction, as far as the structure of the set cement is concerned, is the fact that much of the aluminosilicate glass does not react, leaving cores of this glass bound together by a metal poly-acrylate gel matrix. As with the silicate cement, each glass particle is surrounded by a siliceous hydrogel, where the $Ca^{2+}$ and $Al^{3+}$ cations have been leached out from the aluminosilicate glass.

## Properties of ASPA cement

These are discussed here fairly briefly since these materials are relatively new and little information is available.

### CLINICAL HANDLING

Essentially the same technique as that employed for silicate cement is used. Again a cooled glass slab is preferred, and the speed of mixing is similarly important, in order to avoid excessive exposure of the liquid to the air, which would result in evaporation of water and an increase in the viscosity. It is essential to use the correct powder/liquid ratio, given as 3 or 3·5 g/ml, if the right consistency is to be obtained. The initial set is typically achieved in 4–5 minutes, which is slightly longer than that of silicate cement. It is important that the material is placed in the cavity at the optimum time to maximize the adhesion, as discussed below, and that it is protected from early moisture contamination.

### AESTHETICS

Early presentations of this material had a somewhat lower translucency than silicate cement and gave a notably less pleasing appearance. However, changes in the characteristic of the glass in later developments have given more satisfactory results in this respect.

### MECHANICAL PROPERTIES

The mechanical properties are not vastly different from those of silicate cement. Typically a one-day compressive strength will be 175 $MN/m^2$ compared to 225 $MN/m^2$, rising to 200 $MN/m^2$ (c.f. 245 $MN/m^2$) at seven days. Again the material is brittle, with a tensile strength identical to that of silicate cement at 13–14 $MN/m^2$.

### THERMAL PROPERTIES

The thermal expansion of the ASPA cement should be comparable with that of silicate cement, making it compatible with dentine and enamel in this respect.

COMPATIBILITY WITH ORAL TISSUES AND FLUIDS

There are some considerable advantages of ASPA cement in this respect.

**a** *Solubility of the cement.* Whilst acid solubility is one of the biggest problems with silicate cements, a greater resistance to acids is a favourable feature of ASPA cement. It will be recalled that the solubility of silicate cement was largely due to the susceptibility of the aluminophosphate gel matrix to acid attack. This occurs because this matrix is an ionically-bound substance which inherently has weak resistance to acids. The ASPA cement, however, has a matrix which contains covalent bonds as well as ionic bonds in the polymeric structure, with the result that acid attack is much slower. The amount of ASPA cement dissolved by acid at pH 4 under standard conditions during seven days is 1·2 per cent compared with 5 per cent for silicate cement.

**b** *Effect of ASPA on enamel.* Since this cement also contains a considerable amount of fluoride ions, it should have the same anti-cariogenic effect as silicate cement.

**c** *Effect of ASPA on pulp.* Several reasons have been quoted as to why ASPA cement should not have the same damaging effect on pulp as silicate cement. First, the polycarboxylic acids used are very much weaker than phosphoric acid. Secondly, the fact that the acid is a polymer means that it will have a much higher molecular weight, and this, together with a physical entanglement of the polymer chains, will limit diffusion along dentinal tubules towards the pulp. Thirdly, there is a strong electrostatic attraction between the hydrogen ions and the negatively charged polymer chain so that there is less tendency for these ions to move away from the polymer, even when the acid is dissociated.

These theoretical arguments seem to be confirmed by the clinical evidence, which suggests that ASPA cement produces little pulpal damage.

**d** *Adhesion.* As discussed in some detail in Chapter 2, cements based on polycarboxylic acids have the rare ability to adhere to dentine and enamel. This is, perhaps, the most important advantage that ASPA cement has over other restorative materials. The adhesion is due to the presence of many free carboxyl groups (—COOH) which facilitate wetting of tooth surfaces because of their ability to form hydrogen bonds between the polymer and the substrate. These hydrogen bonds are progressively converted into stronger ionic bonds as calcium, aluminium, and other metal ions displace the hydrogen.

Thus, whereas the strength of bond between either dentine or enamel to silicate cement is effectively zero, a strength of 4 MN/m$^2$ and 3 MN/m$^2$ may be achieved between ASPA cement and enamel and dentine respectively. The greater degree of adhesion of ASPA cement to enamel than to dentine is due to stronger bonds formed with the inorganic substrate, as explained in Chapter 2.

It is important to note a few features of the clinical handling of the ASPA cement related to the adhesion. First, a strong bond will only form if proper wetting takes place, and this is dependent on the availability of the —COOH groups. The cement must, therefore, be applied to the tooth surface before the setting reaction has proceeded too far, that is, whilst there are still sufficient —COOH groups available. Any delay in placing the cement will reduce the wetting and the adhesion.

Secondly, good adhesion relies on sound, clean surfaces. Pre-treatment of the tooth surface may therefore be recommended before use of the ASPA cement. A 50 per cent solution of citric acid is used when the ASPA material is used as a fissure sealant, but is not recommended for large areas of exposed dentine, where hydrogen peroxide solution is preferred.

### Summary of clinical performance of glass-ionomer cement

Clearly these cements possess some very desirable properties and have considerable potential for dental use. The ASPA cement is used successfully in erosion cavities in the restoration of deciduous teeth where it has been difficult to prepare a mechanically retentive cavity, and in certain class III cavities that do not involve labial enamel. The material is also used successfully as a fissure sealant and a fine-grained version is widely used as a luting cement. In these situations, it must be remembered that the cement is weak in tension, which places some restrictions on its use, and that it suffers from the same problem as the silicate when it comes into premature contact with water, so the material must be protected.

## COMPOSITE FILLING MATERIALS

Composites represent an entirely different approach to the problems of anterior restorative materials. The setting reaction in this case involves polymerization, which implies a totally different set of characteristics and properties when compared with those of the cements.

As reviewed in Chapter 1, a composite material is one which contains two or more distinct components of quite different character. In particular, useful composite materials are designed so that their properties reflect the good characteristics of their components but eliminate the undesirable features. Composite restorative materials usually consist of a resin matrix with a ceramic as the dispersed second component. The nature and proportions of these components are chosen to maximize their contribution to the properties of the resulting composite.

In order to fully appreciate the structure of these materials, it is necessary first to discuss briefly the use of an unfilled resin, acrylic resin, as a restorative material, which preceded the development of the composites.

### Acrylic resin as a restorative material

Polymethyl methacrylate, generally known in this context as acrylic resin, will be discussed fully in Chapter 11 because of its major use in dental prosthetics. The use of acrylic resin in that situation largely arose through its ease of preparation. Since the polymerization of methyl methacrylate is as readily achieved chemically (i.e. at room temperature) as it is thermally, it was logical to use it as a filling material, especially since there are, even now, so few polymers that can be formed under intra-oral conditions. It is not necessary to review the chemistry of the polymerization process here; it is sufficient to note that the addition polymerization of methyl methacrylate is achieved by a free radical process involving the initiator benzoyl peroxide, which has to be activated by some suitable means. With heat-cured acrylic, activation of the peroxide is achieved simply by raising the temperature. In cold or self-cured acrylic, this is done by a chemical, usually a tertiary amine. It was this cold-cured acrylic that was introduced as a restorative material around 1950. The material was prepared by mixing one part of methyl methacrylate monomer containing the activator and 2–3 parts of powdered polymethyl methacrylate containing the peroxide.

Although there are some very useful properties associated with this acrylic filling material, it also has some serious disadvantages. These properties are enumerated below with reference to the requirements of a tooth-coloured filling material and the need for improvement.

*Clinical handling.* Although in principle straightforward, the technique of placing an acrylic restoration is complicated by two factors. First, and most important, the polymerization process is associated with a great degree of shrinkage. Techniques have therefore been devised to minimize the effects of such shrinkage; if these are not adopted there is a high risk of marginal leakage. Secondly, although the polymerized resin is inert, volatile and reactive substances are present while polymerization is taking place, and care has to be taken to avoid reaction between these and other substances, especially lining materials. Zinc oxide/eugenol linings cannot be used, for example, because of their reaction with the filling material.

*Dimensional changes on setting.* Reference to the polymerization process shown diagrammatically in Figure 1.20 shows that this process is inevitably associated with some contraction, as discussed in detail in Chapter 1. This arises because weak, long-range forces holding the molecules of the monomer together are largely replaced by covalent bonds to give either a solid, or a liquid of higher molecular weight. The smaller the monomer molecule and the larger the polymer molecule, that is the greater the number of molecules joined together, the greater will be the total shrinkage. Since methyl methacrylate has a relatively small molecule, the shrinkage is high. For the direct polymerization of methyl methacrylate, the total shrinkage is about 21 per cent by volume. With a powdered polymer/liquid monomer ratio of around 3:1, the shrinkage of dental acrylic is in the region of 5–6 per cent. This is quite appreciable and would clearly contribute to marginal leakage as discussed below.

This is an inherent defect in a system which relies on the addition polymerization of large numbers of small molecules. In practice, the effect is minimized, as mentioned above, by using the appropriate method, such as the pressure technique, where excess material is forced into the cavity under pressure, or the incremental technique, which involves the placement of successive layers to build up the restoration.

*Aesthetics.* Very good initial aesthetic properties can be achieved with acrylic resin. However, it wears badly and readily collects plaque and may soon discolour by surface staining. Furthermore the appearance may also change over a period of time, due to discoloration caused by the instability of amine-cured acrylic under ultraviolet light.

*Mechanical properties.* One of the most serious deficiencies in acrylic resin is the lack of strength. Although the tensile strength at about 30 MN/m$^2$ may be twice that of silicate cement, the compressive strength is much lower than that of silicate, at about 70 MN/m$^2$. The modulus of elasticity and the proportional limit are also low, indicating that elastic and then plastic deformation occur readily. The hardness of the resin is considerably lower than that of any other filling materials, giving very poor abrasion-resistance. Large restorations are therefore susceptible to loss of anatomical form.

*Physical properties.* As noted earlier, polymers, as well as ceramics, are good insulators, and therefore thermal conductivity presents no problems. On the other hand, polymers often have a high coefficient of thermal expansion. Acrylic resin has an expansion coefficient of about $81 \times 10^{-6}/°C$ compared with the $11·4$ and $8·3 \times 10^{-6}/°C$ for enamel and dentine respectively. Bearing in mind the figure of only $8 \times 10^{-6}/°C$ for silicate cement, the significance of the high coefficient in relation to marginal leakage is readily appreciated.

*Compatibility with oral tissues and fluids.* In direct contrast to the cements, polymers, such as acrylic resin, are virtually insoluble in oral fluids. There is a tendency to absorb small amounts of water, the significance of which is discussed later. Acrylic resin does not contain any fluoride and therefore has no beneficial effect on enamel solubility. As far as the pulpal response is concerned, although the pH is physiologically acceptable, free monomer present at the time the filling is inserted is quite irritant. This monomer may readily penetrate the dentinal tubules and produce adverse effects in the pulp. It is also possible for the temperature rise associated with the exothermic reaction to produce pulpal damage. Finally, no adhesion is achieved between acrylic resin and tooth structures.

It will be clear from this brief description that although acrylic resin has a few very desirable features to offer as a filling material, especially the good initial aesthetics and the ease of finishing and insolubility, it also possesses several disadvantages which make long-term success hard to achieve. These disadvantages are largely inherent in the polymeric structure and the polymerization process, which result in relatively poor mechanical properties, high polymerization shrinkage, high thermal expansion, and chemical irritation from the monomer.

The reasoning behind the development of composite filling materials, initially based on acrylic resin, was as follows. First, if there are certain undesirable physical properties associated with the resin, it may be possible to dilute the resin with components which do not have these features but which produce a composite structure that retains the good and desirable properties of the resin. Secondly, to obtain an improvement in the mechanical properties, the second component may be a hard material finely dispersed in the matrix to give the classical composite structure discussed in Chapter 1. Thirdly, it may be possible to modify the resin to give better properties within the composite.

The structure of a composite restorative material is therefore similar to that illustrated in Figure 5.6. Typically 70–80 per cent of a fine dispersion of ceramic will be contained within the resin matrix. Assuming for the moment that the resin used is acrylic, and the filler is a ceramic, such as quartz, representing 75 per cent by volume of the composite, then such a structure will offer three specific improvements.

1 Since resin occupies only 25 per cent of the volume, the polymerization shrinkage will be only 25 per cent of that associated with pure resin.
2 The coefficient of expansion will be considerably reduced, not to 25 per cent of the original, since the filler expands and contracts a measurable amount, but nevertheless to a figure approaching that amount. For example a filler with a coefficient of expansion of $10 \times 10^{-6}/°C$ compared with $80 \times 10^{-6}/°C$ for the resin will give a coefficient in the composite of $27.5 \times 10^{-6}/°C$ when used in the 75–25 per cent ratio.
3 Provided that there is sufficient resin to give a coherent matrix, the composite structure may give much better mechanical properties, with improvement in tensile strength, compressive strength, proof strength, elastic modulus, and hardness. The reasons for this have been discussed in Chapter 1.

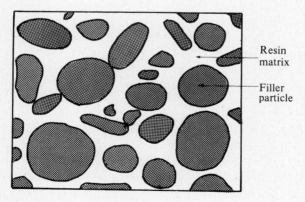

Resin matrix

Filler particle

**Fig. 5.6** Microstructure of a composite filling material.

Thus, by the simple expedient of adding to the resin an inert filler, which neither takes part in the reaction nor has any of the undesirable physical properties of the resin, most of the serious disadvantages can be obviated, or at least reduced. Careful choice of the filler will ensure that the good aesthetic qualities are not lost, and may even be improved in terms of the translucency.

Although some of the first commercially available composite restorative materials did use acrylic resin as the matrix, a different resin is now employed in the majority of materials. This is because acrylic resin itself has one of the highest values of polymerization shrinkage amongst polymers of this type, and because it exhibits no adhesion to tooth structure. Most of these composite materials have, in fact, used a resin which is usually termed 'BIS–GMA resin' on account of its derivation, or alternatively, 'Bowen resin' after its innovator. Composites based on this resin are now discussed in detail before going on to consider some later modifications.

## BIS–GMA RESIN COMPOSITES

### Composition

A large number of BIS–GMA composites are commercially available, and each may have a slightly different formulation. All, however, use the BIS–GMA resin as the major constituent of the matrix, with 60–75 per cent of a ceramic as the dispersed filler. A coupling agent is generally used to promote bonding between the filler and resin.

*Resin.* The BIS–GMA resin represents a compromise between attempts to produce an adhesive resin with one that could harden within the oral environment. Some of the early attempts to produce a suitable resin for a composite were concerned with epoxy resins which have good adhesive properties and harden with minimal shrinkage. However, it was not possible to utilize these resins in suitable composite restorative materials, partly because adhesion to hard tooth substances was poor after prolonged exposure to water and partly because of the difficulty of obtaining a suitable polymerization reaction.

A typical epoxy molecule is shown in Figure 5.7a. It is the oxirane group which is characteristic of the epoxy structure but which, for dental use is replaced by a group more amenable to polymerization under the appropriate conditions. Since one of the most desirable features of the acrylic resin is the ease of polymerization with the methacrylate structure, such methacrylate groups have been used to replace the oxirane groups. Thus the molecule shown in Figure 5.7b is a hybrid consisting of part of the epoxy molecule but terminating at each end with a methacrylate group. It is this molecule that is called the BIS–GMA monomer. It has been given this name because in one of the methods used to synthesize the monomer, bisphenol A reacts with glycidyl methacrylate as illustrated in Figure 5.7c.

Although this resin is derived from an epoxy resin, the oxirane groups

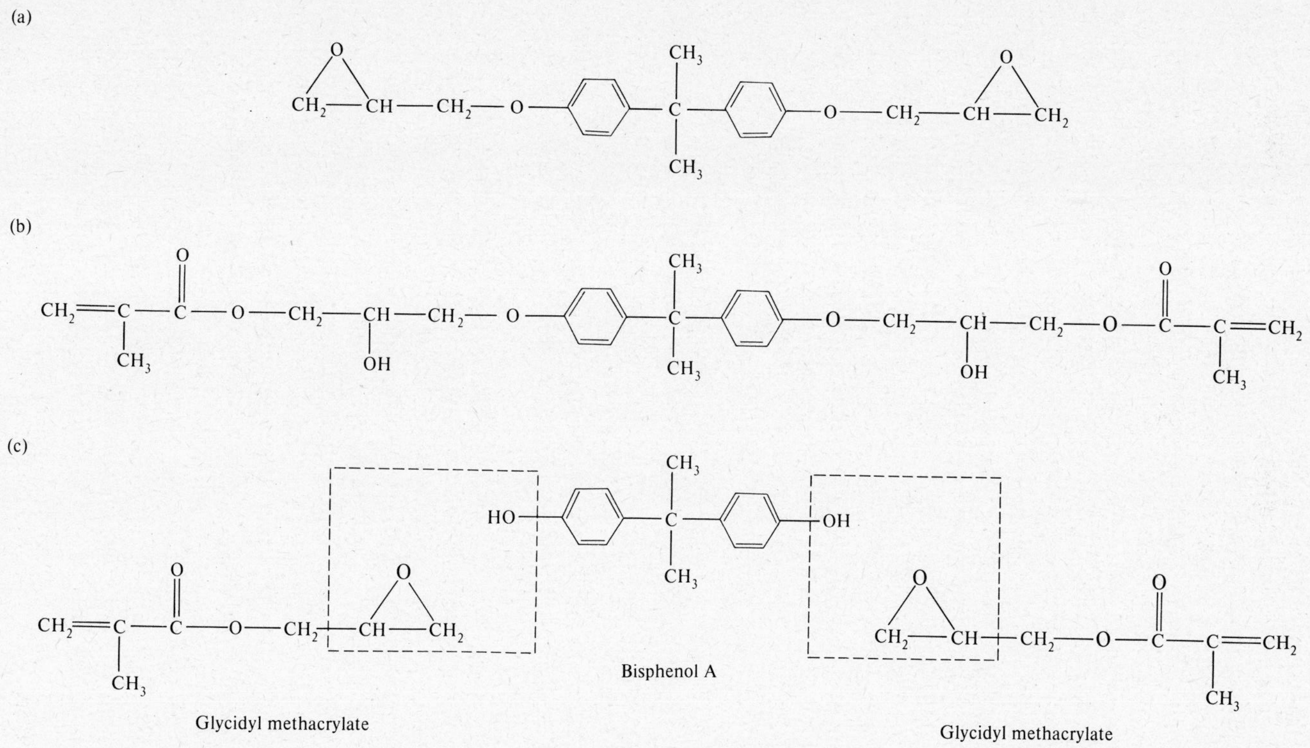

**Fig. 5.7** (a) Typical epoxy molecule; (b) epoxy molecule terminated at each end with a methacrylate group; (c) reaction between Bisphenol A and glycidyl methacrylate to give the BIS–GMA molecule.

have been replaced, so that technically the term 'epoxy' should not be used. Instead it may be described as a 'dimethacrylate resin' or more specifically as an 'aromatic dimethacrylate'.

This BIS–GMA monomer is too viscous to be used alone in the matrix, and several other monomers have been employed as thinners to reduce the viscosity. These have usually been other methacrylate monomers, such as methyl methacrylate, or, more commonly, tetraethylene glycol dimethacrylate.

Polymerization is achieved via the methacrylate groups as discussed below. This may be activated chemically, in which case the benzoyl peroxide–amine system is the most common. The benzoyl peroxide may be dispersed with the filler or dissolved in the monomer at a total concentration of 0·5 per cent. Although the dimethyl-p-toluidine activator has had widespread use, others, such as dimethyl-sym-m-xylidine, are more common as they result in less discoloration of the resin. Alternatively the benzoyl peroxide may be activated by ultraviolet light. In these products a suitable ultraviolet light absorber, such as benzoin methyl ether, is added. A very small amount, measured in parts per million, of an inhibitor will also be present. The nature of the inhibitor is not normally disclosed, although hydroquinone, the monomethyl ether of hydroquinone, and butylated hydroxytoluene have all been used. The inhibitor prevents the spontaneous and premature hardening of the resin.

*Filler*. Several different kinds of filler have been employed in these BIS–GMA composites. Quartz and borosilicate glass are common, but others include lithium aluminium silicate and various aluminosilicate glasses. The use of lithium aluminium silicate is particularly interesting as it has a negative coefficient of expansion and hence reduces the coefficient of the composite even further.

Radiopacity is a desirable feature of a restorative material, and the need for a filler has provided a means for incorporating a radiopaque component into the resin. This has been achieved to a certain extent by the use of heavy metal-containing glasses, and especially barium fluoride glasses, but problems have been encountered in retaining suitable optical properties whilst increasing the radiopacity. Many commercially available composites do, however, contain fillers such as these, usually in combination with a conventional non-radiopaque filler to achieve the right balance of properties.

The filler may be in the form of rods, beads, irregular particles, or platelets, and may vary in size up to 40 or even 60 $\mu$m. There is a tendency, however, to reduce the size so that a mean particle diameter may be in the region of 10–20 $\mu$m. Typically 70–75 per cent of the filler will be present, although values as high as 80 per cent are claimed for some products. This represents the maximum filler content of a composite with a dispersed phase of this type.

*Coupling agents*. For maximum benefit to be achieved with a composite structure, there has to be a good bond between the matrix and the filler. This is necessary both to produce the best mechanical properties and to prevent penetration of water along the filler–matrix interface. Organo-functional silanes have been universally employed as coupling agents in composite restorative materials, although information on the type of silane used in any one product is not generally available.

*Formulation.* It is usual for the chemically cured composites to be presented as a two-paste system, the base or universal paste containing the activator, and the catalyst or reactor paste containing the benzoyl peroxide initiator. A representative composition of such a system is given in Table 5.3. With an ultraviolet-light-cured material, no mixing is necessary and it is supplied as a single paste, containing the ultraviolet light absorber.

**Table 5.3** Composition of a typical two-paste composite filling material

|  | Base or universal paste % | Catalyst paste % |
| --- | --- | --- |
| BIS–GMA resin | 22 | 22 |
| Quartz filler | 76 | 76 |
| Dimethyl-*p*-toluidene | 1 | — |
| Benzoyl peroxide | — | 0·5 |
| Pigments | trace | trace |
| Ultraviolet absorber | 1 | 1 |
| Inhibitor | trace | trace |

## Setting reaction

As mentioned above, the polymerization of the BIS–GMA resin can be achieved through the use of either an ultraviolet light or chemically activated initiator in much the same way as with an acrylic resin. This process is discussed in both Chapter 1 and 11. It is important to note that the ultraviolet light and the amine just provide two alternative methods for producing the free radicals from the benzoyl peroxide. The polymerization process itself is therefore independent of the method of activation since it is initiated by these free radicals.

Polymerization takes place via the methacrylate ends of the BIS–GMA molecule and the dimethacrylate comonomer, such as triethylene glycol dimethacrylate, that is present. Typically there will be about 25 per cent of such a comonomer in the resin. The one important difference to note between this polymerization and that of the simpler methyl methacrylate monomer is that large parts of the molecule in the BIS–GMA are non-functional in this respect so that considerably fewer double bonds are broken during the process, leading to reduced polymerization shrinkage. This is discussed later in relation to dimensional stability. The polymerization process commences once the two pastes have been mixed in the chemically cured composites, but does not do so until the light source has been applied to the material with the ultraviolet-cured systems. This allows the operator to place the material in the cavity and contour the restoration before initiating the polymerization.

## Properties of BIS–GMA composites

It is more difficult to give clear statements about the properties of these composite restorative materials than it is about silicate cements since they have not been in use for so long and since there are now many different BIS–GMA composites commercially available with potentially differing properties. However some generalizations may be made and are dealt with here under the headings used earlier.

### CLINICAL HANDLING

**a** *Mixing.* As noted above, ultraviolet-light-cured composites need no mixing and are supplied as a single paste.

With the chemically cured composites, presentation may be either as a powder and liquid, as a paste and a liquid or as a two-paste system. The last is the most common. Mixing is achieved easily as proportioning is not considered to be critical. Although manufacturers' instructions should always be followed carefully, slight errors in proportioning will not usually result in significantly reduced properties. This provides an advantage over the silicate cements for which handling characteristics are far more critical.

It is important to avoid using a metal spatula for mixing composites as it can be abraded by the hard ceramic filler and may therefore give a grey colour to the material. Plastic spatulas are usually provided. It is also very important to avoid any cross-contamination between the two pastes at this stage either by taking care to use different spatulas in each jar or different ends of the same spatula. Many manufacturers supply spatulas with ends of different shape, or that are clearly marked to assist in dispensing. Any contamination could result in hardening of the resin remaining in the jar.

In order to achieve the right colour-match it may be necessary to add tints to the paste. In a two-paste system the tint is added to the universal paste. Since the universal paste is mixed with an equal amount of reactor paste, the former has to be tinted to a slightly darker colour than that of the tooth to produce the correct shade in the mixed material.

**b** *Mixing time.* Again a single-paste, ultraviolet-light-cured composite offers an unlimited working time, as polymerization is not initiated until the light-source is applied after placement in the cavity.

The working time with the chemically cured materials varies from one product to another but generally is relatively short. Typically 20–30 seconds is allowed for spatulation, following which there is a working time of 1–1·5 minutes. This will depend to a certain extent on the temperature, a hot surgery causing a reduction in this time. It is, of course, important that any tinting is done before the catalyst is added to the universal paste.

c *Placement of the restoration.* Placement of the composite in the cavity is easily achieved, the materials having quite suitable viscosities. Plastic instruments may be used to avoid contamination of the composites from metal instruments. Care must be taken to ensure good packing of the composite in the cavity, since there is a tendency to produce voids which result in weakening of the restoration and reduced retention. The best surface finish is obtained with the use of a plastic matrix band. However, celluloid matrices react slightly with BIS–GMA composites, giving a duller surface, and therefore other materials, such as cellulose acetate are used.

d *Setting characteristics.* It has been noted earlier that the ideal restorative material should set by a reaction which is readily activated, which will go to completion if necessary, and which is not significantly influenced by variables such as temperature and humidity. With the chemically cured BIS–GMA resin these requirements are quite adequately met, the polymerization being readily achieved under the imposed conditions. There is no problem of completing the curing or of hardening, if the correct mixing procedure has been used, and although temperature does have an effect on the rate of polymerization, this should not present any difficulties in the handling of the material. Variations in humidity have a negligible effect on the reaction. Although the presence of water does not significantly influence the setting, care must be taken to avoid contamination of the restoration with water.

The use of ultraviolet light for activating the setting reaction does have some advantages, notably the freedom from the constraint of placing the restoration in the cavity whilst the reaction is taking place. In this case the uncured composite is placed in the cavity and can be contoured before the ultraviolet light source is applied. Manufacturers of these composites supply special ultraviolet lights for use with their material. As illustrated in Figure 5.8, this is usually a hand-held, gun-shaped instrument, the body of which contains the light source. The ultraviolet light is transmitted along a rod or light guide, usually of quartz, which may be shielded by some protective covering to prevent scattering of the ultraviolet light. Filters may be incorporated in the instrument to control the wavelength, and especially to remove the short-wave radiation.

It is possible that the ultraviolet light has harmful effects on both patients and operators. It is difficult to give an unequivocal statement on this matter as little in the way of valid scientific data is available. The main cause for concern is the damage to eyes that can be induced by the light. It is sensible to take precautions to avoid exposure of the eyes directly to the ultraviolet light, and some manufacturers of light sources shield the guide, as noted above. Many operators also take the precaution of shielding their own eyes and those of the patient with sun glasses.

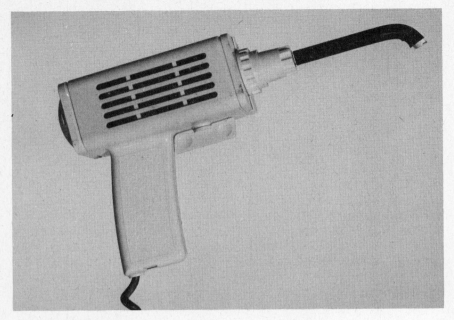

**Fig. 5.8** Ultraviolet light source.

For efficient activation of the resin system, the tip of the rod has usually to be placed in very close proximity to the surface of the restoration and held there for the required period of time, which will vary with the product and the type of restoration. One very important point here is that the extent of the polymerization is dependent on the amount of ultràviolet light energy that is absorbed. If, in a given volume of material, too little energy is absorbed, then the polymerization will be incomplete. This has several implications. First, it is important to follow the manufacturer's instructions concerning the distance between the tip of the probe and the restoration and the time the light is applied, since these both directly control the amount of energy reaching the restoration. The thickness of the restoration is also significant, since the total energy required to produce the right degree of polymerization is dependent upon the volume. For a depth of 1–2 mm this presents no real problems. However, difficulty may be experienced with thicker layers which may necessitate the building up of the restoration in smaller increments and, in the case of most Class IV restorations, exposure from both labial and lingual sides. Finally, ultraviolet light sources do deteriorate, and the amount of energy available from a source will decrease with time with no obvious indication that this is taking place. It is essential, therefore, to ascertain the useful working life of any type of instrument that is used.

**e** *Setting time.* As with the working time, this will vary slightly from one product to another, but generally it is of the order of 3 minutes. It is essential that the restoration should not be disturbed during this time, after which the matrix band and any flash may be removed. A futher 2 minutes or so is then necessary before any gross reduction or finishing processes can be carried out, should they be necessary.

These various stages in the polymerization can be explained as follows. During mixing the activator starts to react with the initiator, causing it to form free radicals, as described earlier. These free radicals cannot initiate the polymerization straight away because of the presence of traces of inhibitor which themselves react with the first free radicals to be produced. This determines the working time. Once all the inhibitor molecules have been consumed in this way, the free radicals are then available to react with the molecules in the resin. Polymerization and cross-linking take place during this setting time, which may also be referred to as the gel time. At the end of these three minutes, or whatever the setting time is for the system, sufficient cross-linking will have occurred to give a reasonably hard material. However, further hardening takes place through a continuation of this process, and especially as a result of the bonding of the filler particles to the resin molecules. After only a few minutes, sufficient strength will have developed to allow any finishing that is necessary to be performed, although the final strength will not have been achieved at this stage.

**f** *Shelf-life.* The shelf-life of composites depends on their presentation and the care exercised during the use of a pack. With the two-paste systems described above, there is a tendency for the benzoyl peroxide to decompose spontaneously to give free radicals at normal temperatures, and since this peroxide is contained within the same paste as the resin, some premature hardening could occur. This slow decomposition of the peroxide will also cause its depletion, with the result that there may not be enough available to give complete polymerization at a later stage. There is, therefore, a finite shelf-life for these materials, typically about one year, which will be stated by the manufacturer of each product, as will be the advice on storage procedures. Generally it is recommended that unopened packs are kept in a refrigerator. This shelf-life is, of course, dependent on there being no cross-contamination, as discussed above.

Since there is a certain ultraviolet wavelength component in daylight, exposure of ultraviolet-cured materials to light may give a decreased shelf-life. All of these products are presented in small light-proof jars to minimize this effect and its consequences.

DIMENSIONAL STABILITY ON SETTING

It will be recalled that the shrinkage accompanying the polymerization of the direct-filling acrylic resin was about 5–6 per cent. Several factors combine to reduce the shrinkage to about one-tenth of this value, typically 0·65 per cent in a BIS–GMA composite. First, there is the high filler content, which reduces the amount of resin available for polymerization to only 20–25 per cent of the total. Secondly, the dimethacrylate molecule of the BIS–GMA resin is much larger than a methyl methacrylate molecule, as shown in Figure 5.9a, so that far fewer steps in the polymerization process are necessary (Fig. 5.9b) than in the former case, leading to a smaller contraction since each double bond broken contributes to the shrinkage.

The important point about this shrinkage is, of course, the effect it has on marginal adaptation. The clinical evidence so far available suggests that the composites do have good marginal adaptation, which must be largely

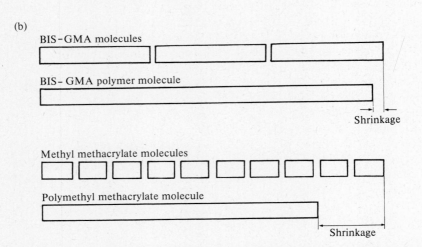

Fig. 5.9 (a) Sizes of dimethacrylate molecule of BIS–GMA and methyl methacrylate; (b) polymerization of BIS–GMA and methyl methacrylate showing amounts of polymerization shrinkage.

due to this low shrinkage. There may, however, be a further factor involved and that is the tendency for these composites to absorb some water, the accompanying swelling counteracting the polymerization shrinkage. A typical figure for water absorption at equilibrium is 1·5 per cent by volume, which translates to a linear swelling of about 0·5 per cent, very similar to the figure given for the polymerization shrinkage.

AESTHETICS

The presence of a ceramic or glass phase within a resin affords considerable scope for varying the optical properties of the composite, and careful choice of the filler in this respect has led to the development of restorative materials with excellent aesthetics. The use of tints has already been discussed, and these allow further matching to the adjacent tooth substance.

Composites are, however, susceptible to changes in their appearance over a period of time. One of the more important reasons for this is the difficulty of obtaining and maintaining a good surface finish on the restoration. This arises because of the heterogeneous nature of the composite, with extremely hard filler particles embedded in a matrix of a very much softer resin. It is extremely difficult to produce a surface finish which is smooth and uniform, as in Figure 5.10a. Problems arise with abrasion of the surface when either the filler particles are plucked out, or the resin matrix is abraded preferentially (Fig. 5.10b). This can occur either during a finishing process itself or during subsequent use.

The best results are obtained with the surface left by the matrix band. If finishing is necessary, it is important to wait until after the gel period before any carving is performed. Shaping may be achieved with either a fine diamond stone or carbide burs and final polishing is performed with appropriate materials, such as fine grit discs or white stones.

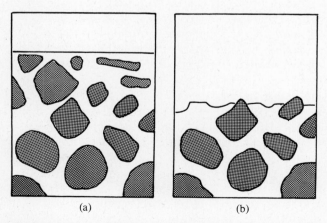

(a)                                   (b)

**Fig. 5.10** (a) Smooth surface on a composite filling material; (b) loss of filler and abrasion of resin, giving rough surface.

The problem with this poor surface finish is, of course, that it encourages plaque accumulation, which may result in superficial discoloration. The resin itself may also discolour, independent of any such surface condition. In early composites, colour changes were associated with oxidation or ultraviolet radiation-induced molecular rearrangements of the amine activator, dimethyl-p-toluidine. Use of other amine activators has reduced this problem but discoloration may also arise from the BIS–GMA molecule itself, parts of which can slowly decompose. All BIS–GMA resin composites are susceptible to discoloration to some extent and although the actual amount varies from one product to another, this is a potential limitation to the life expectancy of these restorations.

MECHANICAL PROPERTIES

As anticipated, the mechanical properties of these materials show considerable improvement over those of the unreinforced acrylic resin and silicate cement. Whereas the acrylic gives figures of about 30 MN/m$^2$ for the tensile strength and 70 MN/m$^2$ for the compressive strength, the composite materials have tensile strengths in the range 40–60 MN/m$^2$ (usually around 45 MN/m$^2$) and compressive strengths of 200–250 MN/m$^2$, occasionally reaching 300 MN/m$^2$. It can be seen that these strengths approach those of amalgam (60 MN/m$^2$ and 300 MN/m$^2$ respectively). However, the abrasion-resistance of composites does not match that of amalgam in clinical practice and loss of anatomical form is a potential problem. This occurs even though standard laboratory tests actually predict superior performance to amalgams.

Thus, even though some authorities state that composite restorative materials of this type can be used in Class II cavities because of their comparable mechanical properties to amalgam, this is not a widely recommended procedure.

PHYSICAL PROPERTIES

The thermal conductivity of composites is similar to that of acrylic resin and hence presents no problems. The coefficient of thermal expansion, however, is quite different. With a 75–80 per cent filler content the coefficient of the composite will be in the region of 24–28 × 10$^{-6}$/°C. Although this represents a considerable improvement over direct-filling acrylic, it is still significantly different from the coefficients of expansion of dentine and enamel. Marginal leakage brought about by percolation is, therefore, still possible with composites. The clinical significance of this is not clear, however, but by use of the appropriate techniques discussed later, this problem appears to be of minor importance.

COMPATIBILITY WITH ORAL TISSUES AND FLUIDS

a *Adverse effects on BIS–GMA composites.* As with acrylic resin, the BIS–GMA resin is virtually insoluble in oral fluids. The presence of the inert filler has little effect, especially if a good bond is achieved with the coupling agent so that there is no significant degradation of the composites in the oral environment.

As noted above, the composites will absorb some water, typically to an equilibrium content of about 1·5 per cent by volume. This may, in fact, have a beneficial effect by counteracting polymerization shrinkage. Very little of this water is taken up by the filler and most is concentrated in the resin matrix. It is undesirable for too much water absorption to take place, however, as it does affect the properties of the composite, especially if it is able to weaken the resin–filler bond. Loss of strength, wear resistance, and colour stability would all result from an excessive water absorption.

**b** *Adverse effects on oral tissues.* The extent of pulpal damage produced by these composites is not clear. The evidence suggests that the irreversible effects on the pulp produced by silicate cement are not found when composites are used. It also appears that composites generally are superior in this respect to direct-filling acrylic, and it has been suggested that BIS–GMA composites produce less damage than acrylic composites because of the lower irritancy of the monomer involved. Nevertheless, the rough surface produced by abrasion does lead to plaque accumulation, which will be harmful to the surrounding tooth substance.

Whatever the merits of the individual products, most, if not all, manufacturers recommend the use of an appropriate lining material to minimize this risk. This matter is discussed further at the end of the chapter.

**c** *Beneficial effects on tissues.* Although attempts have been made to incorporate fluoride into these composites, this has not met with any real success, because of the inability of any such fluoride to diffuse out of the resin and into the tooth substance. Thus there is no beneficial effect on tooth substance arising from the use of these materials. It is true to say, however, that the incidence of secondary caries is very low even in the absence of such an effect, presumably as a result of the good marginal adaptation and resistance to percolation.

**d** *Adhesion.* Although it was hoped that the BIS–GMA resin composites would show some adhesion to tooth substances, this has not been found to occur in practice and there is no real improvement over any other material. However, there is an extremely important point in this context concerning the use of the acid-etch technique for improving the adaptation of restorative materials to tooth substance. This technique has been developed simultaneously with the evolution of the composites, and is widely used in conjunction with them, and therefore, although adhesion itself has not been improved, the use of composites in association with the acid-etch technique has led to a considerable improvement in the marginal seal and retention obtained with restorations, and this has, in turn, produced some changes in the practice of conservative dentistry. The principles of acid-etching have been discussed in Chapter 2, but the application of the technique to anterior restorations will be described at the end of this chapter.

It can be appreciated from these last few pages that the BIS–GMA composites offer considerable advantages over other forms of anterior restorative materials. They are still not ideal, however, and do have some disadvantages, notably the difficulty in obtaining a good surface finish, the relatively poor abrasion-resistance, and the tendency to stain and discolour. Before reviewing the clinical uses of these materials, therefore, certain modifications to the BIS–GMA resin composites will be described, to give some indication of developments that may lead to more satisfactory materials.

## MODIFIED COMPOSITE RESTORATIVE MATERIALS

It is not possible, of course, to pre-empt each development by describing all possible modifications to this basic BIS–GMA system that could be made. A number of trends have become evident, however, and are worthy of discussion.

### SIMPLE MODIFICATION TO THE BIS–GMA MOLECULE

The BIS–GMA molecule, as shown in Figure 5.7b, contains hydroxyl groups which, it has been claimed, are partly responsible for the water-absorption characteristics of the resin. Similar molecules have already been produced without these hydroxyl groups, and the water uptake has been found to be very much less, possibly around 0·1 per cent. Although this is desirable from the point of view of preventing deleterious changes to the mechanical properties, it is as yet uncertain whether the absence of swelling will give poorer marginal adaptation.

### ALTERATIONS TO FILLER SIZE AND COMPOSITION

One of the most interesting developments of the composites has been the use of much finer particle sizes for the filler. The general theory of composite structures shows that, up to a limit, the finer the particle size the greater the increase in strength; and some commercially available composites have particle sizes much less than 1 $\mu$m instead of the 10 to 40 $\mu$m range discussed earlier. It is claimed that the mechanical properties of these materials are equal to or better than those of amalgam, and that abrasion-resistance should also be improved. Of special importance is the ability of these materials to take a higher polish, since there are no large particles to give surface roughness. It remains to be seen whether the superiority that this indicates is substantiated in practice.

Attempts have also been made to alter the nature of the filler particles. For instance, in one material, finely divided silica is mixed with BIS–GMA resin, which is then polymerized. The resulting product is then prepared as a filler and used with further BIS–GMA resin in the composite structure. This certainly gives a good surface finish, but the effectively higher total resin content may prove to give poorer resistance to marginal leakage.

## MODIFIED RESINS

Several manufacturers have produced resins that are substantially, although not completely, different from the aromatic dimethacrylate, BIS–GMA resin. One type of resin that has been extensively investigated, and which is the basis of at least three commercially available dental restoratives, is the urethane dimethacrylate. Many different types of urethane dimethacrylate are possible, but a representative molecule is given in Figure 5.11. $R^1$ and $R^2$ are different radicals, the nature of which controls the characteristics of the material. At least two different types are used in dental composites. It can be seen that the end groups of the molecule are the same as with the BIS–GMA resin, so that polymerization may be achieved in the same way. Again, some suitable comonomer may be used to reduce the viscosity. The clinical handling characteristics, and mechanical, physical, chemical, and biological properties of these composites do not appear to differ significantly from those of the normal BIS–GMA composites.

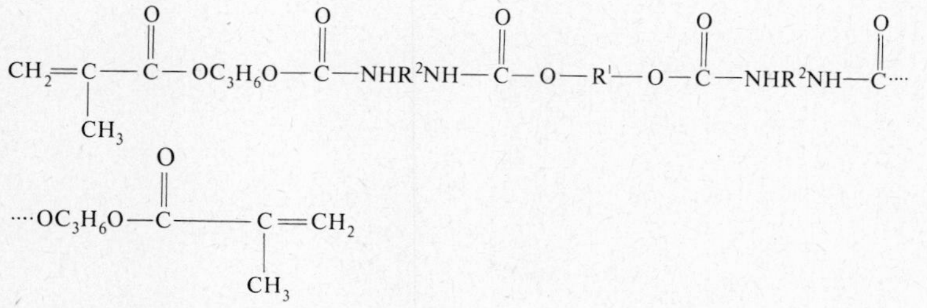

$$CH_2{=}C{-}\overset{\overset{O}{\|}}{C}{-}OC_3H_6O{-}\overset{\overset{O}{\|}}{C}{-}NHR^2NH{-}\overset{\overset{O}{\|}}{C}{-}O{-}R'{-}O{-}\overset{\overset{O}{\|}}{C}{-}NHR^2NH{-}\overset{\overset{O}{\|}}{C}\cdots$$
$$\underset{CH_3}{|}$$

$$\cdots OC_3H_6O{-}\overset{\overset{O}{\|}}{C}{-}{-}C{=}CH_2$$
$$\underset{CH_3}{|}$$

**Fig. 5.11** Urethane dimethacrylate molecule.

## VISIBLE LIGHT-CURED RESINS

The advantages of a single-pack, ultraviolet-light-cured composite system over the two-paste systems have already been discussed. The use of ultraviolet light does have its disadvantages, however, with the potential dangers from the light itself and potential difficulties with depth of cure. This has led to the development of a visible-light-cured system. The composite currently available which utilizes this curing method is, in fact, a urethane dimethacrylate–radiopaque filler composite. The use of the light-curing method instead of the chemical or ultraviolet methods does not influence the choice of resin, however, as these methods are solely involved with the activation of the process by the generation of free radicals. Once these have been formed, the process follows a very specific route, which is then independent of the method of their production.

The real difference, therefore, lies in the catalyst system. In this case an α diketone and an amine are used. These do not interact in the absence of light. However, the ketone absorbs energy in the presence of blue light, with a wavelength in the region of 440–480 nm, transferring to the 'excited' state (Fig. 5.12). This ketone then extracts electrons from the amine to produce two free radicals, one derived from the ketone and one from the amine, and these initiate the polymerization.

A visible light source is supplied with the material. This is cheaper than an ultraviolet-light source and has none of the dangers of ultraviolet light (a filter removes any ultraviolet light from the spectrum).

The shelf-life of this type of composite appears to be very good. In the unopened jar, the α-diketone itself acts as an inhibitor of polymerization provided there is no light. It is only in the presence of high-intensity light of a suitable wavelength that it acts as a catalyst. A shelf-life of two years or so is possible. Care must be taken with opened jars, however, since ordinary daylight can initiate the reactions after prolonged exposure. No obvious deterioration will result if the manufacturer's instructions relating to the use of the material are followed carefully.

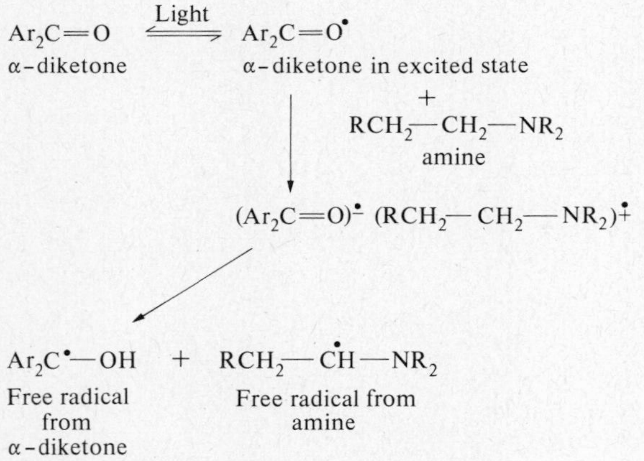

$$Ar_2C{=}O \xrightleftharpoons{\text{Light}} Ar_2C{=}O^{\bullet}$$

α-diketone       α-diketone in excited state

$$+$$
$$RCH_2{-}CH_2{-}NR_2$$
amine

$$(Ar_2C{=}O)^{\underline{\bullet}} \; (RCH_2{-}CH_2{-}NR_2)^{\ddagger}$$

$$Ar_2C^{\bullet}{-}OH \;\; + \;\; RCH_2{-}\overset{\bullet}{C}H{-}NR_2$$

Free radical       Free radical from
from                amine
α-diketone

**Fig. 5.12** Action of catalyst in light-cured resin.

## SCOPE AND APPLICATIONS OF COMPOSITE RESINS

Composites may be used as tooth-coloured restoratives in all the situations previously treatable with silicate cement. However, superior mechanical properties have led to their use in larger cavities where restorations are more susceptible to damage. Anterior restorations involving the incisal edge can be managed satisfactorily with composite resins.

As mentioned earlier, the use of composites in posterior teeth has been suggested. There are a number of short-term practical problems involved, and the durability of such restorations is suspect. It is difficult to condense composites into proximo-occlusal cavities, when a matrix band has been previously placed, without leaving deficiencies in the gingival region. For the most satisfactory results the matrix should completely surround the composite during setting to compress it and aid in its contouring. In posterior teeth this necessitates the use of a conventionally trimmed band with an extra, pre-moulded occlusal portion. Matrix systems made up of two components are difficult to manage and occlusal trimming of the restoration is invariably necessary.

While many composites now contain radiopacifiers, those that do not are difficult to assess radiologically. Thus, overhangs of material and deficiencies at the gingival margin may be difficult to detect by this method and there is no way of recognizing recurrent caries. Most significantly, composites used in the occlusal situation in posterior teeth wear rapidly with a loss of anatomical form. Important features, such as marginal ridges, are gradually lost.

As there is little specific adhesion between the resinous matrix of these materials and tooth substance, it is necessary to ensure adequate mechanical retention for the restoration by appropriate cavity design or perhaps the use of pins. However, the development of the acid-etch technique, discussed below, has led to much improved mechanical adhesion with these restorations.

### Acid-etch technique

If the surface of enamel is treated with an appropriate acid, the mineral phase is differentially etched. In this way an irregular surface is produced, which enhances mechanical adhesion. This technique is now widely applied in clinical practice to assist in the retention of restorations and to improve the seal between them and the tooth.

Different acid formulations have been used, but 50 per cent phosphoric acid is typical. Applied to the previously polished enamel surface it results in the formation of many small channels into the tissue. Etching is usually carried out for one minute. Ideally the enamel prisms are dissolved leaving the inter-prismatic substance intact (Fig. 5.13a and b). The resulting channels are about 5 $\mu$m across and extend from 25–50 $\mu$m into the enamel. Under different conditions etching may be confined to the inter-prismatic substance leaving the prisms (Fig. 5.13c), and on occasions both components of the enamel are attacked to the same extent (Fig. 5.13d). This last feature is usually observed when the duration of etching has been unduly prolonged and clearly nothing is gained by such a result. Several factors influence the etching pattern achieved, including the orientation of the enamel prisms in relation to the surface, the concentration of acid, and the duration of its application.

From the previous paragraph there would not appear to be any point in etching the walls of many conventional cavities, as these involve the longitudinal sectioning of the prisms. This supposition is confirmed by the occurrence of microleakage adjacent to fillings in cavities treated in this way.

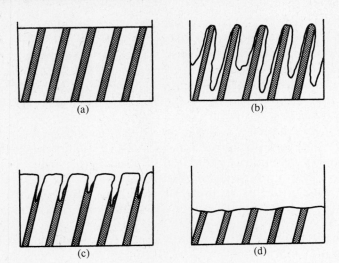

**Fig. 5.13** (a) Unetched enamel surface; (b) etching of prisms; (c) etching of inter-prismatic substance; (d) etching of both prisms and inter-prismatic substance.

Orientation of the enamel prisms is therefore an important consideration in the clinical application of the acid-etch technique.

Having established channels in the enamel, it is clearly important to ensure their effective filling with extensions of the resin, which will then display a series of protruding tags. To ensure that this occurs, several presentations provide a low-viscosity resin, similar in nature to the composite matrix, but devoid of filler particles. In the majority of products the filler particles would be too large to enter the etched channels and might even obstruct their penetration by the matrix. Low-viscosity intermediate resins form a layer that extends into the channels and unites chemically with the matrix of the overlying composite (Fig. 5.14a).

It has been suggested that these intermediate resins may be unnecessary, since the resin from the composite paste does, in fact, fill the channels, leaving the filler particles in the main bulk adjacent to the etched surface (Fig. 5.14b). In this situation the bond strength, which may be as high as 31 MN/m$^2$, is the same as that observed when an intermediate has been used. There is some concern, however, that the durability of the bond may be reduced if the low-viscosity intermediate is omitted. The bond strength is so good that failure is likely to be cohesive in either the composite or the enamel.

MECHANISM OF ADHESION

Several factors may contribute towards the adhesion of acid-etch composites. It is broadly accepted, however, that the mechanical locking of the resin tags into the etched enamel is the most important. The surface area of contact

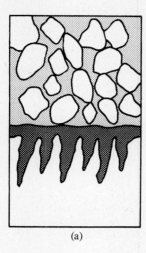
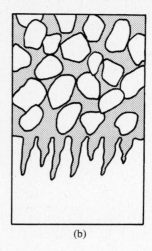

(a)                                    (b)

**Fig. 5.14** (a) Use of intermediate resin with composite on acid-etched enamel; (b) composite without intermediate resin.

between the resin and the tooth is greatly increased as will be appreciated from Figure 5.13. Acid also helps to debride the surface and may expose more reactive tissue with which some slight specific adhesion can occur. Improved wettability of the surface, by encouraging good interfacial contact, could enhance this effect.

APPLICATIONS OF THE ACID-ETCH TECHNIQUE

The first popular application of the acid-etch technique was in fissure sealing, and this is described in detail in Chapter 13. Here the potential for good retention was recognized and developed into a system for the restoration of fractured anterior teeth. The fractured surface in these situations, however, rarely offers an end-on view of the enamel prisms and it is necessary to utilize the adjacent enamel surface for etching. This means that a thin flash of restorative material must be placed beyond the fractured margins and may make the tooth slightly bulbous (Fig. 5.15a). Restorations of this kind are, nevertheless, very successful from a retention point of view, and cases have been reported where a second blow has led to a fracture of the tooth close to the original one, the interface between the restoration and tooth remaining intact. In the management of young children the technique has the obvious advantage of not requiring any tooth preparation. Some operators, however, suggest a shallow reduction of the enamel to prevent subsequent over-contouring by the restoration (Fig. 5.15b). This reduction is called a half-enamel preparation.

Any factors improving the adhesion between a restoration and the tooth will tend to reduce microleakage between the two. For this reason acid-etch

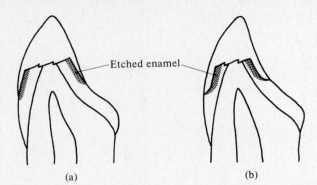

**Fig. 5.15** (a) Cross-section through acid-etched fractured incisor restoration showing a thin flash beyond the fractured margin; (b) half enamel preparation.

techniques have been recommended prior to the placement of otherwise conventional composite fillings. The problems of prism orientation in these circumstances have already been mentioned. Improvements in marginal seal may be achieved if some adjacent surface enamel is involved as in the restoration of the fractured tooth. Again, some restorative material must be placed beyond the cavity margin, and this is generally considered undesirable. Two successful methods of reducing microleakage between a composite restoration and its cavity using a low viscosity resin are shown in Figure 5.16. The coverage of the entire surface of composite restorations with low viscosity resins has been suggested as a way to improve the surface finish. It is likely, however, that this superficial layer would be rapidly lost by abrasion.

Several miscellaneous uses have been found for acid-etch composite techniques. These include splinting teeth, fabrication of long-term temporary bridges, alteration of tooth morphology for prosthetic purposes, and the attachment of orthodontic appliances. The management of cervical abrasion and erosion cavities is limited by the fact that these are primarily in dentine, which does not respond as effectively to the technique as enamel.

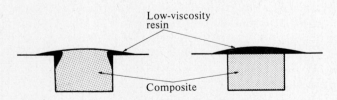

**Fig. 5.16** Use of low-viscosity resin to reduce microleakage.

## SELECTION OF LINING MATERIALS FOR USE WITH COMPOSITES

Most manufacturers recommend the use of a lining material beneath composite resins. There is potential chemical irritation from free monomers and other constituents before polymerization, and in some products there is an appreciable rise in temperature during this process. However, the evidence suggests that these materials are not as irritant as silicate cement and it may be clinically expedient not to line a very shallow cavity rather than prejudice retention and aesthetics by so doing.

Lining materials containing essential oils would plasticize resins and are therefore incompatible with composites. Zinc oxide/eugenol and its modifications, including EBA cements, should not be used. Indeed, it is a generalization that zinc oxide/eugenol should not be used under any tooth-coloured filling material. All the other lining materials are compatible with composites but the two-paste calcium hydroxide presentations are undoubtedly the most convenient. While they are weak, they do not have to withstand high compressive stresses on insertion of the restoration. It has been suggested that calcium hydroxide preparations containing chloroform should not be used under composites based on acrylic resin, as the former dissolves the latter. As so few composites are now based on acrylic resin this is not a major problem. Indeed, it is unlikely that the amount of free chloroform available when the lining has set is great enough to have any appreciable effect.

# 6

# Impression materials

The preparation of a model or cast of the patient's mouth or dentition is an essential part of the construction of many dental restorations and prostheses. In order to achieve this, a mould or impression of the mouth is made using an appropriate material. This is called an impression material, which on insertion into the mouth is in a fluid state and is usually supported in a tray. In the mouth it hardens, normally by means of a chemical reaction, but sometimes because of a change in temperature. After it has set, the impression is removed and a model prepared by casting or pouring into it a suitable material, the nature of which will depend on the particular procedure being undertaken. Models produced in this way are used in the preparation of tooth restorations, dentures, splints, and orthodonic appliances. In addition, it is often useful to have study models as an aid to case assessment and treatment planning.

### Requirements of impression materials

Precision technical procedures involving the use of a model of the mouth and dentition demand great accuracy. This may only be achieved in the technician's working model if the impression material produces correspondingly accurate results. Accuracy may be considered under the two headings of surface reproducibility and dimensional stability. The former relates to the degree of detail recorded by the material and is largely a function of its viscosity. The need to reproduce fine surface detail varies with the procedure. Impressions of teeth prepared to receive inlays or crowns require greater accuracy in this respect than those of the edentulous jaws for which full dentures are to be constructed. Different types of impression material have different capacities to reproduce detail, and an appropriate material is chosen for the particular task in hand.

An impression material with good dimensional stability is one which maintains its size and shape for an extended period. In practical terms an impression material with good dimensional stability can be stored for 24–48 hours with minimal distortion. It is desirable that there should be little or no change in dimension until the impression is poured in, whatever model material is to be used. Clearly if an impression is to be dispatched to a laboratory some distance away, days may elapse before the model is made. If, however, the impression may be poured in the surgery, dimensional stability may be slightly less critical. When considering dimensional stability it is often considered that the time following the removal of the impression from the mouth is the most important. However, dimensional changes occurring in the mouth while the material hardens or sets are of obvious importance and it is desirable that changes in dimension occurring at this time should be minimal.

Problems of dimensional stability may be associated with the setting reaction of the material, changes in temperature and humidity, and the loss or gain of substances by the final impression. Changes in the impression consequent upon the degree of elasticity of the material and its particular clinical application will be discussed in the appropriate sections that follow.

Ideally an impression material should have sufficient elasticity to allow its removal from undercut areas without any permanent distortion. The impression material may engage undercut in many regions of a patient's mouth, particularly around the gingival half of the crowns of the teeth. If a material of sufficiently low viscosity is used it will flow interdentally to record the narrow spaces between the teeth. On removal of the impression these narrow strips of material tend to tear. The impression material needs to be of the right strength to rupture at one point only, allowing it to be removed from the mouth without leaving any fragments behind.

For the convenience of both patient and dentist, impression materials should harden or set rapidly after application to the mouth. However, it is also necessary to have an adequate working time to allow mixing, loading into an impression tray, and insertion into the mouth. During this last procedure the material must be of sufficiently low viscosity to allow its close adaptation to the tissues. Some impression techniques in conservative dentistry are more complex, and additional working time is useful to permit their completion before the material sets. These two ideals are, of course, generally contradictory and a compromise is usually accepted. In addition to the time factor, patient acceptability is also increased by a pleasant taste and smell and the capacity to use the material in minimal bulk.

Impression materials must be compatible with the model materials that are to be poured into them, not interfering with their setting reaction or final physical properties, and not reacting with them. The impression should be easily removed from the final model. For some technical procedures it is desirable to increase the surface hardness of the resultant model by electroplating the impression, for example with silver or copper, before pouring it. In these cases an impression material must be selected that can be treated in this way.

As impression materials come into contact with extensive areas of oral mucosa it is important that they are neither toxic nor irritant, and indeed most currently used materials satisfy this requirement. Some patients, however, appear to be hypersensitive or allergic to some types of impression materials, and clearly these materials should be avoided in these particular cases.

Finally it is advantageous to use materials that are cheap, easy to use and that have a long shelf-life. Impression materials in use at the present time vary widely on all these counts as will become apparent in the sections that follow.

## Classification of impression materials

Although impression materials may be classified in several different ways, the distinction between elastic and non-elastic materials is most frequently used as the basis, as shown in Table 6.1.

**Table 6.1.** Classification of impression materials

| Non-elastic | Elastic |
|---|---|
| Plaster of Paris | Hydrocolloids |
| Composition | — irreversible |
| Zinc oxide/eugenol | — reversible |
| Waxes | Synthetic elastomers |
|  | — silicone |
|  | — polysulphide |
|  | — polyether |

## NON-ELASTIC IMPRESSION MATERIALS

By definition non-elastic impression materials set to a rigid consistency displaying little or no elasticity. If such a material engages undercuts, perhaps in the gingival region around the necks of teeth, it is impossible to remove the impression without it distorting or fracturing. This property severely limits the scope of these materials and they are most commonly used to take impressions of edentulous mouths prior to the construction of full dentures. Even in this situation severe hard and soft tissue undercut may make removal of the impression difficult. Usually, however, the soft tissues may be displaced to allow the removal of the impression.

### Plaster of Paris

COMPOSITION AND SETTING REACTION

The chemical and physical properties of plaster of Paris are described in Chapter 7. Plaster for impression purposes is based on calcined calcium sulphate hemihydrate, which reacts with water to form a hard mass of calcium sulphate dihydrate. This reaction is normally associated with expansion of about 0·3 per cent, but it may be as much as 0·6 per cent. While these values may not appear to be high, expansion of this order in material confined within a rigid impression tray may lead to distortion of the impression with a significant reduction in accuracy.

The addition of salts, such as potassium sulphate, in concentrations of about 4 per cent, reduces expansion to about 0·05 per cent. Potassium sulphate, however, accelerates the setting reaction to an unacceptable degree and retarders must be added. Borax is commonly used and its concentration varies, depending on the desired rate of reaction, from 0·4 to 1·0 per cent.

Impression plasters usually contain a pigment, such as alizarin red, which may be present to about 0·04 per cent to impart a pink colour to the mixed material. This makes it easier to distinguish between the impression and the model produced from it. The constituents of a typical impression plaster are given in Table 6.2.

**Table 6.2** Constituents of a typical impression plaster

Calcium sulphate hemihydrate
Potassium sulphate
Borax
Alizarin red

Other additives may be present, such as gum tragacanth, zinc oxide, or polyvinyl acetate, which are used to improve the cohesion of the mixed material, flavouring, and starch. When plaster containing starch is placed in boiling water the starch swells and the impression disintegrates making removal from the hardened model easier. Presentations of this kind may be referred to as 'soluble' plaster.

The additives may be included in the plaster powder, which is mixed with water, or they may be presented in aqueous solution which is added to the pure plaster at the time of mixing. Such solutions are referred to as 'anti-expansion', or AE, solutions and they may be graded depending on their concentration of borax and thus the setting time they exhibit when mixed. Proportioning is important as deviations from the manufacturer's directions will affect the consistency of the mix, the rate of reaction, and the strength of the set material. A typical mix would be 100 g of powder to 50–60 ml of water or AE solution. After a 30–40 second mixing time a low viscosity consistency results which has adequate working time and a relatively well defined hardening point after 2–3 minutes.

PROPERTIES

The dimensional stability of plaster is good provided extreme drying of the impression is avoided. If this occurs differential loss of water leads to distortion. When mixed as described above, the low viscosity consistency results in an impression with good surface reproduction, and the displacement of soft tissues is minimal. The thin mix produces an impression with low strength, as does the presence of potassium sulphate. In view of the lack of elasticity of plaster this is desirable as impressions engaging undercut must be fractured for removal and reassembled subsequently. The compressive strength of impression plaster is 2–5 $MN/m^2$ and, if correctly mixed, the resulting fracture is clean.

To prevent bonding between a plaster impression and the model material poured into it a separating medium is required. Many different agents have been employed, including alginate mould seals, varnishes, soap solutions, and liquid paraffin. The use of some of these may lead to a slight reduction in surface detail. Plaster is a relatively cheap material and has a good shelf-life provided it is stored in a dry, airtight container.

APPLICATIONS

With the advent of satisfactory elastic materials plaster has undergone a reduction in popularity. Its principal use is in the impression of edentulous mouths where undercut problems are least severe. Plaster may be used to correct or perfect a basic impression in a material, such as composition, with poor surface reproducibility. Here the plaster is applied to the fitting surface of the first impression, which is then returned to the mouth to produce a wash impression. However, if the underlying impression distorts, the plaster will fracture, and it is recommended that impressions made in this way are poured early. For patients, the drying of the mouth experienced and the heat evolved during the setting reaction are unpleasant.

In bridgework separate components of the bridge seated on the prepared teeth may be temporarily united or located in the mouth by means of a small plaster impression using a tongue spatula to support it. The relationship of the components, one to another, is maintained accurately on removal from the mouth. Following investment and removal of the plaster the restorations may be soldered together. Impressions used in this way are referred to as locating impressions. There is a danger with this technique that water absorbed by the spatula may result in its distortion, which can crack the impression.

## Impression compound

Impression compound, often referred to as composition and occasionally abbreviated to 'compo', is a thermoplastic material. On warming, it becomes semi-fluid and is placed in the mouth to record the impression. Hardening occurs on cooling to mouth temperature and the impression is removed. This process does not involve a chemical reaction.

CONSTITUENTS

A wide range of substances has been included in impression compounds and manufacturers rarely disclose the precise contents of their products. However, constituents fall into three main categories—thermoplastic materials, lubricants, and fillers.

The principal thermoplastic components are generally combinations of waxes and resins. In earlier products substances such as beeswax, paraffin wax, carnauba wax, gutta percha, shellac, and Kauri resin were employed in addition to stearin and stearic acid as lubricants or softeners. Impression compound based on beeswax is brittle, and shellac and gutta percha are added as plasticizers. The combination of stearin and Kauri resin leads to the latter being plasticized excessively by the former and fillers are added to counteract this. In more recent preparations commercial stearic acid has replaced stearin. This is a mixture of stearic, palmitic, and oleic acids, which can be pro-portioned in a controlled fashion. Oleic acid lowers the strength and the softening temperature while palmitic acid acts as a hardener. Stearic acid is a plasticizer and aids in the dispersion of the filler. There has been a tendency to replace the natural resins with synthetic ones, such as the cummerone indene type, which may be prepared more readily and are more predictable in their behaviour.

Fillers are added to improve the consistency of the compound, reduce flow and improve its strength. Commonly used fillers are French chalk, talc, and pumice. Softeners or lubricants such as stearin, stearic acid, and glycerine provide a good working consistency at temperatures compatible with use in the mouth. Finally, manufacturers usually include a colouring agent to distinguish between different varieties of preparation.

SOFTENING TEMPERATURE

Impression compounds may be broadly classified into two groups depending on their softening temperature. The most widely used group has a relatively low fusion temperature and is used to achieve impressions of the mouth in the conventional sense. There is, however, a group of products with a higher softening temperature that may be used to form or modify an impression tray for use with another impression material such as zinc oxide/eugenol paste or plaster of Paris. These materials are harder and more rigid at mouth temperature to impart greater stability to the final impression. The former group soften at temperatures between 55 and 65 °C while with the latter materials the softening temperature approaches and may exceed 70 °C.

It is important that impression compound should be sufficiently fluid to record the impression at a temperature that will not cause damage to the tissues or discomfort to the patient. In the case of an impression of the prepared tooth, thermal trauma to the pulp could occur. At the same time the material should be rigid at mouth temperature, exhibiting minimal flow, in order to prevent distortion of the impression on its removal.

Figure 6.1 shows a cooling curve for impression compound. While a horizontal zone can be seen, the transition temperature is not clearly defined as the different constituents behave differently. The horizontal portion prob-ably represents the point at which the crystalline components solidify. Below this temperature the material does not flow sufficiently to record surface detail adequately. However, hardening is not complete until the temperature approximates that of the mouth as the non-crystalline constituents solidify at lower temperatures. It is important, therefore, to ensure that the material is heated above the apparent transition temperature while the impression is taken but also to ensure that it is cooled well below it before the impression is disturbed or removed.

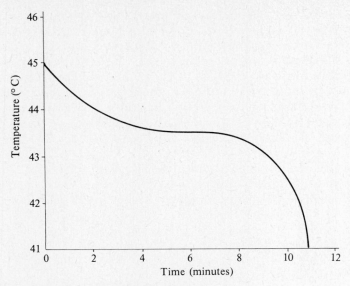

**Fig. 6.1** Cooling curve for impression compound.

THERMAL PROPERTIES

Impression compound has a high coefficient of expansion, which may result in a contraction of up to 0·3 per cent when removed from mouth to room temperature. Error induced in an impression of the edentulous jaw in this way can lead to significant distortion of the impression. This problem may be partially overcome by reheating the surface of the impression and reseating it in the mouth. In this way part of the contraction error is corrected and the thickness of the composition involved in the reheating process is so small that the error similarly produced at this stage is very slight in absolute terms. On the same basis the use of a small bulk of impression compound in thin section minimizes the overall error.

The thermal conductivity of impression compound is low and therefore care must be taken to ensure uniform heating throughout the entire mass. If this is not achieved softening will not be consistent and internal stresses will arise within the impression, which may subsequently lead to distortion.

DIMENSIONAL STABILITY

Impression compound has relatively poor dimensional stability and impressions made in this material tend to distort if left for prolonged periods. It is essential to minimize internal stresses, as stated above, by warming the material throughout to a temperature above the transition temperature of the higher softening point constituents. The impression must be supported lightly during the period of hardening until a temperature closely approximating that of the mouth is achieved. Above this temperature composition still has the tendency to flow, and distortion may result if an attempt is made to remove the impression.

As impression compound is a non-elastic material it will distort if removed from undercut areas, and the greater the flow the greater will be distortion in such situations. The flow should be at least 85 per cent at 45 °C but not more than 6 per cent at 37 °C (Fig. 6.2). As composition impressions always tend to distort it is advisable to pour the models soon after they have been taken.

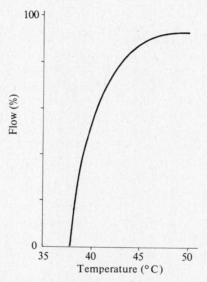

**Fig. 6.2** Effect of temperature on the flow of impression compound.

SOFTENING

Impression compound may be softened by dry heat over a flame or by immersion in warm water. When small amounts are being used, as in the copper ring impression of a single tooth, the material can be adequately softened throughout over a flame. It is important, however, not to overheat the compound as the more volatile constituents may be lost and extremely hot material may damage the pulp. In addition, overheating may lead to the impression sticking to the tooth. To ensure this does not happen, even at the correct temperature, a thin film of a separating medium on the tooth should be used. Teepol or saliva are satisfactory for this purpose.

The larger bulk of material employed for denture impressions is not heated uniformly or efficiently over a flame and is best softened by immersion in a warm water bath at 50–60 °C. Such a bath should be lined with a dental napkin to prevent the composition adhering to its walls. When the material is removed from the bath, water on its surface is generally incorporated as it is kneaded before placement in the impression tray. Water plasticizes impression compound and increases its flow. While this may improve surface reproducibility it will also increase the chances of distortion on removal of the impression. Generally a certain degree of plasticizing in this way is desirable to achieve optimal handling conditions. Compound that has been in water for a prolonged period may be severely affected and should be discarded. In this situation there will also be a loss of soluble constituents, which may lead to altered properties.

APPLICATIONS

Impression compound is most widely used in the preparation of impressions for full dentures. The surface reproducibility is not as good as other materials and its relatively high viscosity tends to allow the displacement of soft tissues to produce what may be described as a muco-compressive impression. Many operators perfect such impressions with a corrective impression material, while some produce a model from the impression on which a special tray is made. This can be used subsequently to take a second impression using a more appropriate material.

Composition presented in stick form is used to modify the periphery of an impression tray for use with other materials. The viscosity that is displayed makes it suitable to carry out muscle trimming. Such products are often referred to as tracing stick. In this and other situations it may become necessary to trim composition with a sharp knife, and a good quality product should allow this without fragmenting.

In conservative dentistry, composition in the form of sticks or small cones may be used to take an impression of a single prepared tooth. For this purpose the material is supported in a hard copper band trimmed in such a way as to minimize the involvement of undercuts. It is important that, after thorough cooling, the band is carefully removed along the path of insertion of the proposed restoration in order to avoid deformation. An advantage of using this material and technique is that the resultant impression may be readily electroplated, usually with copper, to produce an individual tooth model with high surface hardness. This model is referred to as a die. Even if this capability is not utilized, composition is compatible with all model and die materials likely to be used.

The use of composition as a tray-forming material has already been described.

Impression compound is non-irritant and non-toxic if used within the recommended temperature range and it has a good shelf-life. Presentations containing shellac may undergo some deterioration if stored for over 4–5 years. Although composition for full mouth impressions can be reused, gradual deterioration takes place. Constituents are leached out, water plasticizes the material to excess and, as sterilization cannot be carried out conveniently, many operators discard impression compound after it has been used once.

### Zinc oxide/eugenol impression paste

The reaction between zinc oxide and eugenol is described in Chapter 3. The basic constituents may both be presented in paste form which, when mixed together, set to a hard non-elastic mass. Setting is by a chemical reaction, although some products are thermoplastic to a limited extent.

CONSTITUENTS

The base contains zinc oxide made into a paste by the addition of inert oils and others such as olive oil, linseed oil, and light mineral oils. Those in the latter group act as plasticizers and, if not present in the base, are generally included in the reactor paste. Hydrogenated rosin accelerates the set, improves cohesion of the final material, and imparts a degree of thermoplasticity. This last property aids the removal of the impression from the hardened model. Other gums, rosins, and waxes have been used to produce similar effects. Eugenol, often present in the form of oil of cloves, which contains 70–85 per cent eugenol, is the principal regent in the reactor paste. In addition accelerators including zinc acetate and sulphate and magnesium acetate and chloride are included (Table 6.3).

**Table 6.3** Constituents of a typical zinc oxide/eugenol impression paste

| Base paste | Reactor paste |
| --- | --- |
| Zinc oxide | Eugenol |
| Inert oils | Zinc acetate |
| Hydrogenated rosin | Fillers |

SETTING TIME

The setting time of impression pastes is of obvious importance. The set must be sufficiently delayed to allow time for mixing, placement in the impression tray, and seating in the mouth with muscle trimming if necessary. After this time the material should harden rapidly to minimize the duration of the impression and the chances of disturbing the tray. Movement of the tray as the paste hardens will lead to a deformed, inaccurate impression. Usually 3–5 minutes is a convenient order of time for the setting reaction.

Products vary considerably in their setting time and therefore in their suitability for the dentist's requirements. The setting reaction may be accelerated by the addition of specific chemicals, such as zinc acetate or water, and slowed by the inclusion of inert oils. In general, however, these practices are inadvisable as lack of uniform distribution of the additives may occur. A degree of variation may be achieved by altering the proportion of the two pastes before mixing. It is clearly necessary to determine which of the pastes contains the accelerators before this can be done. Proportioning should not be varied too far beyond the manufacturer's directions as alterations will occur in the physical properties of the mix and final set. It is probably safer for a dentist to select a product with a setting time suited to his requirements and personal preference, rather than to attempt to adjust an unsuitable presentation. The increased temperature and humidity in the mouth increase the rate of setting of zinc oxide/eugenol impression pastes. Altered atmospheric conditions in the surgery may bring about a similar result.

ACCURACY

The surface reproducibility of these materials depends on the viscosity and flow of the mixed paste, and presentations vary considerably. Low viscosity products reproduce details well with minimal displacement of soft tissue. However, as they are used in thin section, usually of 1–2 mm, some tissue displacement is inevitable as pressure is transmitted from the impression tray. Pastes that have high viscosity when mixed displace tissues to a greater degree and record less detail. In addition, some products have a tendency to adhere to dental stones. Small amounts of material, by remaining on the surface of the model, will bring about a corresponding loss of detail.

Dimensional stability of these pastes is good. A shrinkage of about 0·1 per cent may occur in the first 30 minutes after mixing but thereafter there is no appreciable change in dimension. It should be remembered, however, that if the underlying tray or basic impression is unstable, distortion will be reflected in the paste impression.

Products set to varying degrees of hardness, some undergoing a distinctive change, giving a brittle material, others merely undergoing a progressive increase in viscosity. All are essentially non-elastic and may not be removed from all but the smallest of undercuts without fracture and distortion occurring.

HANDLING AND APPLICATIONS

The base and reactor pastes are usually presented in contrasting colours and are constituted in such a way that strips of equal length, mixed to a uniform colour, produce the optimal mix. This is most conveniently carried out on a paper pad, as glass slabs are difficult to clean. Indeed the material adheres effectively to any dry surfaces including impression trays and skin. It is advisable to protect the skin around the patient's lips with petroleum jelly to prevent this occurring, and special solvents are available.

Surface imperfections in a zinc oxide/eugenol impression may be corrected by making an addition of freshly mixed material and returning the impression to the mouth. This can be done, in the majority of cases, without detriment to accuracy. With the possible exception of adhesion in rare instances, the impressions are compatible with dental stones and plaster which are the model materials likely to be used, and removal is aided by warming the impression in water to 60–65 °C when some softening occurs. The shelf-life of zinc oxide impression pastes is good.

As with other non-elastic impression materials the most suitable application is in making impressions of the edentulous jaws. Ideally these are taken in closely adapted special trays constructed for the purpose. Used correctly, the paste can be applied to a composition impression to achieve an apparently similar result. However, distortion of the composition will always put the accuracy of the completed impression at risk. Zinc oxide/eugenol is valuable in achieving a corrective impression in the patient's dentures prior to their being relined. While these pastes have been used in crown and bridgework to register the occlusion and to relocate separated components they generally lack the strength and rigidity desired in these situations.

NON-EUGENOL PRODUCTS

A number of patients experience discomfort in the form of a burning or tingling sensation during an impression with zinc oxide/eugenol pastes. This tendency is reduced in most presentations by the use of oil of cloves rather than pure eugenol, and the effect is masked to some extent by the presence of other oils. There are also some patients, and indeed some dentists, who display a true allergy to eugenol. In these cases preparations devoid of eugenol may be used. There is not a wide choice, and such materials are based on the reaction between a carboxylic acid, such as $o$-ethoxybenzoic acid, and zinc hydroxide resulting from the hydrolysis of the zinc oxide which leads to the production of an insoluble 'soap'.

## Impression waxes

Waxes possessing a range of softening temperature may be used singly or in combination to achieve a corrective impression. These products are generally a combination of low fusing waxes and synthetic resins, and as they cool to mouth temperature their flow decreases. However, at mouth temperature they continue to flow to a greater or lesser extent, up to as much as 80 per cent. As with impression compound, there is no chemical setting reaction.

Advantage may be taken of the continual flow to achieve a functional impression. Here an attempt is made to compress or displace soft tissues to a similar degree to that expected during the application of occlusal forces via the denture. This is achieved during a relining process by allowing the patient to occlude on the dentures which carry the impression wax on their fitting surfaces. The result may be enhanced by using a wax with a relatively higher softening point that flows less at mouth temperature.

Impression waxes have a high coefficient of expansion and therefore a proportionately high degree of contraction occurs on removal from the mouth. In absolute terms, however, the error induced in this way is small as the material tends to be used in thin layers. Softening of the wax is most effectively achieved by storing the materials in containers, the temperature of which is thermostatically controlled. Here the wax remains in liquid form ready for use, and when required it is painted on to the fitting surface of the denture. Removal of the impression must be undertaken with care as distortion will readily occur at mouth temperature. The involvement of undercuts will clearly lead to a distorted impression. If immediate pouring is not possible, the impression should be stored at a low temperature, preferably near 0 °C, to minimize distortion.

The principal application of impression waxes is in the relining of dentures, and they are particularly useful in correcting the tissue fitting surface of lower free-end saddle dentures. In this situation, following a corrective impression, the denture may be relined prior to its initial fitting. With the development of a wide range of synthetic elastomeric impression materials with great variation in viscosity it is possible to achieve a muco-compressive impression in the first instance. This has led to the less frequent use of impression waxes. Nevertheless, waxes are still useful in patients unable to tolerate conventional impressions.

## ELASTIC IMPRESSION MATERIALS

Elastic impression materials have the capacity to be withdrawn from undercuts with minimal permanent deformation. While it would be ideal for no permanent distortion to occur, this is not achieved in the materials presently available. Therefore, an important factor in the comparison of products is the degree of permanent deformation that results. This is usually expressed as a percentage of the total deformation that occurs on removal from the undercut, and the lower the value the better. The effect of permanent deformation on accuracy will depend on the degree of undercut involved and the bulk of material used when taking the impression.

A process of elastic recoil or recovery brings about a return to the original shape after the impression has been removed from undercut. This does not occur immediately but takes a varying period of time and the longer the impression is left the more complete elastic recovery will be. However, other factors are generally influencing the dimensional stability of the impression and an optimal time should be selected to pour the impression. In practice there is a period in which pouring the model will result in acceptable reproduction, but this varies in duration depending on the material used.

It should be possible with a completely elastic impression material to pour a series of dimensionally identical models from one impression, allowing a period of elastic recovery to occur after each removal. With a degree of permanent deformation occurring, however, the models would become progressively inaccurate. Nevertheless, some impression materials will allow two models to be produced with acceptable results. This capacity is useful in certain disciplines, such as bridgework, where a second reference model is helpful.

By definition, an elastic impression material has to transform from a fluid state to a highly elastic solid state under the conditions of the oral environment. Consideration of the structure of fluids and elastic solids, as outlined in Chapter 1, will show that this is not easily achieved, because their characteristics are quite different. A fluid consists of molecules which have very little affinity for one another and are free to move about. A highly elastic solid, on the other hand, must have strong inter-atomic bonds but with a molecular geometry and just the right number and type of inter-molecular bonds to allow large elastic displacements, a structure typified by the coiled molecular arrangement in elastomeric solids. The process of transforming a fluid into a highly elastic solid must therefore be one of establishing the desired type of inter-molecular bond and it is this that is involved in the setting reaction of an elastic impression material (Fig. 6.3). The most significant limitation is that this process has to occur within a suitable time range under the imposed conditions of temperature, pH, and so on. In practice two systems are used. The first involves a change, at mouth temperature in the characteristics of colloids where bonds are established between the individual components of the dispersed phase. The second involves elastomeric polymers where the setting reaction produces an optimal amount of cross-linking between the molecules.

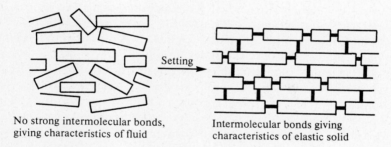

No strong intermolecular bonds, giving characteristics of fluid

Setting

Intermolecular bonds giving characteristics of elastic solid

**Fig. 6.3** Cross-linking and rearrangement of structural units during the setting of an elastomeric impression material.

## Hydrocolloids

### THE COLLOIDAL STATE

A colloid is a two-phase system in which one substance, usually a solid, is dispersed in another, usually a liquid, but where the two phases are microscopically indistinguishable. This colloidal state can be considered as a compromise between a solution and a suspension. In a solution, solute particles of small molecular or ionic dimensions have a mutual attraction for those of the solvent, they are free to move throughout the solution and are uniformly distributed in it. A suspension consists of larger particles that may be detected with the microscope, or even with the naked eye, dispersed in a medium. Unlike the solution, which has only one phase, the suspension is a two-phase system.

In the colloid, molecules or aggregates of molecules, known as the dispersed phase, are present in a dispersion medium. If the dispersion medium is water the material is called a hydrocolloid. The particles are larger than those in solutions and range from 1–200 nm. The distinction between colloids, solutions, and suspensions is often unclear and there may appear to be a degree of overlap.

Colloids with a liquid as the dispersion medium can exist in two different forms, known as 'sol' and 'gel'. A sol has the appearance and most of the characteristics of a viscous liquid. A gel, on the other hand, is a semi-solid, and is produced from a sol during the process of gelation by the formation of fibrils of the dispersed phase which become interlocked to give the characteristic 'jelly-like' consistency. Most of the dispersion medium is held between the fibrils by capillary forces.

The transformation from the sol to gel state, known as gelation, may be brought about in one of two ways. Lowering the temperature, by reducing the thermal energy of the molecules, allows inter-molecular forces of attraction to operate more effectively. These are secondary valence forces and probably result from dipole interaction (Chapter 2). Such a change may be reversed by raising the temperature when liquefaction recurs. The liquefaction temperature is considerably higher than the gelation temperature and this property is known as hysteresis. Gelation may also be induced by a chemical reaction. Here the dispersed phase of a sol is allowed to react with a substance to give a different type of dispersed phase, the characteristics of which result in a gel structure rather than a sol. The process is not reversed by an increase in temperature. These two mechanisms form the basis of the reversible and irreversible hydrocolloid impression materials. Impressions in such materials are inserted in the mouth in the sol state and are removed after gelation has occurred.

The strength of a gel depends on the concentration or density of the fibrillar structure and the concentration of any inert fillers that may have been added. Filler particles become trapped in the fibrillar network and their size, shape, and density are important in determining their effectiveness. The addition of fillers also leads to an increase in the viscosity of the sol. In reversible hydrocolloids, the lower the temperature the greater the strength, as gelation is more complete.

As hydrocolloids are based on water as the dispersion medium they are prone to dimensional change resulting from its loss or gain. If left in a dry atmosphere, water is lost by evaporation, and if the material is immersed in water, any such loss is recouped by a process known as imbibition. The reversible hydrocolloids do not imbibe more than their original content following loss by evaporation, but the process is probably associated with some distortion and must, therefore, be considered undesirable in a material used for impression purposes. The irreversible materials, however, continue to imbibe water beyond this point, which results in swelling and distortion. In addition, moisture may be lost by a process of exudation known as syneresis, which also involves the loss of some of the more soluble constituents. Syneresis results in the formation of small droplets of exudate on the surface of the hydrocolloid and the process occurs irrespective of the humidity of the surrounding atmosphere. Moisture loss by evaporation and syneresis is less in hydrocolloids containing a high concentration of dispersed phase.

Hydrocolloids for dental use may be reversible or irreversible, but as the latter are more widely used they will be considered first.

## Irreversible hydrocolloids—alginates

Irreversible hydrocolloid impression materials are presented as a powder. When mixed with water a viscous sol is produced, which is placed in the mouth in a suitable tray. After a delay, which varies from product to product, an elastic gel forms and the impression may be removed. The main constituents of these materials are salts of alginic acid, which is derived from seaweed, and they are therefore referred to as alginates.

### CONSTITUENTS

The principal reagent is a soluble salt of alginic acid such as sodium, potassium, or ammonium alginate. Sodium alginate is perhaps the most frequently used and is present in the powder to about 12 per cent. This reacts with calcium ions to produce insoluble calcium alginate. The source of these ions is calcium sulphate, which is also present to about 12 per cent. To prevent immediate gelation on mixing with water, a retarder is present. Various salts are used, including sodium and trisodium phosphate. These react preferentially with calcium sulphate according to the equation

$$2Na_nAlg + nCaSO_4 \longrightarrow nNa_2SO_4 + Ca_nAlg_2$$

Therefore calcium ions are not available to react with the sodium alginate until the retarder has been exhausted. A concentration of 2 per cent trisodium phosphate results in a delay which gives the clinician adequate working time. Calcium sulphate is used as a source of calcium ions because it is only sparingly soluble and liberates the ions slowly. A more soluble salt, such as calcium chloride, would lead to almost immediate and uncontrolled gelation.

To improve the cohesion and reduce the tackiness of the mix, a high proportion (up to 70 per cent) of an inert filler is present. Diatomaceous earth is used in this way. Diatomaceous earth consists of the siliceous remains of small aquatic plants called diatoms. As will be explained later some alginates have a detrimental effect on the surface hardness of dental stone models, and most modern alginates contain a small amount of model hardener. Fluorides and silico-fluorides are used in this role. In addition, most products contain colouring and flavouring agents. Table 6.4 lists the constituents of a typical alginate impression material.

**Table 6.4** Constituents of a typical alginate impression material

Sodium alginate
Calcium sulphate
Trisodium phosphate
Filler
Model hardener
Colouring and flavouring

SETTING REACTION AND GEL STRUCTURE

On mixing the powder with water a hydrocolloid sol is produced which commences to gel when no retarder is left to react with calcium sulphate. Gelation involves the production of insoluble calcium alginate.

$$2Na_nAlg + nCaSO_4 \longrightarrow nNa_2SO_4 + Ca_nAlg_2$$

The gel fibrils produced by this reaction become progressively cross-linked by bridges established by calcium ions reacting with functional carboxyl $(COO^-)$ groups on adjacent chains. At the time the impression is removed from the mouth the gel fibrils have encapsulated unreacted sol, filler particles, reaction by-products, and excess water. Calcium alginate is, in itself, a brittle substance but the resultant mass retains its elasticity by virtue of the entrapped sol in combination with the fibrillar gel structure. It is the cross-linking of the fibrils via calcium ions that causes elastic recoil of the impression to its original shape following removal from undercuts.

While a definitive point of gelation can generally be identified clinically, the reaction between sodium alginate and calcium sulphate is a continuing one. Eventually the entire mass is converted to calcium alginate, which is relatively hard and brittle. This can be appreciated by examining an alginate impression that has been exposed to air for a few hours. Continued formation of calcium alginate is associated with slight contraction. The identification of gelation is easier in some products as the transition is well defined, whereas in others the process appears more gradual. The sudden transition is probably the more desirable, since error due to premature removal of the impression is less likely. Since it is important that the impression should not be disturbed during gelation, a short gelation is an advantage.

SETTING TIME

As with any impression material, the setting time of alginate must be carefully controlled to combine adequate working time with a short duration in the mouth. This is largely in the hands of the manufacturers, who control the concentration of retarders and recommend the powder/water ratio. Modifications to this ratio are best avoided as they are generally associated with alterations to the consistency of the sol and final properties of the impression. The clinician can influence the rate of setting by altering the temperature of the water with which the powder is mixed. An increase in the temperature

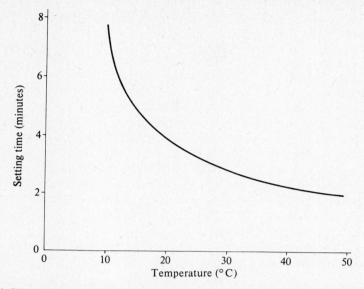

**Fig. 6.4** Effect of water temperature on the setting time of an alginate impression material.

increases the rate of setting (Fig. 6.4). A not uncommon problem is for the set to occur too rapidly because warm water has been used. Manufacturers' calculations are generally based on the use of water at room temperature. As with zinc oxide/eugenol impression pastes, a range of products with different setting times is available, and the dentist is recommended to choose one that suits his particular requirements. A setting time of 2–5 minutes is usually acceptable, although some products set in less than 2 minutes.

As the incorrect handling of alginate impression materials can have marked effects on their properties it is convenient to consider these in the context of clinical manipulation.

PROPORTIONING AND MIXING

Manufacturers determine the powder/water ratio that gives optimal results and generally provide the means for attaining this conveniently. Presentations may include measures to proportion the water and powder by volume. While this may be done for the water with some degree of accuracy, the degree of compaction of the powder will cause some variation in the amount of powder used. Variation in the powder/water ratio will effect the viscosity of the sol, and therefore its handling characteristics, and may lead to a reduction in strength of the final impression. However, such minor variations attributable to the use of powder measures are unlikely to be of any clinical significance. The greatest accuracy is clearly achieved by weighing the powder, and sachets containing pre-weighed portions are available for use with a measured volume of water. Water-soluble sachets are the simplest and most convenient to use.

Uniform distribution of all the constituents of the powder is important throughout the making of an alginate impression. This is primarily achieved by the manufacturer, but should be confirmed clinically by shaking the tin before dispensing the powder, and by thorough mixing with water. Alginate should be mixed in a flexible plastic bowl with a large spatula and both these implements must be thoroughly clean. Contamination with plaster, for example, could accelerate the set by contributing additional calcium to the mix. Rapid spatulation against the side of the bowl should be carried out for the recommended time, which is usually about one minute. Under-mixing results in inadequate wetting, lack of homogeneity, and reduced strength in the final impression. Overmixing also leads to a reduction in the final strength as the gel fibrils are destroyed as they form, and there is also a reduction in the working time.

### THE IMPRESSION TRAY

Impression trays for use with alginate should be rigid, and of sufficient size to allow an adequate bulk of material to be used. A thickness of at least 3 mm should be allowed and ideally the material should be of uniform thickness throughout the impression, although this latter condition may be difficult to achieve with stock trays. It is important to retain the impression evenly against the tray, especially when it is withdrawn from the mouth. This may be achieved using a perforated tray or an adhesive designed for the purpose, and indeed both methods may be employed together for maximum efficiency. Perforations should be large enough to allow an adequate thickness of material to penetrate to reduce the risk of tearing as the impression is removed. Holes about 2 mm in diameter are optimal, and they should be distributed closely throughout the tray. Failure of the tray to retain the material completely results in distortion of the impression.

### INSERTION AND REMOVAL

The material should be placed in the mouth before gelation occurs. If gelation has commenced, stresses will be incorporated in the impression which may lead to subsequent distortion. The increase in viscosity associated with gelation will also reduce the surface reproducibility and fine details will not be recorded. Care should be taken to avoid moving the impression as gelation occurs, so as to prevent disruption of the fibrillar structure and the development of stresses.

There is an increase in the strength and elasticity for a few minutes following gelation and therefore the impression should not be removed until about 2 minutes after gelation, as determined clinically by a reduction in tackiness. From the foregoing statement it can be appreciated that premature removal of the impression may lead to tearing, particularly if the material is in thin section. During the entire procedure the tray should be lightly supported without applying undue pressure. Some products use a pH indicator which causes a change in colour as the various stages of gelation are reached. Their action is based on pH changes associated with the gelation process and an indicator that displays a change in colour at the beginning and end of gelation is the most advantageous.

The impression should be removed with one swift movement, since hydro-colloids display the best elastic qualities under such circumstances. Slow removal involving longer periods of distortion should be avoided as the fibrillar network becomes altered preventing complete elastic recoil. In this respect continued rocking movements are the most damaging. With a 'snap' removal rapid elastic recoil occurs.

The recently removed impression should be washed with water to free it from saliva before being poured.

STORAGE OF THE IMPRESSION

With the techniques described above, where moderate undercuts have been involved, it is best to pour the impression as soon as possible, ideally within a few minutes. If large undercuts were present, the greater distortion produced on removal requires a little time to recover. In any event the impression should be poured within an hour.

The dimensional stability of alginate impression materials is poor. Water loss by evaporation and syneresis is the major factor involved. Continued conversion of sodium to calcium alginate also plays a part in causing contraction. Exposure to air for as little as 30 minutes can lead to great inaccuracy, and care should be exercised if storage is necessary. Immersion in water tends to cause swelling and distortion and the best results are achieved by keeping the impression in an atmosphere of 100 per cent humidity. A humidor may be used or the impression may be wrapped in damp dental napkins. Initially there may be a slight expansion on removal from the mouth and this is thought to be due to the further imbibition of free water encapsulated in the gel.

COMPATIBILITY WITH MODEL MATERIALS

The model materials most frequently used with alginate impressions are dental stone and plaster. Hydrocolloid materials, especially the alginates, may display a lack of compatibility with some makes of dental stone. The resultant model may show reduced surface hardness, and possibly surface irregularities and roughness. In extreme cases the surface of the stone may be powdery, making the model quite unusable. There may be a number of factors or mechanisms involved.

High molecular weight constituents of the impression materials retard the setting of the gypsum adjacent to them and syneresis probably increases their contamination superficially. Some alginates undergo a continuous change in pH following gelation and this is different from those associated with the setting of gypsum. The latter occurs between pH 6 and 7, the former may be as high as 10. Alteration to the pH of the gypsum in this way may interfere with its setting. If an alginate impression is left in a dry atmosphere following pouring, drying will occur and the impression may draw water from the setting stone to compensate, so interfering with its setting reaction. When there is free water in the impression at the time of pouring, the stone mix is diluted and is consequently weakened. If on the other hand, a thin mix of stone is used the slow rate of setting allows time for syneresis to occur. This can lead to surface imperfections in the model in the regions where the exudate is produced.

To overcome these problems modern products contain accelerators to bring about a rapid set of the model stone adjacent to the impression. At one time this effect was produced by soaking the impression for a few minutes in an accelerator, such as 2 per cent potassium sulphate or potash alum, before pouring in the model material. These accelerators may also reduce syneresis by affecting the superficial layer of the impression.

It is, of course, important to avoid damaging or distorting an alginate impression while pouring it. Large volumes of stone should not be applied at once or the more fragile components of the impression, such as the extensions of material between the teeth, may be displaced. To ensure the stone has hardened completely the impression should be left for at least 30, and preferably 60, minutes before it is removed. If, after the initial set of the stone, the model and impression are stored in a humid atmosphere, drying will be minimal and the impression may be easily removed from the model. If drying has occurred, parts of the model, for example single standing teeth, may be fractured at this stage. The surface reproducibility of the alginates is reasonably good but is dependent on the initial viscosity of the sodium alginate sol. This in turn is governed by the concentration and molecular weight of the sodium alginate and these factors are clearly decided by the manufacturers.

MISCELLANEOUS PROPERTIES

Alginate impression materials are non-toxic and non-irritant. Provided the powder is stored in a dry atmosphere at room temperature the shelf-life is good. Clearly, if a tin of powder is contaminated by moisture the contents will not produce satisfactory results. In this context the storage of tins of alginate powder in the refrigerator should be undertaken with caution. On removal, condensation on the powder may have the same undesirable side effect. Alginate is a relatively cheap impression material.

APPLICATIONS

Alginate is a widely used impression material. Its primary use is in the construction of partial and full dentures, but it is also used extensively in orthodontic practice and for the production of study models. Alginate may be used as a corrective impression material to record the fine detail missing from a basic impression in a material such as composition. It is important to ensure that an adequate means of adhering the alginate to the basic impression is used.

In advanced conservative dentistry alginate lacks the necessary dimensional stability and its surface reproducibility is not as good as that of other materials available. It is also weak in thin section and tends to tear from between the teeth. This is often a critical area for inlay, crown, and bridge impressions. Alginate can be used as an overall impression to relate a die or copper ring impression to the rest of the arch. However, the poor dimensional stability makes its use in this way suspect in a great many situations.

## Reversible hydrocolloids

Reversible hydrocolloids undergo the transition from sol to gel on cooling. The hydrocolloid, supplied as the gel, is heated above its liquefaction point, cooled to a temperature compatible with the oral tissues and placed in the mouth. Gelation occurs as the tray continues to cool, after which the impression is removed and poured. Reversible hydrocolloid impression materials are based on water and agar, which, like alginic acid, is derived from seaweed.

**Table 6.5** Constituents of a typical reversible hydrocolloid

| |
| --- |
| Agar |
| Water |
| Borax |
| Potassium sulphate |
| Filler |

CONSTITUENTS

The constitution of a reversible hydrocolloid is given in Table 6.5. The principal colloid constituent is a polysaccharide, agar, which is present from 12–17 per cent. Agar is the sulphuric ester of a galactan complex with a complicated structural formula. Water, acting as the dispersion medium, makes up the greatest part of the material, on average about 84 per cent. In addition, many presentations contain about 0·2 per cent borax, which improves the strength of the final gel. However, borax inhibits the setting of dental stone and an accelerator, such as 2 per cent potassium sulphate, is generally included to counteract this effect. Different products contain a variety of additives, most frequently in the form of a filler. Zinc oxide, diatomaceous earth, silica, and powdered wax may be used for this purpose and impart a better consistency to the sol and increased strength to the gel. A further increase in strength may be achieved by the inclusion of cellulose fibres. As reversible hydrocolloids may be reused, some products include an antimicrobial agent, such as thymol or alkyl benzoate, to minimize the growth of micro-organisms on the surface of the gel.

### GELATION

It is necessary to heat reversible hydrocolloids to as much as 100 °C to produce the sol. On cooling, as the material nears mouth temperature, an increase in viscosity occurs. Increased viscosity at a higher temperature would make the introduction of stresses more likely as the impression is taken. A sudden transition from sol to gel is desirable at a temperature a little above that of the mouth (Fig. 6.5). It is obviously necessary to maintain a low viscosity at a temperature that can be tolerated by the patient in order to achieve good surface reproducibility. On the other hand, if gelation occurs at a temperature too close to that of the mouth, cooling the tray and its contents adequately and uniformly may be difficult. It is necessary, therefore, for gelation to occur somewhat above mouth temperature.

As cooling of the impression occurs more rapidly adjacent to the tray, it is necessary to leave it in the mouth for sufficient time to ensure that gelation takes place completely, especially in the material adjacent to the tissues. Here the higher temperature delays gelation, unlike the situation with alginate where the raised temperature accelerates gelation.

### PROPERTIES

Many of the properties and handling considerations are similar to those of alginate.

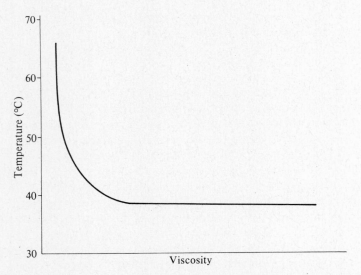

**Fig. 6.5** Changes in viscosity of reversible hydrocolloid with temperature. Sudden gelation occurs close to mouth temperature.

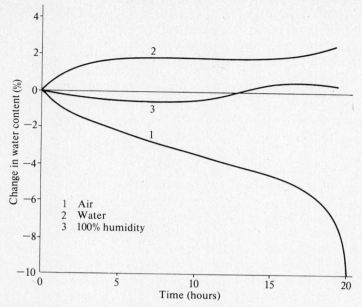

**Fig. 6.6** Effect of storage environment on the water content of reversible hydrocolloids.

The reversible hydrocolloids are potentially accurate materials offering good surface reproducibility, better than that of alginate, but they share similar problems of dimensional stability. Exposure to a dry atmosphere leads to a loss of moisture by evaporation and syneresis, which results in shrinkage and distortion of the impression. Again, if storage is necessary, a humid atmosphere is the most suitable environment (Fig. 6.6). For the best results, however, the impression should be poured immediately after withdrawal from the mouth. If drying has occurred, immersion in water will bring about an almost complete return to the original dimensions. However, some slight deformation does take place, perhaps sufficient to prejudice the fit of the final restoration. Different products behave differently in this respect, probably because of structural and density variations in the fibrillar network and the modifying effects of different fillers. As agar distorts there is also a progressive loss of elasticity.

With alginate impressions the material in contact with the oral tissues sets most rapidly and there is always a risk of distortion being introduced in this layer by movement of the tray while waiting for the rest to set. As the opposite situation occurs with the reversible hydrocolloids the tendency for distortion to occur in the agar adjacent to the tissues, which is the last to gel, is reduced. Accuracy in the latter materials is therefore potentially better.

It is recommended with some products that they should be immersed in a die or model-hardening solution before pouring the impressions. These solutions, having a similar osmolarity to the hydrocolloid, also tend to inhibit syneresis, and better dimensional stability is achieved in the agar. Reversible hydrocolloids are compatible with most model and die stones after the use of hardening or fixing solutions.

Although reversible hydrocolloids are non-irritant and non-toxic, the temperature extremes involved in their manipulation may upset some patients. Initially the material may be very warm on placement in the mouth and is cooled by cold water directed over the tray or through cooling channels within it.

MANIPULATION

Reversible hydrocolloids are usually presented in foil tubes containing the gel. The most effective way of producing the sol is by heating to between 75 and 100 °C in a thermostatically controlled water bath designed for the purpose. Before insertion in the mouth the agar must be cooled to 45–60 °C and this is achieved in a similar tempering bath. The loaded tray should be left for some minutes in this environment to allow an even temperature to be achieved throughout its mass. After insertion in the mouth the tray is cooled. Specially designed trays containing ducts through which cold water may be circulated may be used. It generally takes between 5 and 10 minutes for gelation to occur under these conditions and the tray should be lightly supported and held still for this time. A sudden 'snap' removal results in the least distortion and the impression may be poured immediately. As adhesives are less effective with agar than with alginate, perforated and ridged trays must be used to retain the material. It is possible to apply agar from a syringe to ensure its close adaptation to prepared teeth during impressions for inlays, crowns, and bridges.

Although reversible hydrocolloids are reusable they cannot be effectively sterilized, and therefore become contaminated. Most operators prefer to discard the material after it has been used once. Provided the agar is stored in sealed tubes the shelf-life is good and the material is cheap compared with the synthetic elastic materials.

APPLICATIONS

Reversible hydrocolloids offer sufficient accuracy to allow their use in conservative dentistry for inlay, crown, and bridgework, and they have been used extensively to produce impressions for denture construction. However, since the development of irreversible hydrocolloids and synthetic elastomers, which are more easily handled and require less specialized techniques and apparatus, reversible materials have been used less and less. Agar products are, however, used in the dental laboratory as duplicating materials.

DUPLICATING MATERIALS

It is sometimes necessary to have an exact replica of a dental stone model for technical purposes. For example, during the construction of a cobalt–chromium partial denture a modified model of the patient's mouth must be duplicated in a refractory investment material that will subsequently withstand the high temperatures involved in the casting procedures. Essentially an impression technique is employed for this purpose. While these products are fundamentally the same as the impression materials they produce a less viscous sol, partly because no fillers are included and partly because a high percentage of water is present. Again the hydrocolloid is cooled well below the liquefaction temperature before being poured around the master model seated in a special flask. Following further cooling, when gelation occurs, the master model is removed with a single sharp movement. The surface of the mould so produced is generally treated with model hardener before the stone or investment duplicate is poured.

These products are reused but in time contamination occurs and there is deterioration in their properties. It is important to confirm that the product is compatible with the investment or stone to be used. Some laboratory duplicating materials are based on irreversible hydrocolloids and clearly these may only be used once.

## Synthetic elastomers

These impression materials are based on synthetic rubber polymers. Initially they are of relatively low molecular weight and are of a fluid consistency but, when mixed with an appropriate reactor, undergo further polymerization and cross-linking to produce a firm elastic solid. Such a transformation from a fluid forms the basis of their use as impression materials. The set structure, with just a limited amount of cross-linking allows considerable elastic deformation, as described in Chapter 1.

In the majority of synthetic elastomers the further polymerization is brought about by a condensation reaction. This leads to the formation of a by-product, and this contributes to the small amount of contraction that occurs during polymerization, especially if the by-product is volatile. As the rubber molecules become more regimented in their orientation owing to polymerization and cross-linking they tend to occupy less space, and this accounts for the remaining polymerization shrinkage. While the contraction produced in this way occurs to the greatest extent during the clinical setting of the material, continued shrinkage does take place over an extended period. Although dimensional changes vary, with materials liberating a volatile by-product displaying more shrinkage, the amount is small in practical terms.

Synthetic elastomers have a relatively high coefficient of thermal expansion. This probably plays a larger part in the dimensional change of impressions than the factors previously considered. Dental impressions may undergo a number of temperature changes. The first occurs when it is transferred from mouth to room temperature, and this is probably the greatest. Subsequent fluctuation in temperature occurs as the impression is dispatched to the laboratory.

Contraction of an elastomeric impression occurs, therefore, for three reasons—continued polymerization shrinkage, loss of volatile constituents or by-products, and thermal contraction. These factors influence the dimensional stability to a certain extent, but not, in general, to a degree that prejudices the use of the materials for impression purposes. The dimensional stability of the synthetic elastomers varies from product to product but is superior, over a long period, to that of the hydrocolloids. If it is not possible to produce the model immediately, or very shortly after taking the impression, the elastomers are a more appropriate choice. Other factors, including ease of handling and patient acceptability, also support the choice of synthetic elastomers for precision impressions.

To minimize the effect of contraction it is important to ensure that the impression material is effectively retained against the tray with an adhesive designed for the purpose. In this way any shrinkage is directed towards the outer surface of the impression. This tends to favour the ultimate fit of many types of restoration. In the absence of adhesion between the tray and the impression, contraction is directed centrally and results in a model with slightly smaller teeth than the original. Consequently the fit of a crown, for example, could be tight. More importantly, contraction with a form as complex in shape as an impression will tend to lead to its distortion. Adhesion to the tray opposes this tendency. The effect of contraction of the impression on the ultimate dimensions of models containing more complex features, such as gold inlay cavities, is not as easy to analyse.

Further limitation of dimensional change may be achieved in absolute terms by using a small bulk of material in the tray. For this reason most elastomeric impression pastes should be used in a closely adapted tray constructed for the particular patient. As the amount of filler used in the pastes is raised to increase the viscosity, dimensional changes are reduced. The fillers do not contribute towards polymerization shrinkage and, in effect, 'dilute' that occurring in the rubber. They also have a lower coefficient of thermal expansion.

The surface reproducibility of synthetic elastomers is very good. Clearly the viscosity of the presentation is important, and this depends on the amount of filler present. Most products provide a low-viscosity paste, and these record greater detail than most model and die materials are capable of reproducing. However, the lack of filler leads to poorer dimensional stability as a result of shrinkage, as explained earlier. Low viscosity presentations should be used in minimum bulk. It is usual for manufacturers to present a range of viscosities for different purposes, and several produce materials in the form of a viscous putty. Although it is necessary to use these in considerable bulk, dimensional changes are low in view of the high concentration of filler.

Elasticity in the rubber impression materials allows them to be withdrawn from undercuts with subsequent recovery. Elastic recovery is incomplete and a small amount of deformation remains after the impression has been removed. Permanent strain varies from one type of material to another but is generally 2–4 per cent. Variation in the degree of undercut and the bulk of material being used also influences this figure. The greater strength of these materials makes tearing less likely than with the hydrocolloids, although again there is variation.

Although synthetic elastomers are, in general, non-toxic and non-irritant, the taste and smell of a few presentations may be objectionable to some patients. The development of hypersensitivity to some products is also possible. Polymerization or setting time varies from 4 to 10 minutes and the use of the slower materials may be uncomfortable in view of this.

The rubber impression materials are compatible with most model and die materials and may be electroplated to produce dies of high surface hardness. Unlike the hydrocolloids they are hydrophobic and should be dried before being poured. Provided they are kept cool, the shelf-life is reasonable but some silicones are less satisfactory in this respect.

Synthetic elastomers may be classified according to the chemistry of their bases. There are fundamentally three groups—silicones, polysulphides, and polyethers. A fourth variety, polythioether, has been introduced more recently. However, this material is used in conjunction with a polysulphide, as will be seen later.

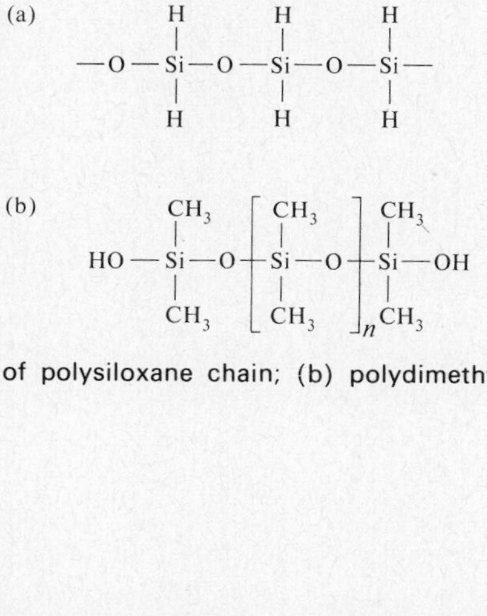

(a)

$$-O-\underset{\underset{H}{|}}{\overset{\overset{H}{|}}{Si}}-O-\underset{\underset{H}{|}}{\overset{\overset{H}{|}}{Si}}-O-\underset{\underset{H}{|}}{\overset{\overset{H}{|}}{Si}}-$$

(b)

$$HO-\underset{\underset{CH_3}{|}}{\overset{\overset{CH_3}{|}}{Si}}-O\left[\underset{\underset{CH_3}{|}}{\overset{\overset{CH_3}{|}}{Si}}-O\right]_n\underset{\underset{CH_3}{|}}{\overset{\overset{CH_3}{|}}{Si}}-OH$$

**Fig. 6.7** (a) Segment of polysiloxane chain; (b) polydimethylsiloxane with terminal hydroxyl groups.

## Silicones

CONSTITUENTS

Silicone rubbers are polymers based on a polysiloxane chain (Fig. 6.7a), the most frequent form being polydimethyl siloxane with terminal hydroxyl groups (Fig. 6.7b). The length of the molecules determines the viscosity of the rubber and the ultimate physical properties of the set material. Longer chain forms exist as a solid, while lower molecular weight forms are liquids. It is these low molecular weight liquids that are used in dental impression materials.

There are several different presentations of silicone impression materials. The silicone base is supplied in the form of pastes of varying viscosity or as a putty. Inert fillers, such as silica, titanium dioxide, and zinc oxide, modify the viscosity. Putties contain a very high proportion of filler. Most frequently the reactor is in the form of a liquid, although paste presentations are available. They contain an activator or catalyst and a cross-linking agent. The former is an organo–tin compound, such as tin octoate or dibutyl tin dilaurate. Different types of cross-linking agent have been employed but most are tetra-alkyl silicates, while early products used organo–hydrogen siloxanes (Table 6.6).

**Table 6.6** Constituents of a typical silicone impression material

| Base paste or putty | Reactor liquid |
| --- | --- |
| Silicone polymer | Tetra-alkyl silicate |
| Filler | Organo–tin compound |
|  | Oils |

SETTING REACTION

Further polymerization and cross-linking of the silicone chains is brought about by mixing with the appropriate amount of reactor. With paste presentations this generally means mixing equal lengths of material dispensed from tubes. With liquid reactors, the number of drops used is dependent on the amount of base paste dispensed, and the manufacturer's directions should always be followed. The presence of an organo–tin compound catalyst induces the union of base molecules via the cross-linking agent. The tetra-alkyl silicates are able to bring three chains together with liberation of an alcohol (Fig. 6.8a). Organo–hydrogen siloxanes unite chains liberating hydrogen (Fig. 6.8b). In earlier products the evolution of hydrogen gas led to the surface pitting of dental stone models poured in the impression. Presentations still using these cross-linking agents overcome the problem by carrying hydrogen acceptors such as aldehydes or chromium oxide.

PROPERTIES

Polymerization shrinkage is greater in silicone pastes than in polysulphide impression materials. However, silicone in putty form is considerably better and displays similar shrinkage to polysulphides. The more recent addition reaction silicone impression materials, to be described later, appear to offer a further improvement with virtually no contraction during polymerization. Silicones display the best elasticity of the synthetic elastomers. Following a 12 per cent strain the permanent deformation is 1–2 per cent, compared with 4 per cent for polysulphides.

Silicone impression materials are clean, pleasant to work with, and have a clinical setting time of about four minutes. It is often difficult to ensure the even distribution of the reactor in the base if the former is a liquid. This problem is most apparent when a liquid reactor is mixed with a putty base.

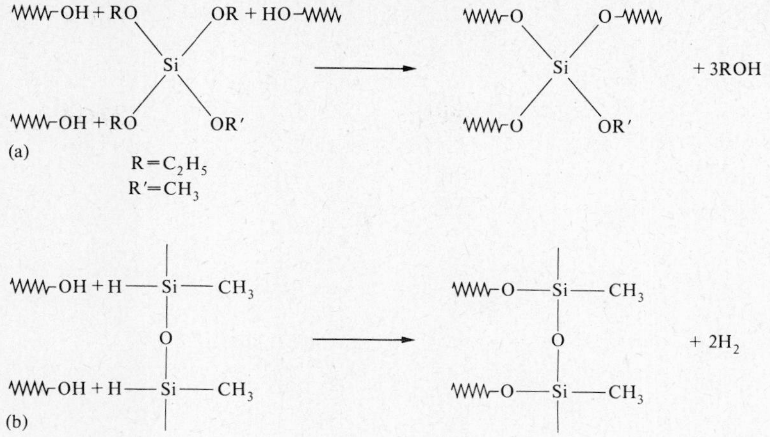

**Fig. 6.8** Setting of silicone impression rubber (a) using tetra-aklyl silicate cross-linking agent; (b) using organo-hydrogen siloxane cross-linking agent.

In such a situation a differential rate of setting may occur in an impression, part setting on time and part being delayed. By incorporating the reactor in a paste of contrasting colour thorough mixing is much more easily achieved. In some preparations the contents of the liquid reactor crystallize in the nozzle of the dispenser. This alters the concentration of the reactor and may also influence the volume of drops dispensed from the bottle. Some organo–metallic compounds are toxic and the reactor should be handled as little as possible. Thorough mixing prevents excess of these compounds remaining free in the impression material when it is in the patient's mouth.

Since some products contain both activator and cross-linking agent in the one liquid or paste, gradual deterioration may occur. This may lead to failure of polymerization when the material is used. Instability of the tetra-alkyl silicate, especially in the presence of the tin activator, is responsible. The base paste may also undergo spontaneous cross-linking following its degredation.

ADDITION REACTION SILICONES

Some silicone impression materials polymerize by an addition reaction rather than by condensation. The organo-tin compound in these materials has been replaced by a platinum-containing catalyst and the silicone molecules

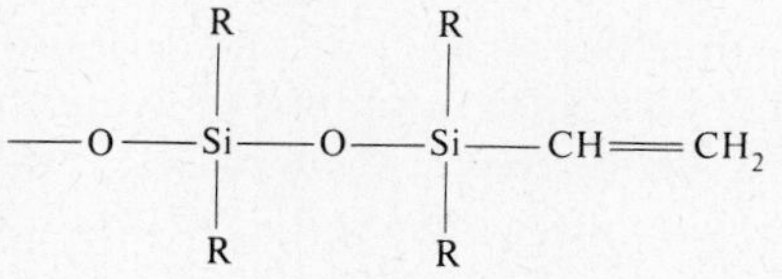

**Fig. 6.9** Segment of addition reaction silicone molecule displaying terminal vinyl group.

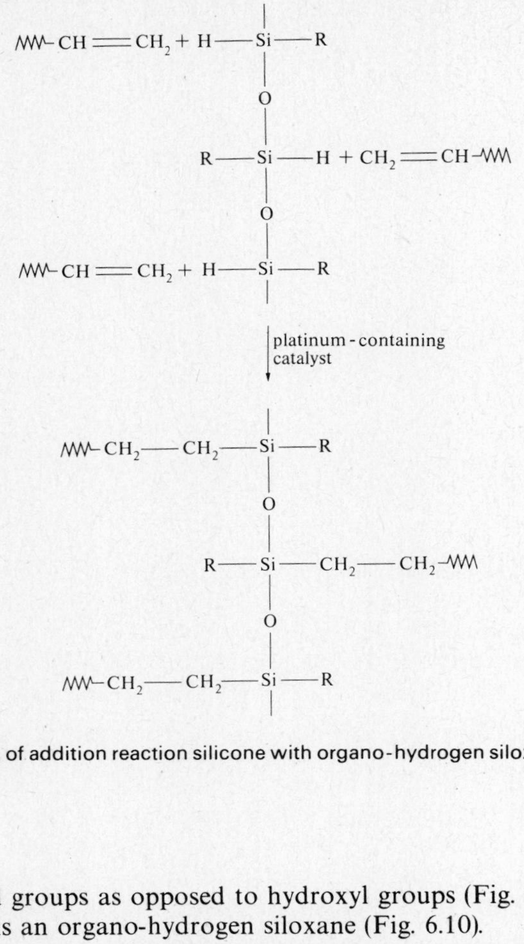

**Fig. 6.10** Setting of addition reaction silicone with organo-hydrogen siloxane cross-linking agent.

have vinyl end groups as opposed to hydroxyl groups (Fig. 6.9). The cross-linking agent is an organo-hydrogen siloxane (Fig. 6.10).

As no by-product is formed there is virtually no contraction on setting and in this respect the dimensional stability is very good. The coefficient of thermal expansion of the rubber is still high, however, and some contraction will occur when the impression is removed from the mouth. Addition reaction silicones are expensive compared with conventional silicone materials.

### Polysulphides

Polysulphide materials are sometimes referred to as Thiokol rubbers after the Thiokol Corporation that developed an early polymer on which these products are based. The term mercaptan may also be applied as the material contains —SH groups. Most frequently, however, these products are given the title rubber base. Two pastes are employed which, when mixed together, set to a rubbery solid. A range of viscosities is usually available but some products supply a diluent to reduce the viscosity of one basic material.

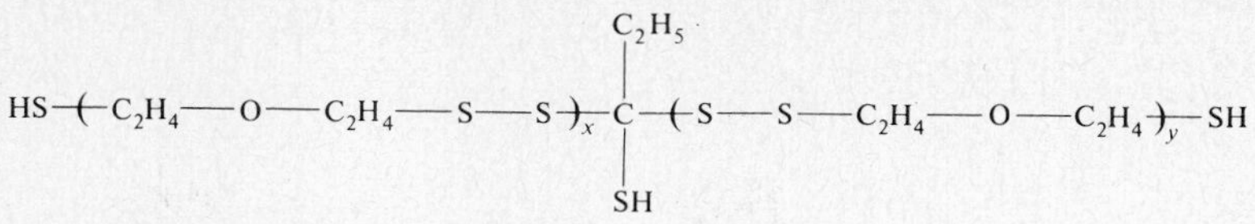

$$\text{HS}\!-\!\!\big(\!\text{C}_2\text{H}_4\!-\!\text{O}\!-\!\text{C}_2\text{H}_4\!-\!\text{S}\!-\!\text{S}\!\big)_{\!x}\!\underset{\underset{\text{SH}}{|}}{\overset{\overset{\text{C}_2\text{H}_5}{|}}{\text{C}}}\!\big(\!\text{S}\!-\!\text{S}\!-\!\text{C}_2\text{H}_4\!-\!\text{O}\!-\!\text{C}_2\text{H}_4\!\big)_{\!y}\!-\!\text{SH}$$

**Fig. 6.11** Structure of typical polysulphide rubber molecule.

CONSTITUENTS

One paste contains the rubber which is itself a polymer (Fig. 6.11). Poly-sulphide rubber is a viscous liquid, and an inert filler, usually titanium dioxide, produces pastes of different viscosity depending on the amount added. Filler may therefore be present in proportions from about 10–55 per cent and gives the paste a white colour. The reactor contains an oxidizing agent, sulphur, and oils to produce a paste. The most frequently used oxidizing agent is lead dioxide. This substance gives the paste its brown colour. In attempts to obviate certain difficulties with lead dioxide other oxidizing agents have been used, although in practice they are no better. Indeed, more serious drawbacks usually result. These include organic hydroperoxides, such as cumene hydroperoxide, and copper salts, which impart characteristic colours to the reactor pastes. The concentration of lead dioxide varies from 52 per cent to 82 per cent. The constituents of the most commonly used type of polysulphide material are given in Table 6.7.

**Table 6.7** Constituents of a typical polysulphide impression material

| Base paste | Reactor paste |
| --- | --- |
| Polysulphide polymer | Lead dioxide |
| Filler | Sulphur |
| | Oils |

SETTING REACTION

On mixing the base and reactor pastes oxidation of the terminal and pendant —SH groups occurs (Fig. 6.12). Initially the reaction is confined pre-dominantly to the terminal groups leading to an increase in the polymer chain length and an increase in viscosity. Later cross-linking via the pendant groups occurs to a greater extent and this leads to elasticity in the set material.

PROPERTIES

The dimensional stability of polysulphide rubbers is good. Only the addition reaction silicones are superior in this respect. Problems occur with materials using reactors other than lead dioxide. Organic hydroperoxides are volatile and their loss from the set material leads to shrinkage and distortion of

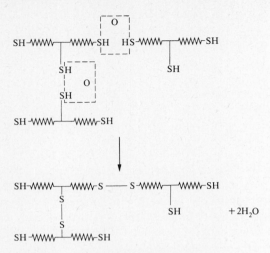

**Fig. 6.12** Setting reaction of polysulphide impression rubber.

the impression. The copper-salt products have good dimensional stability, but the final set is unstable. The elasticity of polysulphides is not as good as silicones and there is variation between products.

Lead dioxide makes the material messy to work with and the rubbery smell is unpleasant for some patients. Further discomfort may be associated with the relatively long polymerization time. This varies from 4 to 8 minutes, but on occasions 10 minutes may be required to ensure adequate setting and gain in elasticity. Heat and moisture accelerate the setting reaction. In warm weather, particularly if the surgery atmosphere is humid, setting and working times are reduced. Under these conditions it is therefore necessary to ensure rapid mixing and early placement of the impression to prevent internal stresses which may produce distortion. While it is possible to reduce the setting time by the addition of a drop of water to the mix, this cannot be achieved in a controlled fashion and is not recommended.

POLYTHIOETHER

Polysulphide impression materials are always presented as pastes. It is not possible to increase the viscosity of the rubber by the addition of fillers to an extent that will allow the production of a putty in view of the initially low viscosity of the rubber polymers themselves. There are certain clinical advantages to putty systems, and these will be discussed later. In order that polysulphides may be used with a putty system a new material has been developed.

This is a sulphur-containing polymer described as polythioether. It is presented as two putties, a base and a reactor, of contrasting colour. When mixed together in measured proportions it sets to a hard and inelastic mass in 2 to 3 minutes. An impression in putty is made in a stock tray and is later used as a 'special tray' in which to take a wash impression in a conventional low viscosity polysulphide rubber. The use of a polythene spacer during the initial impression limits the flow of the putty around the teeth, which allows room for the wash impression. This is helped further if the basic impression is taken before the teeth are prepared. Additional space in the important areas becomes available after the reduction of the teeth. Chemical union occurs between the polythioether and polysulphide rubber. The former should not be considered as an integral part of the impression, but rather as a means of converting a stock tray into a special tray. This is in contrast to the silicone putty systems where the putty forms an important part of the impression and may even record part of the surface. Here the low viscosity silicones are used to perfect the basic impression to a high degree of accuracy.

Clinically the polythioether system produces good results in crown and bridgework. It is important, however, to ensure extremely thorough mixing of the putties if they are to set uniformly. The shelf-life of the product is shortened by prolonged exposure to air, which allows spontaneous polymerization. As with addition reaction silicones, polythioether is an expensive product.

### Polyether

This material is presented as two pastes, a base and reactor. It is mixed and handled in an essentially similar way to polysulphide impression materials.

CONSTITUENTS AND SETTING REACTION

The base is an unsaturated polyether with terminal imine groups (Fig. 6.13) made into a paste of suitable viscosity by the addition of a filler and plasticizer. An aromatic sulphonate is the reactor, also prepared as a paste with a plasticizer and inorganic filler. This induces polymerization of the polyether via the imine groups.

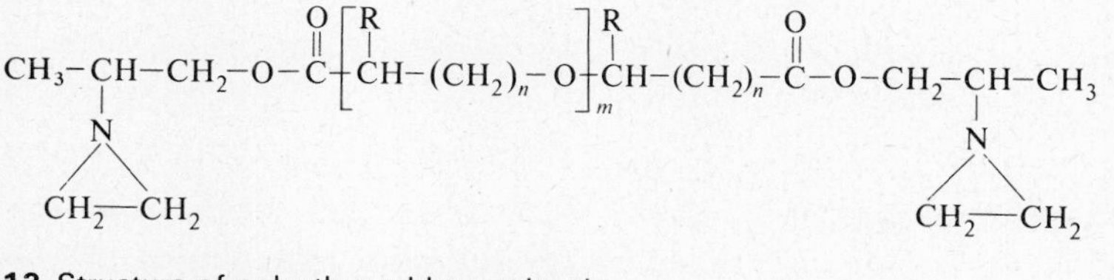

$$CH_3-CH-CH_2-O-\overset{O}{\overset{\|}{C}}\left[\overset{R}{\underset{}{CH}}-(CH_2)_n-O\right]_m\overset{R}{\underset{}{CH}}-(CH_2)_n-\overset{O}{\overset{\|}{C}}-O-CH_2-CH-CH_3$$

Fig. 6.13 Structure of polyether rubber molecule.

PROPERTIES

The two pastes are of contrasting colour, which helps efficient mixing. Elasticity develops rapidly from the time of mixing. It is therefore important that the impression should be seated as soon as possible and held undisturbed until set in order to avoid introducing stresses that would lead to distortion. Polymerization is complete in 5 minutes, at which time the material is relatively hard, and difficulty may arise in removing the impression. In areas of pronounced undercut it is advisable to allow for a greater thickness of material in the tray to facilitate removal. Continued increase in hardness occurs and removal of the impression from the cast model may also be difficult. At this stage it is possible to fracture teeth from the model.

The dimensional stability of this product is potentially good if storage of the impression is undertaken with care. Absorption of water is high and the impression should be kept dry or it will swell and distort. Direct sunlight also has a detrimental effect on the dimensions of the impression.

The manufacturers warn that skin contact with the reactor may induce sensitization, and contact should therefore be avoided. Presumably this type of sensitivity may also occur following contact with the oral mucosa. Some patients complain that the material has an unpleasant taste.

### Applications of synthetic elastomers

While synthetic elastomers are used extensively in prosthetic dentistry their properties make them ideally suited for crown and bridge impressions. Here an elastic material of great accuracy is required, as a very small error may make the fit of a restoration quite unacceptable. Generally these impressions are made using a combination of low and high viscosity pastes in order to achieve good surface reproducibility, contributed by the former, and improved strength and dimensional stability from the latter. Techniques for achieving impressions in this way are outlined in the next section.

In denture construction the synthetic elastomers may be used in virtually every situation. The range of viscosity available offers materials for use in very thin section, as would be required in relining techniques. Conversely high viscosity preparations will produce tissue compression to a varying degree if this is required. Clearly, in complex partial dentures with cast alloy skeletons great accuracy is required and here the good dimensional stability of the elastomers is of benefit. However, many impressions in prosthetics may be produced satisfactorily with much cheaper materials, such as alginate.

SYNTHETIC ELASTOMER TECHNIQUES IN CONSERVATIVE DENTISTRY

Impressions of inlay and crown preparations are generally made using materials of varying viscosity. Most products include these in their presentations.

A two-stage technique is the most widely used, and can be applied to the majority of materials. The first stage involves the application of the low-viscosity paste to the prepared teeth. This is conveniently carried out with a syringe, which allows the paste to be positioned under pressure to ensure close adaptation to the preparations. Immediately following this a tray containing a paste or putty of higher viscosity is placed over the arch and the combined impression is allowed to polymerize. In presentations offering only one viscosity paste this may be used in both syringe and tray using the same technique.

The silicone materials with a putty presentation allow an alternative technique. Again there are two stages. A basic impression is prepared using the putty in a stock tray, and this is perfected in the second stage with a low-viscosity paste. The basic impression is modified before this by cutting escape channels from the region of the prepared teeth to the periphery to allow excess perfecting paste to escape freely. It is also necessary to remove the thin pieces of putty from between the teeth to ensure that the impression may be reseated accurately and easily in the mouth. The basic impression is thoroughly washed and dried before the addition of the perfecting paste to the region of the prepared teeth. The surface of the final impression is recorded largely by the perfecting paste, albeit in very thin section, but also by the underlying putty in some places where adaptation of the basic impression to the tooth is complete.

The latter technique is more time-consuming as the impression has to be placed in the mouth for two periods of polymerization. Errors may easily arise during the second stage unless great care is taken. There is a risk that the impression may not be fully seated in its original position, which would lead to the production of a step at the junction of the paste and putty. This may also result if the paste has too high a viscosity at the time of insertion, which limits its flow. It may be necessary with some products to use less reactor in the perfecting paste to give a longer working time in order to overcome this problem. These disadvantages do not arise with the first technique.

Too much pressure applied to the tray as the synthetic elastomer polymerizes can lead to the generation of stresses in the impression with resultant distortion. This danger exists with any technique, and impression trays should only be lightly supported. Dimensional changes consequential to thermal changes may be reduced in absolute terms by minimizing the bulk of material used. For this reason special trays that allow the use of about 2 mm of material are recommended for the paste presentations. Putties must be used in larger bulk, but as they have a high filler content their coefficient of expansion is lower. Special trays should be constructed from a rigid material, such as acrylic resin, rather than a thermoplastic product. The latter is unstable and can lead to distortion of the impression as a result of warping.

One of the most important, and at the same time most difficult, areas of preparations to record is the gingival margin. Here the impression must be clear and unambiguous if the technician is to trim the die with precision and achieve an accurate fit of the restoration. Where the margin of the preparation is level with or below the free gingival margin, retraction should be used to hold the free gingivae away from the tooth and reduce exudation and bleeding from the tissues while the impression is taken. This may be achieved using a combination of gingival retraction cords and solutions. They contain a variety of chemical agents to achieve these objectives including vasoconstrictors, such as adrenaline, and styptics, such as aluminium trichloride. Careful gingival retraction is an essential stage in the production of most crown and bridge impressions.

Developments in impression materials, particularly in the synthetic elastomers, have improved their accuracy to a high degree. Impressions of the most complex bridge preparations may now be undertaken with a high rate of success, which minimizes costly failures and remakes. It should be remembered, however, that many of the well established materials described in this chapter will produce perfectly satisfactory results for certain varieties of work, generally at a fraction of the cost of the more sophisticated products.

# 7
# Model and die materials: waxes

The discussion of impression materials in Chapter 6 explained the need for models of the patient's mouth and dentition as an essential aspect of many forms of treatment. The construction of dentures and many other forms of prostheses must be carried out on such models. The technical preparation of inlays, crowns, and bridges requires an individual model of each prepared tooth. These individual replicas are referred to as dies. In addition to these fundamental applications model materials are used in many less demanding technical situations.

### Desirable properties of model and die materials

The great dimensional accuracy and surface reproducibility of impression materials would be of little value if they were not matched by similar properties in the resultant model. It is important, therefore, that dimensional change on and after setting is minimal and that the material is capable of reproducing fine detail. Both of these properties are of more critical significance in the construction of restorations for prepared teeth than, say, in the manufacture of full dentures for the edentulous jaw. Hard tooth substance is virtually unyielding, and the dimensions of the restoration must approach perfection if a satisfactory fit is to be achieved. On the other hand, the displacement of the soft tissues by a denture will allow a certain degree of latitude.

Model and die materials should have good strength and hardness. The technical procedures involved in the production of dentures demand that considerable pressures are applied to the denture base material via the model on which it is being moulded. The compressive strength is the more important and is the parameter most frequently assessed. Surface hardness, which relates to abrasion-resistance, is particularly important in dies. These are generally employed to produce wax patterns and the use of a carving instrument close to the die surface, especially around the margins of the preparation, must not lead to abrasion of the die. Similarly the burnishing of a platinum foil matrix prior to the construction of a porcelain jacket crown must not damage the die (Chapter 9).

Model materials must be compatible with impression materials and any other substances, such as waxes and separating media, which are likely to come into contact with them during the technical procedures. Thus, there must not be any interaction that would adversely affect their setting reaction or final properties. They should be insoluble in water, since washing of the models, sometimes in boiling water, is necessary in some technical procedures.

It is helpful if the colour of models contrasts clearly with those of materials, such as waxes, to be used on them. As model materials are used in considerable bulk by a dental laboratory they should be cheap and have a long shelf-life.

Among the most widely used and most successful model materials are the gypsum products. These also form the basis of impression plaster (Chapter 6) and investment materials to be considered in the next chapter, and their chemistry and setting reaction are discussed below.

## GYPSUM PRODUCTS

CHEMISTRY

Gypsum is calcium sulphate dihydrate ($CaSO_4 . 2H_2O$), which is a naturally occurring mineral. It is also an industrial by-product. The application of heat to gypsum leads to the formation of calcium sulphate hemihydrate (($CaSO_4)_2 . H_2O$) which can exist in a number of forms, depending on the method of heating. Of direct relevance to the use of gypsum products in dentistry is that heating in air to about 120 °C leads to the formation of calcined calcium sulphate hemihydrate, whilst heating under steam pressure yields autoclaved calcium sulphate hemihydrate. These different forms are chemically identical but differ in their structure, the calcined material being more porous with larger, irregular particles. Because of this the two forms react differently with water and since this is the basis of the setting reaction of gypsum products, each must be handled differently.

This setting reaction can be represented by the equation

$$(CaSO_4)_2 . H_2O + 3H_2O \longrightarrow 2(CaSO_4 . 2H_2O).$$

The reaction is exothermic and there is no chemical distinction between the dihydrates produced from the different types of hemihydrate. Continued exposure of the hemihydrate to a high temperature leads firstly to the production of a soluble anhydrite and later to an insoluble anhydrite.

The setting reaction of gypsum products can be visualized in the following stages.

**a** The hemihydrate, on mixing with water, dissolves sparingly to give $Ca^{2+}$ and $SO_4^{2-}$ ions. At room temperature the solubility is about 0·8 per cent.

**b** As the solubility of calcium sulphate dihydrate is only 0·2 per cent, the solution becomes supersaturated with respect to this and crystallization occurs.

**c** Crystallization initially takes place around dihydrate crystals already in existence. These may have remained at the end of production of the hemihydrate by the manufacturer but are sometimes added specifically. Small foci of dirt and other impurities may also act as nuclei. As the dihydrate crystallizes, more hemihydrate dissolves and the reaction continues. The result is a hard mass of calcium sulphate dihydrate.

DIMENSIONAL CHANGE ON SETTING

The setting reaction of gypsum products is associated with apparent expansion, which is real in practical terms. As crystals of the dihydrate grow outwards from the nuclei, they eventually impinge on one another and exert a pressure. The result is separation of the nuclei with an apparent increase in the volume (Fig. 7.1). It is important to realize, however, that the set material consists of pores as well as crystals and that the real volume of the crystals is, in fact, less than the volume of the original hemihydrate. It is the combination of dihydrate crystals and voids that gives the apparent expansion.

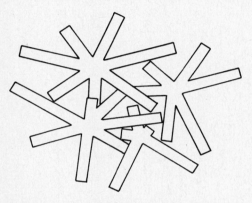

**Fig. 7.1** Impingement of growing dihydrate crystals, which results in their separation.

Different forms of hemihydrate produce different degrees of expansion, which may be further controlled by the use of chemical additives. For example, a small amount of potassium sulphate can reduce the setting expansion in plaster from 0·4 per cent to 0·05 per cent. Often the additive that controls the expansion also influences the rate of reaction, the potassium sulphate tending to increase this rate. Under these situations a retarder has to be added to counteract this effect.

If gypsum products are allowed to set under water the expansion occurring is greater than in air. This is referred to as hygroscopic expansion. As crystal growth occurs small voids are produced in the mesh, which contain the excess water required to mix the material. In air, as water is used up, the nuclei of crystallization are drawn together by surface tension of the water. In water, however, as hydration of the hemihydrate occurs, more water is available and the nuclei remain the same distance apart. Thus the expansion may be double that observed in air. Hygroscopic expansion does not have any useful application in the production of models and dies, but may be of benefit in the handling of gypsum-bonded investments. These are described in detail in Chapter 10.

## Dental plaster

Dental plaster as an impression material has already been described in the previous chapter. Plaster for dental models and general laboratory use is essentially similar but additives are present in different proportions to achieve different objectives.

CONSTITUENTS

The principal constituent of dental plaster is calcined calcium sulphate hemihydrate which constitutes 75–85 per cent of the total. This is prepared by heating the dihydrate in air to 120–130 °C which drives off some of the water. Between 5 and 8 per cent gypsum is usually present to contribute foci or nuclei of crystallization. The amount will clearly have a bearing on the rate of the setting reaction. Often the soluble anhydrite is included in similar proportions, and since this reacts rapidly with water it tends to increase the rate of reaction. However, if stored for a long period this reverts to the hemihydrate by reacting with moisture in the atmosphere. Plaster in this condition is said to have matured. A number of impurities are generally present and may make up as much as 4 per cent of the product.

In addition to these basic constituents a number of specific chemical agents are included to modify the setting rate, expansion, and strength. Potassium sulphate reduces the setting expansion to an amount that is negligible but accelerates the setting reaction. Retarders are therefore added, such as borax or potassium citrate. Accelerators probably increase the solubility of calcium sulphate hemihydrate while retarders may act in the opposite way. Retarders may also act by poisoning the nuclei of crystallization by depositing a layer over the surface of the crystals. Some retarders, such as sodium citrate, also help reduce setting expansion. When gypsum products contain both accelerators and retarders they may be referred to as balanced. The constituents of a typical dental plaster are listed in Table 7.1.

**Table 7.1** Constituents of typical dental plaster

| |
| --- |
| Calcium sulphate hemihydrate |
| Calcium sulphate dihydrate |
| Soluble calcium sulphate anhydrite |
| Potassium sulphate |
| Borax |

SETTING TIME

Many factors influence the setting time of dental plaster. Some are dependent on the ingredients and the method of manufacture, others on the handling technique of the dentist or technician.

The proportion of gypsum included in the presentation alters the setting rate. By presenting more nuclei for dihydrate crystallization an increase in the amount of gypsum leads to a more rapid rate of reaction. Gypsum is generally added to the hemihydrate in controlled amounts following its production, although incomplete calcination may result in a higher concentration. Over-calcination leads to an increased amount of soluble and insoluble anhydrite. The former is fast setting and increases the rate of reaction of the product while the latter, sometimes referred to as dead-burnt plaster, has the opposite effect.

Grinding of the product to a powder with controlled particle size is undertaken by the manufacturer. The smaller the particle size the larger will be the surface area and this leads to an increased reaction rate. In addition, grinding splits the crystals of gypsum into smaller units all of which act as nuclei for crystallization with the same result on setting time.

The role of specific accelerators and retarders has already been discussed.

Handling techniques may also have an influence on the setting rate and indeed on other properties to be discussed later.

**a** *Water/powder ratio*. An increase in this ratio, that is the production of a thin mix, tends to retard the setting reaction as fewer nuclei of crystallization are present per unit volume. Theoretically the amount of water required to react with a given amount of powder can be calculated from the equation of the setting reaction. In practice, however, it is necessary to use an excess of water in order to wet the powder adequately and ensure a smooth workable mix. For dental plaster 100 g of powder are generally mixed with 50–60 ml of water.

**b** *Duration of mixing*. A mixing time of 1·0–1·5 minutes is usually sufficient to ensure thorough wetting of the powder, absorption of the water by the powder, and the production of a creamy lump-free mix. Mixing beyond this time serves to break up forming crystals, fragments of which act as additional nuclei of crystallization. Hence the setting rate is increased and a stage can be reached when the material sets as soon as mixing is stopped.

**c** *Mixing temperature*. The temperature of the water with which the plaster is mixed does not have the effect that might be expected, certainly below 50 °C. An increase in temperature leads to a reduction in the solubility of calcium sulphate hemihydrate and therefore the concentration of $Ca^{2+}$ and $SO_4^{2-}$ ions is also reduced. However, a raised temperature increases the diffusion of ions through the developing dihydrate crystals. This tends to increase the availability of ions at nuclei of crystal growth. These two factors have opposite and almost equal effects and the setting rate remains virtually unaltered.

Distinct stages in the setting reaction of dental plaster may be detected by gross observation of the setting mass. If the mix has been correctly executed, the result should be creamy and capable of being poured. Subsequently a stage, sometimes referred to as the initial set, is reached where the plaster can be carved with a knife but not moulded. Eventually the mass becomes hard and difficult to carve. This is called the final set. The time intervals between mixing and the attainment of the initial and final sets can be determined by needle penetration tests but the results are not of direct practical significance.

STRENGTH

Plaster is a relatively weak material and is unable to withstand the compressive forces in many technical procedures. Its strength, however, depends on several factors, including the way in which it is handled and the conditions under which it is tested.

The ultimate strength and hardness of set plaster are determined by its porosity. Compared with the dental stones, to be discussed later, the hemihydrate particles of plaster are large, irregular, and porous. In view of this, a higher water/powder ratio must be used to ensure efficient mixing. As a result more residual water is present in the set material and there are larger voids between the dihydrate crystals, accounting for the relative weakness of dental plaster. If an unnecessarily high water/powder ratio is used this situation is exaggerated, giving an even weaker material. The same happens if insufficient water is used, since inadequate wetting of the powder leads to the production of an incoherent crystalline structure.

The mixing time can also affect the strength of the set plaster. Inadequate mixing has much the same result as described above as the dihydrate crystals are not formed uniformly. Over-mixing tends to break up crystals as they form, giving a weaker material. As explained earlier the setting and working times are also reduced under these circumstances.

Set plaster that has been allowed to dry out displays greater compressive strength than plaster that has been kept moist (Table 7.2). Slight dissolution of the dihydrate crystals in the residual water at their junctions may occur (Fig. 7.2) allowing slight movement of crystals in relation to one another when the material is stressed. This does not happen when thorough drying out has occurred, and greater strength is achieved. The wet and dry compressive strengths of dental plasters and stones are generally quoted in promotional literature. Over the first two hours following the final set there is a considerable increase in strength.

Additives to dental plaster to modify its rate of setting and its setting expansion usually reduce its strength.

**Table 7.2** Compressive strengths of dental plaster and stones under wet and dry conditions

|  | Compressive strength (wet) MN/m² | Compressive strength (dry) MN/m² |
|---|---|---|
| Plaster | 10 | 24 |
| Stone | 35 | 70 |

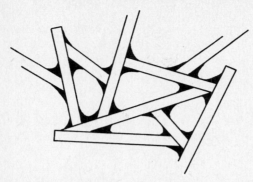

**Fig. 7.2** Residual water associated with the junctions between dihydrate crystals.

Comments have already been made concerning the water/powder ratio and its influence on the setting time, setting expansion, and strength. With experience, it is not necessary to weigh the powder for each mix as this can be gauged with reasonable ease. However, having decided upon a water/powder ratio, attempts should not be made to alter this when mixing has begun. The addition of powder to a mix that is too thin causes uneven setting and a heterogeneous material results. If water is added in an attempt to dilute a thick mix the crystal mass is weakened and broken up. The set plaster will tend to be crumbly and weak.

Mixing is carried out in a flexible rubber bowl with a broad spatula, care being taken to minimize the inclusion of air. Air voids weaken the set material and if they involve the surface of a model they detract from its accuracy. A conventional hand spatula may be used to mix plaster or a hand-operated mechanical system may be used. The latter probably produces a more uniform mix, but there is a danger that overspatulation may occur. Apparatus is available to allow the mixing of plaster in vacuum. All mixing utensils should be kept clean as a mixing bowl contaminated with set plaster debris will tend to accelerate the setting reaction by contributing additional dihydrate nuclei of crystallization.

If an impression is being poured in plaster a vibrator should be used. This brings incorporated air to the surface by encouraging settling of the mixed material. By adding the plaster in increments and allowing each to travel gradually around the impression, air incorporation is virtually eliminated.

STORAGE

Provided dental plaster is stored with care it has an indefinite shelf-life. Clearly if the powder is kept in a damp or humid atmosphere the hemihydrate will tend to revert to the dihydrate. Initially these dihydrate crystals appear on the surface of the hemihydrate powder particles. Here they act as additional nuclei of crystallization and the setting time is reduced as a result. Later the entire surface of the hemihydrate particles becomes covered and this, by reducing the access of water to the surrounded hemihydrate, retards the setting reaction. If plaster is stored in very hot, dry conditions the gypsum included by the manufacturer is slowly converted to hemihydrate. By reducing the concentration of nuclei for crystallization the setting time is prolonged. It is unlikely that the extreme conditions required to bring this about will be present in most dental laboratories.

APPLICATIONS

Plaster has many clinical and technical uses in dentistry. While the dimensional stability and surface reproducibility are good enough for its use as a model material, its strength is relatively low. Models are therefore apt to be damaged easily, especially in certain technical procedures that involve the application of a high compressive stress. In these situations the stronger dental stones are more appropriate. Plaster is used in flasking and packing acrylic resin dentures and for mounting dental stone models on articulators.

Following flasking and packing, remnants of plaster or dental stone are often difficult to remove from the completed denture. Gypsum is only sparingly soluble in water but a 30 per cent solution of ammonium citrate buffered to pH 8 is useful in removing these traces. Repeated exposure to boiling water does result in some dissolution of gypsum and there may be some loss of surface detail from models treated in this way. Boiling off wax should therefore be undertaken with care.

As outlined in Chapter 6 plaster is a useful impression material in certain circumstances, and, being white, it contrasts with the dental stones generally used as the model material. Plaster is compatible with most impression materials. However, some hydrocolloids reduce the surface hardness of plaster and stone models.

## Dental stones

Most of the comments made in the previous sections may be applied to dental stones. In this section the differences between dental stones and plaster will be discussed.

PREPARATION OF DENTAL STONES

Dental stones are based on calcium sulphate hemihydrate which, when mixed with water, sets to a hard mass of calcium sulphate dihydrate. Chemically, therefore, the setting reaction is the same as for dental plaster. However, the hemihydrate is prepared by a different method. The exact technique of preparation determines the nature of the hemihydrate and the physical properties of the final set material.

By autoclaving gypsum at 120–130 °C a form of hemihydrate is produced which is sometimes referred to as Hydrocal. On reacting with water a material with physical properties superior to plaster is produced. A further improvement in physical properties is achieved if the hemihydrate is prepared by boiling the gypsum in a 30 per cent solution of calcium or magnesium chloride. The product may be called Densite, improved dental stone or die stone. Another variety is formed by autoclaving gypsum at 140 °C with a small amount of organic acid or salt. The differences between these types is dependent on the shape, size, and size distribution of the hemihydrate particles. As better packing is achieved, less water is required for the reaction and the strength is improved. There is also reduced setting expansion, which improves the accuracy. In practice, however, it is unlikely that the differences between the categories of dental stone will be significant enough to warrant separate consideration.

Additives are present to control the setting time and expansion in much the same way as for dental plaster. Certain stones contain substances designed to increase the strength of the set material. The use of polymers, such as polyesters, polystyrene, acrylic, and epoxy resins have been suggested. Wetting agents have also been used. These allow the powder to be wetted by a smaller volume of water; the density of the set material, and therefore its strength, is increased. Lignosulphonates, derived from wood, are used in this way. An increase in the concentration of accelerator is necessary when these strengthening agents are used as they tend to increase the setting time and expansion. The setting expansion of dental stones should be 0·06–0·12 per cent.

Generally pigments are present to produce a colour contrast between the stone and dental plaster that is often used in conjunction with it.

COMPARISON WITH PLASTER

Compared with plaster the hemihydrate particles of dental stones are smaller and more regular in size and shape. They are virtually non-porous whereas plaster is porous to a considerable degree. Porosity influences the amount of water required to produce a satisfactory mix of the material. A product of high porosity requires more water for the mix and more excess water remains trapped between the resultant dihydrate crystals, and the final set is therefore weaker. For this reason plaster requires more water than stone and is not as strong. Dental stones require 22–35 ml of water per 100 g of powder, depending on the type, to produce an optimal mix.

Unlike dental plaster the reduced water/powder ratio used with dental stones should be carefully controlled and the powder should be weighed rather than estimated. Deviation from the ideal leads to a set stone of markedly reduced strength. It is possible, by mishandling the material in this way, to produce a model of lower strength than one made from plaster. Too much water in a mix of dental stone also results in greater setting expansion. The setting time of dental stone is 5–8 minutes.

## DIE MATERIALS

As explained earlier, a die is a model of a single tooth generally used in the construction of inlays, crowns, and bridges. It is used in conjunction with a model of the relevant dental arch, from which it is normally removable. The requirements of die materials follow closely those outlined in general at the beginning of the chapter but certain properties are worth emphasizing.

While the strength is important, surface hardness is of great significance as it relates to abrasion-resistance. Repeated application of instruments to the die surface may gradually alter its dimensions if the abrasion-resistance is low. This is particularly likely to occur around the margins of the preparations, where the carving of a wax pattern, for example, must be undertaken with great care. A number of techniques are specifically designed to improve the surface hardness of the die.

The need for great accuracy in the construction of the die has already been emphasized, and both dimensional stability and surface reproducibility should be good. It is desirable for dies to have a low thermal conductivity to prevent the rapid heat-loss from wax patterns prepared from them. If this does occur, differential cooling of the wax may induce internal stresses in the pattern that could result in its distortion.

Colour contrast with materials to be used on dies makes handling easier at the margins of the preparation as the technician can clearly see the junction to ensure accurate adaptation to the cavity. Unfortunately when good contrast is established with inlay waxes, which are generally dark blue or green, poor contrast exists with the tooth-coloured porcelains.

Several techniques and materials may be used in the construction of dies. To a certain extent the choice is dependent, or at least limited, by the impression material that has been employed.

### Die stones

These have been considered in the previous section. A thick mix is produced, according to the manufacturer's instructions, and vibrated into the impression. If this is of a synthetic elastomer the entire arch is usually poured in the stone and the model produced is based in a softer dental stone or plaster. With impressions of single teeth, such as a copper-ring/composition impression, the stone may be used to prepare the die that is then located in the major model which may be of a softer dental stone. Die stones should be left for 24 hours to gain their maximum hardness, although the impression may be safely removed one hour after pouring.

The abrasion-resistance of stones is not as high as with other systems, and hardening solutions may be used. Some of these can be substituted for water during mixing and may be either a resin solution or aqueous colloidal silica. Alternatively the surface of a completed stone die may be treated with liquids or varnishes. With the latter technique the surface becomes impregnated with, for example, a polymer, such as polymethyl methacrylate or polystyrene, or a liquid epoxide that subsequently polymerizes. By applying a light mineral oil to the die surface the action of the instruments is lubricated and abrasion is less likely to occur. However, these oils tend to reduce surface hardness. The presence of oil facilitates the removal of wax patterns from stone dies.

These products are usually pale in colour and contrast well with inlay wax. Porcelain is sometimes rather more difficult to distinguish from the die.

### Electro-plated dies

By electro-plating impressions prior to pouring in a material, such as a stone or resin, the resultant die displays a metallic surface. This markedly improves the surface hardness. Impressions may be copper or silver plated.

a *Copper*. This is ideally suited to composition impressions in copper rings. The surface of the impression is dried and made conductive, usually by the application of colloidal graphite or a fine metallic dust. The impression is placed in a plating bath where it acts as the cathode while the anode is copper. An acidic solution of copper sulphate is the electrolyte and a typical formulation is given in Table 7.3. Sometimes organic additives, such as ethyl alcohol or phenol, are present to increase the hardness of the deposited copper. A direct current of 2–12 V at up to 100 mA is used and plating takes 10–15 hours. Any areas not to be plated are masked with wax beforehand.

**Table 7.3** Copper plating electrolyte

| | |
|---|---|
| Copper sulphate | 212 g |
| Potassium alum | 12 g |
| Sulphuric acid | 31 ml |
| Distilled water | to 1 l |

The resulting die surface tends to be rather dark and may be discoloured by the graphite. This makes contrast poor with inlay wax, but good with porcelain. Surface hardness and reproducibility are good. Silicone impressions may be copper plated but the electrolyte reacts with polysulphide. Although this problem may be overcome using a two-stage technique, it is not usually considered satisfactory. It has been suggested that the prolonged period of plating may allow dimensional change to occur in elastomeric impressions.

b *Silver*. Silver plating is applied to the synthetic elastomers but is becoming less popular because of the toxic hazard associated with the cyanide employed. Impressions are rendered conductive by the application of a fine silver dust to the surfaces where plating is required. The composition of the electrolyte is given in Table 7.4 and the anode is silver. A current of 10 mA per tooth is used to deposit the initial layer of silver after which the current is increased to accelerate plating which takes 4–8 hours. Before the impression is poured it is thoroughly washed to remove all traces of electrolyte.

**Table 7.4** Silver plating electrolyte

| | |
|---|---|
| Silver cyanide | 36 g |
| Potassium cyanide | 60 g |
| Potassium carbonate | 40 g |
| Distilled water | to 1 l |

Impression compound reacts with the electrolyte and may not be plated with silver. Again the surface qualities are good, but the contrast with porcelain is not as satisfactory as that with the darker inlay waxes.

The electrolyte is highly poisonous and, if contaminated with acid, hydrocyanic acid fumes are liberated. In view of this serious toxic hazard the entire procedure should be carried out with extreme caution in a fume cupboard. Many laboratories do not employ this technique in view of the potential danger involved.

## Alternative die materials

RESINS

Various filled and unfilled resins may be used in die construction. They tend to have reasonable abrasion-resistance but all contract on polymerization to a greater or lesser extent, unfilled resins being worse in this respect.

**a** *Acrylic resin.* Cold-cure acrylic resin may be used to fill an electroplated die, but it is inaccurate as a result of contraction. A thin mix has to be prepared that can be dripped into the impression. The addition of powdered fillers, such as silver, copper, and porcelain offers some improvement, but not sufficient to recommend the general use of these materials.

**b** *Epoxy resins.* Products based on epoxy resin display less contraction than acrylic resin, as little as 0·1 per cent. However, they react with polysulphide impression materials.

**c** *Polyester resins.* These have a powder/liquid presentation. The powder contains a high proportion (95 per cent) of filler, such as bronze or quartz, and a benzoyl peroxide hardener. A polyester resin is present in the liquid together with an amine and dimethylanaline as an accelerator. On mixing a viscous paste is produced which has to be adapted to the impression as it cannot be poured. Polymerization is complete in about one hour but appreciable shrinkage occurs. These resins are suitable for use with silicone and composition impressions.

CERAMICS

Two types of ceramic material may be used for die construction. After mixing and placement in the impression both undergo an initial set in under an hour and are fired. One is heated to 600 °C for 8 minutes to produce maximum hardness and is quenched in light mineral oil. The second is placed in the

furnace and raised from 650 to 1015 °C at 20° per minute, after being preheated at the furnace entrance for 5 minutes. Slow cooling on the bench
should follow. This latter product allows the construction of porcelain crowns
without the use of a platinum foil matrix (Chapter 9).

## CEMENTS

These are similar to dental cements, such as the silico–phosphate cements.
These are no longer widely used in dentistry but were used as tooth-coloured
filling materials. They were, in effect, products combining some of the constituents and properties of both phosphate and silicate cements.

The dies produced have a high surface hardness but shrinkage occurs on
setting. As with silicate cement, these materials must not be allowed to dry
out if their optimal properties are to be retained. Dies should be stored in
oil.

## AMALGAM

Amalgam is discussed in detail as a filling material in Chapter 4. To produce
a die, amalgam must be condensed into the impression. Clearly if the
impression is not rigid this cannot be achieved effectively and if the shape
of the impression is complex difficulty is also encountered. Therefore amalgam
can only be used safely in simple copper-ring/composition impressions.
A 10–12 hour period should be allowed for hardening. As explained in
Chapter 4, amalgam is prone to dimensional change on setting and a
distorted die could result because of this. Amalgam dies are hard and have
good surface reproducibility provided condensation has been adequate. As
the metal has a high thermal conductivity rapid cooling of inlay wax may
occur. Warming the die slightly reduces this problem.

## BISMUTH–TIN ALLOY

A technique was developed whereby a molten bismuth–tin alloy could be
sprayed directly on to the surface of impressions. The melting-point of this
alloy is 138 °C, and great care must be exercised if it is to be applied to
impressions in thermoplastic trays. It is maintained that with care the alloy
may be used with composition impressions in copper rings without loss of
surface detail.

Coated impressions are poured in dental stones. The surface hardness of
the dies is not great and care must be taken if damage by abrasion is not
to occur. Precautions should be taken to avoid the inhalation of the metallic
spray. Because of this danger and the specialized equipment required for the
technique, this method is not widely used.

While many products have been developed, each with its own claimed
advantages, the dental stones are by far the cheapest and most effective
material for producing dies for the construction of inlays, crowns, and bridges.

## WAXES

The use of waxes as impression materials was described in the previous chapter. Clearly waxes used in this way require certain properties if they are to be successful. There are many varieties of wax for use in dentistry, both in the surgery and the laboratory, and each has very particular requirements depending on its role. While the basic constituents employed in each preparation are essentially similar, their exact proportioning is important in determining their final properties.

Laboratory procedures in the construction of dentures and many other appliances make use of wax as a modelling material. Different types of wax are used to produce patterns for alloy castings. A similar procedure for the preparation of gold crowns and inlays involves the production of a wax pattern which is subsequently reproduced in metal. This pattern may be achieved directly in the mouth or from a die in the laboratory. While these are very specific and major applications of wax, there are a great many miscellaneous uses that make it a material of considerable importance.

### VARIETIES OF WAX

Waxes occur naturally in a great many forms from animal, plant, and mineral sources. Paraffin and microcrystalline wax are distillation products of petroleum and are both hydrocarbons. Paraffin wax tends to be brittle at room temperature whereas microcrystalline wax is less so. Among the waxes from vegetable sources are carnauba and candelilla waxes. These are natural esters and are comparatively tough substances. Adhesive qualities are imparted to some preparations by the addition of natural gums and resins, such as dammar resin, and the resultant wax is also tougher. Beeswax is included in many dental waxes and tends to reduce the brittleness.

The major problem with natural products is that they are not consistent in their composition, and therefore their properties. To overcome this, synthetic waxes have been increasingly used. These can be carefully prepared under controlled conditions to give a standardized and predictable result. They may be based on polyethylene, nitrogenous derivatives of fatty acids, or may be produced by the modification of natural substances, such as petroleum. Most modern dental waxes are therefore made up of a combination of natural and synthetic products.

Waxes have a number of important properties in relation to their dental use. These properties represent the summation of those of the various constituents and their proportions in any particular material. Although different applications require different properties, waxes for the production of inlay patterns probably require the most careful balance and will serve to illustrate the more important general properties. They will therefore be considered in some detail.

## Inlay wax

The lost-wax casting technique is described in Chapter 10. In order to prepare a gold restoration a wax replica or pattern must first be produced. This may be achieved by filling the prepared cavity with wax, which is carved to the desired shape and removed. Alternatively an impression of the prepared tooth may be used to produce a model on which the wax pattern is made. The former method is called the direct technique, the latter the indirect technique.

### COMPOSITION OF INLAY WAX

The main constituent of inlay wax is paraffin wax, which makes up 40–60 per cent. Most products contain carnauba wax and dammar resin, and may have beeswax and candelilla wax in addition to some synthetics. Pigments are included to produce colour contrast with tooth substance. The exact proportions of these constituents is of great importance in determining the final properties of the product, but this information is not disclosed by manufacturers. Paraffin wax is used to establish the melting-point, as different varieties, each with a different melting-point, can be produced. Dammar resin toughens the inlay wax and makes it smoother and more resistant to flaking. Surface finish is improved by carnauba wax, which also decreases the flow at mouth temperature as it is hard and has a relatively high melting-point. In some products synthetic waxes, compatible with paraffin wax, replace some of the carnauba wax. By appropriate proportioning of the constituent waxes a product that fulfils, as far as possible, the desirable properties of inlay wax is achieved.

### REQUIREMENTS OF INLAY WAX

**a** *Thermal properties.* Waxes have relatively high coefficients of thermal expansion. Therefore, on removal of a wax pattern from mouth to room temperature contraction will occur to as much as 0·6 per cent. This should be minimized in order to reduce dimensional error from this source. It is not possible to eliminate this effect, and techniques to compensate must be employed during investing and casting (Chapter 10). Clearly when inlay wax is used by the technician during the indirect technique the pattern is handled at room temperature throughout and contraction is correspondingly reduced.

In order to ensure thorough and uniform softening of the wax prior to insertion into the cavity or die it must be heated evenly. Wax has a low thermal conductivity and adequate time must be allowed for this to happen.

**b** *Changes on heating.* As wax is warmed it undergoes progressive softening and its flow consequently increases. With continued warming the melting-point is reached and the wax liquefies. The temperature at which a wax begins to soften and flow is referred to as the solid–solid transition temperature. Between this and the melting-point the wax can be moulded without flaking or tearing. Within this temperature range the crystalline structure is altered from a more stable, orthorhombic crystal lattice to a less stable hexagonal form. The transition temperature for dental waxes is not clearly defined, as the individual constituents have their own different transition temperatures, and gradual softening of the wax occurs as more components reach their transition temperature. The cooling curve of a typical inlay wax is shown in Figure 7.3.

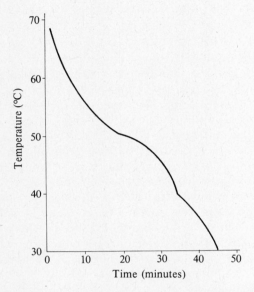

**Fig. 7.3** Cooling curve for a typical inlay wax. The 40–50° range displays the transition temperatures of the constituent waxes.

With inlay wax it is essential that maximum flow should be achieved at a temperature a few degrees above that of the mouth. If flow is inadequate the wax will not record the fine detail of the cavity surface. At the same time, flow should be minimal at mouth temperature to prevent distortion of the pattern on removal from the tooth. Ideally all the constituents of the wax should have transition temperatures above, and some close to, that of the mouth. Wax can safely be placed in the mouth without damaging the tissues at 45 °C and therefore optimal flow should be available at this temperature.

**c** *Carving qualities.* The constitution of inlay wax should be such that it can be carved with an unheated instrument at mouth temperature without flaking and distortion, even when it is in thin section. The accurate carving of the margins of patterns for gold crowns and inlays is facilitated by good colour contrast between the wax and the tooth or die. Inlay waxes are therefore generally dark blue or green.

**d** *Residue on heating.* The invested wax pattern is placed in a furnace and raised to a high temperature before casting is carried out. This results in expansion of the investment, which compensates to some extent for contraction of the wax pattern and casting. As the temperature of the furnace is gradually raised the wax within the investment melts and eventually ignites. It is important that no residue remains at this stage either in the mould cavity, where loss of detail in the casting would occur, or within the surrounding investment, which would reduce its porosity. At 500 °C no more than 0·1 per cent of the original weight of the pattern should remain.

Inlay waxes are sometimes used to prepare patterns for restorations such as acrylic jacket crowns. There is a danger that as the wax is boiled out of the mould some of the pigments remain behind. These could affect the appearance of the crown. Tooth-coloured inlay waxes are therefore available, and they are termed non-residual wax.

MANIPULATION OF INLAY WAX

For maximum reproduction of the internal features of the inlay cavity the wax must exhibit high flow at the time of insertion. As explained earlier, this is achieved by ensuring thorough and uniform softening of the wax. Without this, distortion of the pattern will follow the release of internal stresses. Inlay wax, which is presented as small sticks, is usually softened directly over a flame. Softening often takes several minutes with this method and there is a danger that the superficial layer of wax may melt completely. If this occurs volatile constituents may be lost, which interferes with the physical properties of the wax. Although uniform softening may be achieved by immersing the wax in warm water this technique is not recommended. Soluble components may be leached out, with consequential changes to the properties of the wax, but perhaps more importantly water may be incorporated. If this occurs it is difficult to achieve a smooth finish and the application of a warm instrument results in a spluttering effect when contaminated areas are involved.

To minimize internal stresses the wax should be allowed to cool gradually to mouth temperature, rather than applying cold water to its surface. Rapid cooling results in differential contraction and the development of internal stresses.

The localized reheating of the wax with a warm carving instrument, especially when pooling occurs, has a similar effect and more distortion may result. For this reason it is often recommended that the carving of wax patterns should be undertaken with a cold instrument. However, in the laboratory, with the indirect technique, a warmed instrument is generally used by the technician.

Theoretically if molten wax was poured into the die and allowed to solidify, very little residual stress would occur. However, the large temperature-drop would result in considerable contraction, with obvious consequences. If molten wax is allowed to solidify under pressure the effects of this contraction can be reduced. By using an inlay wax with a softening temperature of 28–32 °C a smaller fall in temperature is involved and less contraction occurs. Clearly this wax may only be used for the indirect technique as it would remain soft at mouth temperature.

Wax patterns should be removed with great care from the tooth or die to minimize distortion. Withdrawal should be in the long axis of the cavity and rocking or tilting movements must be avoided. It is usual to remove wax patterns from the die with the sprue. This is a piece of wire or tubing to which the pattern is attached for investment. Before the inlay is cast the sprue is removed and gold enters the investment mould through the resulting channel (Fig. 10.3). The configuration of the pattern and its orientation in the mouth often allows it to be removed from the cavity on the sprue with the direct technique. To facilitate removal of the pattern from the die, a separating medium, such as a dilute detergent or a light oil, is used. In the mouth a thin film of saliva is just as effective. Sprues are inserted into the pattern in the region of greatest bulk to allow the rapid and unimpeded flow of alloy into the mould.

Having withdrawn the wax pattern from the cavity it should be invested as soon as possible. Inevitably some internal stresses are present and these result in distortion. The longer the pattern is left the greater will be the relaxation of these stresses. Stress release occurs more readily at higher temperatures and wax patterns should be kept in a cool environment to minimize distortion. By far the most effective way of achieving this is to invest the wax pattern immediately after its removal from the tooth or die. In patterns of more complex restorations even a slight distortion will result in a poorly adapted casting.

### Sheet casting wax

This presentation is in the form of thin sheets which are available in different gauges to allow the technician to produce castings of known dimensions. Usually each different thickness has its own characteristic colour for easy identification in the laboratory. Clearly the advantages of such a system are easily lost if the product is mishandled. Great care should be taken not to overheat or over-compress the wax as its thickness will be altered. To avoid overheating, the wax should be softened in warm water, not over a flame. As with inlay wax, there should be no residue in the investment mould prior to casting.

### Sticky wax

Sticky wax is a hard brittle product and, as its title suggests, it has some adhesive qualities. It is based on beeswax and resins, the latter contributing to its stickiness. At room temperature sticky wax has minimal flow and its melting-point is 60–65 °C. On cooling it should not undergo excessive shrinkage. There are several miscellaneous uses of sticky wax, mainly in the laboratory. Separate components of bridges may be located together rigidly prior to being invested and soldered together. The wax should therefore boil or burn out leaving no residue.

### Carding wax

Carding wax displays high flow at room temperature, and can therefore be moulded without heat. Manufacturers supply denture teeth attached to cards with this wax and this practice gave rise to the title. Carding wax is used mainly in the laboratory where a common application is the boxing in of impressions prior to pouring in dental stone.

### Modelling wax

Modelling waxes are used extensively during denture construction for the production of registration blocks and try-in dentures. For this reason they are coloured pink to impart some basic aesthetic quality. Paraffin wax is the main constituent, making up 70–80 per cent. The remainder is a combination of waxes, but beeswax and carnauba wax are generally present.

When softened, modelling wax should be mouldable without tearing or flaking. The softening temperature is 49–58 °C and the product should be hard, exhibiting little flow at mouth temperature. Repeated softening should be possible without detriment to the physical properties, and the wax should be carvable. As modelling wax is used as a pattern material for dentures it must not leave a residue on boiling out of the plaster mould.

Although small dimensional changes in denture modelling waxes do not have the same consequences as those occuring in inlay wax they should nevertheless be minimized. Therefore little change in dimension should occur from mouth to room temperature. Thorough and uniform softening is again important if internal stresses are not to lead to distortion.

### Alternative baseplate materials

When greater strength and rigidity than that offered by modelling wax is required to support registration blocks and try-in dentures other baseplate materials may be employed.

Cold or heat-cured acrylic resin may be used (Chapter 11). A carefully constructed heat-cured acrylic resin baseplate may be subsequently incorporated in the completed denture.

Shellac resin, used with added fillers, is a thermoplastic material with a higher softening temperature than waxes. It is therefore more stable at mouth temperature. However, it is important to ensure adequate softening during construction to minimize the formation of internal stresses that would distort the overlying registration block or wax denture. Shellac with metallic fillers may also be used to produce special trays for impressions.

# 8
## Casting alloys in conservative dentistry

Inlays, crowns, bridges, and, indeed, partial dentures, are restorations that can be made entirely or partly from metals and are fabricated outside the mouth. They therefore have to be made very accurately to fit the shape of the prepared teeth. The availability of metallic materials for such applications is extremely limited because of the very specific requirements involved. These may be grouped as follows.

### Requirements of casting alloys

**a** The metal must have the ability to be shaped very accurately to a model, which clearly will be different for each patient. The restoration is generally small and may be of complex shape so that casting is the only production method that is suitable. This involves melting the metal and pouring it into a mould preformed to the exact size and shape required. Many factors govern the ability of a metal to be cast the most important of which are:

**i** *The melting-point.* High melting-points require complex equipment, and although dental laboratories are very versatile, it is impractical to use materials with melting-points greater than about 1400–1450 °C, and preferable to work at temperatures closer to 1000 °C.

**ii** *The reactivity in the molten state.* Many molten metals are highly reactive, either with the atmosphere or with the refractory mould material. Either non-reactive metals have to be chosen or a vacuum or inert atmosphere used for their protection.

**iii** *The melting range.* As noted in Chapter 1, alloys with grossly different component metals may exhibit large differences between their liquidus and solidus, giving a wide melting range. This poses difficulties in casting for it is not always easy to detect complete melting in this situation. Furthermore, considerable segregation, or coring, may occur on cooling.

**iv** *The casting shrinkage.* All metals contract as they freeze and then cool to room temperature, but it is desirable, both to facilitate the production of accurate castings and to prevent porosity, that shrinkage should be kept to a low level.

**v** *The surface finish.* Castings usually have a fairly rough surface and ideally the metal should be amenable to finishing processes.

**b** The metal must have good mechanical properties. The exact requirements will depend on the nature of the restoration. Generally the strength required, both in terms of the proportional limit and the ultimate tensile strength, increases with their size and complexity, from simple inlays to large bridges or partial dentures. A degree of ductility is required, which presents some problems, as cast metals are normally quite brittle. This is most relevant in the case of partial dentures which will be discussed in Chapter 10.

The optimal elastic modulus is a matter of some controversy. Clearly there are many parts of a restoration that need to be rigid and in which a high modulus is required. As noted later, this is not necessarily the case with clasps on partial dentures and it is often suggested that an elastic modulus equivalent to that of enamel or especially dentine is appropriate for a restoration. It is not possible, therefore, to specify the required elastic modulus, although it is usual to assume, at this stage, that a reasonably high modulus is the most desirable.

c Some of these restorations are clearly visible and should therefore have a good appearance. It is, of course, impossible to produce metals with the colour of the natural dentition and so the main criterion is the ability of the material to retain a high lustre. This is related to corrosion and tarnish-resistance.

d It is important that these metals are resistant to tarnish and corrosion, for three reasons. First, a tarnished surface is usually less pleasing than a polished one; secondly, corrosion could affect the mechanical properties; and thirdly, the released corrosion products could elicit an undesirable reaction in the adjacent soft tissue.

e As with all restorative materials, these casting alloys must be easily tolerated by the oral tissues. All of the usual features of biocompatibility have to be considered, especially hypersensitivity, since many metals, including nickel and cobalt, are known sensitizers. It is important that, where complex alloys are used, all the constituents are considered in this way.

f Some metals are very expensive; and quite frequently it is the expensive metals that possess the necessary properties for application in the oral environment. Costs, therefore, do have some significance, as discussed later.

g Although a metallic surface is aesthetically acceptable to some people, most restorations involving anterior teeth are made from a tooth-coloured material. For crowns this is usually porcelain. As discussed in Chapter 9, it is common practice to bond porcelain to a metallic substructure to provide a strong and aesthetic restoration. In these situations it is essential that a bond is established between the metal and the porcelain, and this is an important factor controlling the composition of the metallic material used.

It will be recalled from Chapter 1 that pure metals have very limited applications because of their lack of strength. Therefore, it is necessary to use alloys rather than pure metals in order to achieve a suitable combination of properties. The requirements of these particular situations are so demanding, in fact, that very few alloy systems could be considered suitable. With the previously mentioned properties in mind, three types of alloy used in the preparation of indirect restorations can be described.

Of the three types, gold alloys are the most commonly used, in spite of their cost. The search for alternatives to gold has led to the development of the so-called non-precious dental casting alloys, one group being based on nickel and the other on cobalt. The latter are more widely used in partial denture construction and are discussed in Chapter 10. The remainder of this chapter concentrates on those alloys used in conservative dentistry, that is for inlay, crown, and bridgework. The techniques and laboratory materials used in the casting of dental alloys are discussed in detail in Chapter 10.

## GOLD ALLOYS

Gold is an obvious choice of metal for restorative dentistry on account of its nobility and colour. The appearance of gold has always been considered pleasing and is associated with quality. The ability of gold to retain a lustre without tarnishing is almost unique. In addition to this it has a suitably low melting-point and appears to have good biocompatibility.

Pure gold has two disadvantages in the context of restorative dentistry. First, it is expensive, and secondly, in common with most pure metals, it is soft and ductile and unsuitable for even moderately stressed conditions. Little can be done about the first of these problems. On the other hand gold can be alloyed with certain elements to give much better mechanical properties without significant detriment to the other properties. Provided, therefore, the expense does not preclude their use, gold alloys are the materials of choice for these applications. Although the non-precious casting alloys discussed later can be considered as alternative materials, they do not give restorations of the same quality. It is interesting to note that any decrease in the use of gold for these restorations has been due to developments in other restorative techniques rather than superior alternative alloys. For example, large restorations in anterior teeth can now be achieved with composite materials, described in Chapter 5, and most patients would prefer the tooth-coloured appearance to that of gold. Similarly pin-retained amalgams are frequently used in posterior teeth where gold inlays might previously have been chosen.

### Composition of gold alloys

Dental casting gold alloys are usually classified according to their mechanical properties, which depend on their composition. Normally four classes of alloy, termed Types I, II, III, and IV are distinguished; the normal range of composition for these groups being given in Table 8.1. It is clear from this table that the amount of gold and the total amount of noble metal generally decreases, while the amount of non-noble metal increases, from Type I to Type IV. The most important factor here is the balance between

**Table 8.1** Range of compositions for Types I–IV gold alloys

| Type | Composition (%) | | | | | |
|---|---|---|---|---|---|---|
| | Au | Ag | Cu | Pd | Pt | Zn |
| I | 80–95 | 2–12 | 1·5–6 | 0–3·6 | 0–1 | 0–1·2 |
| II | 73–83 | 7–14·5 | 5·8–10 | 0–5·6 | 0–4·2 | 0–1·4 |
| III | 71–80 | 5–13·5 | 7–12·5 | 0–6·5 | 0–7·5 | 0–2·0 |
| IV | 62–72 | 8–17·5 | 8·5–15 | 0–10 | 0·2–8·2 | 0–2·7 |

the appearance, nobility, and castability of the gold and the strengthening effects of the alloying additions. In general the greater the amount of these alloying elements the greater the strength, but this is also associated with a lower corrosion-resistance, a poorer aesthetic appearance, and, in some cases, increased difficulty in casting. The range of alloys available allows the correct balance to be chosen for any particular situation.

It should be noted here that some gold alloys are available which deviate considerably from the composition given in Table 8.1 but which conform to the mechanical property specifications of these groups. These are the so-called white gold alloys, which are considered separately.

The significance of the elements present in casting gold alloys is as follows.

*Gold.* As noted above, gold as the parent metal provides the corrosion and tarnish-resistance, the biocompatibility, and the desirable appearance. With a melting-point of 1063 °C, the casting is easily achieved in the dental laboratory.

*Copper.* Copper is added to increase the strength of the gold. The gold–copper phase diagram is illustrated in Figure 8.1, which shows that a solid solution is formed at all compositions. The slightly differing atomic sizes of these two elements should give a small solid solution hardening effect, by the mechanism described in Chapter 1. A much more significant increase in strength is achieved under certain conditions when the AuCu ordered phase shown in Figure 8.1 becomes stable. This strengthening mechanism is an extremely important factor in the properties of dental casting gold alloys and is considered in detail later.

It will be noted from Figure 8.1 that the addition of copper up to a composition of 20 per cent by weight decreases the melting-point and, since there is very little temperature difference between the liquidus and solidus, casting should still be straightforward. The reddish colour of copper is imparted to the alloy, which places a limit on the amount that can be added. Simultaneously the copper decreases the tarnish-resistance to such an extent that, for acceptable properties, it has to be kept below about 16 per cent. It is generally agreed that the total amount of noble metals present should not be lower than 75 per cent if satisfactory corrosion and tarnish-resistance are to be maintained.

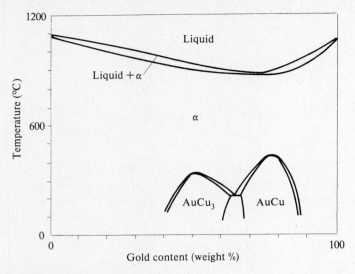

**Fig. 8.1** Simplified gold–copper phase diagram.

*Silver.* Silver is the other major alloying element. This plays only a small part in the strengthening process, the gold and silver being so similar that a solid solution is formed over the whole range of composition with little solid solution hardening. In the presence of other elements it may form dispersed phases and contribute to the precipitation hardening effects discussed below. The main virtue of the silver concerns the appearance of the alloy, as it tends to counteract the reddish colour of the copper. In large amounts silver has a harmful effect on the tarnish-resistance.

*Platinum and palladium.* Platinum is added to the gold–copper–silver alloy to give further improvement to the strength. This is achieved by the precipitation of a platinum-rich phase. The presence of such a second dispersed phase gives a much more significant strengthening effect than with solid solution hardening alone, as described in Chapter 1. The more effective precipitates are produced when copper is present in the alloy.

The potential strengthening effect is quite considerable in this system, but the amount of platinum that can be incorporated into the alloy is limited by several factors. First, it is expensive and generally increases the cost of the alloy. Secondly, it has a high melting-point and would increase the melting-point of the alloy considerably if present in large amounts. Thirdly, there is a large gap between the liquidus and solidus in the gold–platinum alloys, as expected from a combination of high and relatively low melting-point metals, so that casting would result in a heterogeneous alloy, especially if the platinum content was greater than 10 per cent.

Fortunately, palladium can be added to the alloy instead of, or in addition to, small quantities of platinum, having a substantial strengthening effect itself and being much cheaper. However, it also has a high melting-point and this limits the proportion that can be incorporated. Both platinum and palladium have a considerable whitening effect on the alloy and tend to counteract the detrimental effect of copper on the tarnish-resistance.

*Zinc.* The function of zinc in these alloys is much the same as its function in amalgam alloys since it is used as a scavanger, preventing oxidation of the metals on melting. It generally improves the castability of the alloys. Indium and possibly tin may also be used in small amounts for the same purpose.

*Other elements.* One of the main problems with many castings is the tendency to produce a coarse grain-size, which reduces the strength of the alloy. This is particularly important where the metal is used in thin section where a single grain cross-section is quite possible. Many manufacturers make small additions, usually much less than 0·5 per cent, of high melting-point elements, such as iridium, ruthenium, or rhenium to give a fine-grained casting.

### Properties of dental gold alloys

These will be dealt with in terms of the requirements outlined earlier.

EASE OF CASTING

The melting-point of a gold alloy depends on its composition but rarely differs from that of pure gold (1063 °C) by more than 150 °C in either direction. Representative figures for the four classes of alloy are given in Table 8.2. The higher values of melting-point are obtained with the higher platinum and palladium content. Generally a gas–air or gas–oxygen torch is suitable for melting the alloys. Technical details of the process are given later.

**Table 8.2** Melting-points for gold alloys

| Type | Range of melting-point (°C) |
| --- | --- |
| I | 1100–1180 |
| II | 920–970 |
| III | 900–960 |
| IV | 880–950 |

Gold is not a reactive metal, even at high temperatures, but there may be a tendency for some of the alloying additions to oxidize. However, the presence of the zinc or other scavengers in the alloy minimizes this tendency. Oxidation is also prevented by the use of fluxes during the melting and by using the reducing part of the flame.

As noted above, the gold–copper and gold–silver alloy systems have only slight differences between liquidus and solidus temperatures, so that the casting should be relatively easy and the result quite homogeneous. However, the presence of higher melting-point metals, such as platinum and palladium, does give a larger gap, and it is generally agreed that an homogenizing anneal is desirable. A temperature in the region of 700 °C, maintained for 10 minutes, is adequate for this purpose.

In common with all metals gold alloys contract on casting, due both to the shrinkage inherent in the solidification process and to the contraction that occurs on cooling to room temperature. The amount of contraction observed varies only slightly with the alloy composition, falling within the range of 1·3–1·6 per cent linear contraction. In theory this can be readily compensated for by the use of appropriate investments, as discussed in Chapter 10. Whilst this should therefore present no clinical problems, inaccuracies do arise from this source and may lead to a poor fit of the restoration.

Finally, gold-alloy castings are readily cleaned and finished to give a bright and smooth surface. This is in contrast to some base metal alloys which are very hard and therefore more difficult to finish.

**Table 8.3** Range of mechanical properties in gold alloys

| Type | Condition | 0·1% proof strength MN/m² | U.T.S. MN/m² | Elongation % | Vickers Hardness Number |
|------|-----------|---------------------------|--------------|--------------|-------------------------|
| I    | As cast   | 60–150                    | 200–310      | 20–35        | 40–70                   |
| II   | As cast   | 150–250                   | 310–380      | 20–35        | 70–100                  |
| III  | As cast   | 180–260                   | 330–390      | 20–25        | 90–130                  |
|      | Hardened  | 280–350                   | 410–560      | 6–20         | 115–170                 |
| IV   | As cast   | 300–390                   | 410–520      | 4–25         | 130–160                 |
|      | Hardened  | 550–680                   | 690–830      | 1–6          | 200–240                 |

MECHANICAL PROPERTIES

The range of mechanical properties obtained with these gold alloys is given in Table 8.3. It is convenient to consider them in two groups. First, in Types I and II, the increased strength compared to pure gold is due primarily to the solid solution hardening effects associated with the copper and silver in the gold lattice and to a lesser extent to the precipitation hardening effect produced by dispersed second phases, such as the platinum-rich phase mentioned earlier. Manufacturers usually supply a range of alloy compositions which conform to the Types I and II specifications but which have a range of strengths depending on the relative proportions of copper, silver, and the other elements. In contrast to Types III and IV alloys these materials cannot be hardened by any heat treatment so that the properties obtained on casting represent the best that can be achieved. A little work hardening may result from extensive burnishing operations. This is not uniform and is not particularly desirable and may be eliminated by an annealing treatment at about 700 °C. These alloys are, therefore, generally used in the soft state.

Types III and IV alloys may be produced with considerably greater strengths. In the as-cast or soft condition, the improvement in their strength compared to Types I and II is due to the higher concentration of alloying elements and especially to the greater contribution from the precipitation hardening effect. They may, however, be hardened by a heat treatment, which alters the arrangement of the atoms in the crystal structure.

*Heat hardening of gold alloys.* It will be recalled from Chapter 1 that the atoms in a substitutional solid solution are randomly dispersed in the lattice. That is, if atoms of element B are added to the crystal lattice of element A, as in Figure 8.2a, they will occupy sites in this lattice at random; there is no particular order to the distribution of the different atoms. The strengthening is achieved by virtue of the slight disruption the B-atoms cause in the A-atom lattice, which makes the relative movement of the atomic layers more difficult. The precise location of the B-atoms does not matter, provided there is a random distribution.

In a few alloy systems the alloying element is not randomly dispersed,

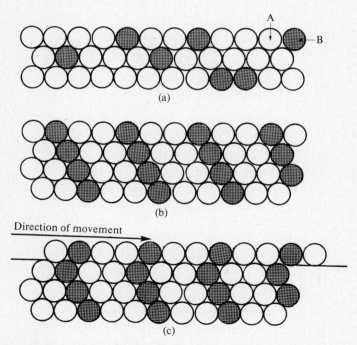

**Fig. 8.2** (a) Random distribution of atoms of element B in lattice of element A, giving disordered, or random, solid solution; (b) ordered distribution of B atoms in A; (c) effect of slip on arrangement of atoms in ordered structure.

giving a situation such as that in Figure 8.2b where the B-atoms now occupy specific sites. To do this, the ordered structure must clearly have a lower internal energy than the random structure. This implies that a certain amount of extra energy will be needed to distort the ordered arrangement. It is, therefore, more difficult to produce plastic deformation in the structure since the applied stress has to supply this extra energy in addition to that normally required to cause movement of the atoms. In Figure 8.2c, for example, the upper rows of atoms have moved under the stress, producing a totally different atomic arrangement at the slip plane. This situation is similar to that with ceramics, discussed in Chapter 1, where the juxtaposition of like ions inhibits plastic deformation.

It follows, therefore, that an ordered alloy structure should be stronger than the corresponding disordered alloy of the same composition. Fortunately the gold–copper system provides one of the few situations where an ordered structure can be produced, and this is the basis of the heat-hardening process in dental gold alloys.

Although the gold–copper phase diagram (Fig. 8.1) shows complete solid solubility, two discrete areas can be identified corresponding to two quite specific ordered phases. Clearly any one ordered structure cannot exist over a wide range of composition as there has to be a certain number of atoms of each type in the lattice. In the gold–copper system, two ordered phases, corresponding to the atomic formulae $AuCu_3$ and $AuCu$ exist. The $AuCu_3$ phase has a lattice in which there are three atoms of copper to every atom of gold, arranged in regular manner. Since this proportion of copper is too high to maintain adequate corrosion-resistance in the mouth, this phase is not normally encountered in dental gold alloys.

On the other hand, the $AuCu$ phase, involving equal numbers of gold and copper atoms, is produced over a composition range of about 65–89 weight per cent gold, and is therefore of interest in these alloys. The gold and copper atoms are arranged in a face-centred tetragonal crystal structure (similar to a face-centred cubic structure, but elongated in one direction) as illustrated by the unit cell in Figure 8.3a. Five copper atoms occupy the corners and centre of the top face and also the bottom face, with gold atoms placed at the centre of the side faces. The arrangement of the atoms in the structure is best seen by extending the unit cell, as in Figure 8.3b, where the equal numbers of gold and copper atoms become evident. In effect the gold atoms and copper atoms form two interpenetrating lattices, to give a structure known as a 'superlattice'. This indicates quite clearly the difficulty of producing deformation in an ordered structure.

It can be seen from Figure 8.1 that at least 11 per cent copper is needed to produce an ordered phase; this is the reason why hardening by this process cannot be achieved in the low-copper Types I and II alloys. Also the phase is produced only below about 400 °C. Therefore, as a Type III or IV alloy cools from the melting-point, it first solidifies as a random solid solution, and only when it cools below 400 °C can it become ordered.

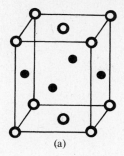

(a)

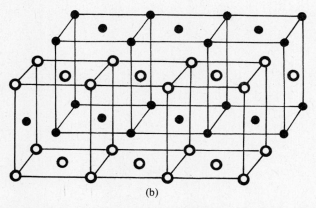

(b)

**Fig. 8.3** (a) Unit cell of face-centred tetragonal crystal structure of AuCu with copper atoms (open circles) at the corners and centre of bottom and top faces and gold atoms at centre of side faces; (b) space lattice in AuCu indicating nature of superlattice.

However, it takes quite a long time for the copper and gold atoms to diffuse from their random sites to their places in the superlattice, even at 400 °C. A random solution at room temperature would never transform, because the atoms have insufficient thermal energy for diffusion. Thus, if the alloy is rapidly cooled, or quenched, it will be retained in the random or soft condition. Values for the properties of these Type III and IV alloys in this condition are included in Table 8.3. In order to produce the ordered phase, the alloys have to be heat treated, technical details of which are given later. Basically this involves maintaining the casting, which has previously been quenched, at a suitably high temperature to allow diffusion of the atoms. This is best achieved at a temperature just below the phase limit, 300 °C for 30 minutes being typical.

Type III alloys have only just sufficient copper to enable heat hardening to be achieved, and, as indicated in Table 8.3, the improvement in strength over the softened condition is not very great. However, with Type IV alloys, the increase is quite substantial, the maximum ultimate tensile strength, approaching 800 MN/m², being very respectable for an engineering alloy.

As with any hardening process, the heat hardening of gold alloys is also associated with a substantial loss of ductility. Nevertheless, the lowest value, of around 9 or 10 per cent appears to be quite adequate.

*Heat treatment of gold alloys.* Although only Type III and Type IV can be heat hardened, it is recommended that all gold alloys should be given an annealing treatment, typically 10–15 minutes at 700 °C to remove internal stresses and homogenize the structure. There are two basic ways of hardening Types III and IV alloys. The first is sometimes described as self hardening, which involves cooling the casting slowly to room temperature rather than giving the more usual rapid quench in water. Although this generally gives satisfactory results, the lack of proper control of the temperature means that the hardening may not be uniform throughout the restoration, especially if it involves a number of units of differing bulk.

The second method, which is more suitable for more complex restorations, involves annealing at 700 °C for 10 minutes, following by quenching, and then reheating to 350 °C for 30 minutes or so to achieve the hardening. This is a more controlled process. A modification of this method sometimes used involves heating to 550–600 °C, corresponding to a dull red heat, and cooling slowly under cover. Obviously there is less control when using this method. It should be noted that with a few alloys care has to be taken to avoid over-hardening by, for example, cooling too slowly, as this would result in a significant loss of ductility. The manufacturer normally warns the user of the product should this danger exist with an alloy.

*Hardness of gold alloys.* It is usual to quote hardness values in addition to, or even instead of, values for the strength of these alloys. These figures are indicated in Table 8.1, from which it can be seen that hardness and strength are directly related, as indicated in Chapter 1. To put these values in perspective, the Vickers Hardness Number of 50 for a Type I and the maximum of 280 for hardened Type IV compare with 70 for dentine and 300 for enamel.

*Elastic modulus of gold alloys.* The variation in elastic modulus of these alloys is small compared with the difference in strength, hardness, and ductility. This is quite usual, for strengthening mechanisms rarely effect the elastic modulus by any appreciable amount. The Young's modulus for Type I alloy is about 75 GN/m² while that of a hardened Type IV alloy is in the region of 100 GN/m².

More significantly, this range of elastic modulus is considerably lower than for many base metal engineering alloys. The cobalt and nickel-based alloys used as alternatives to gold for dental castings have moduli between 200 and 250 GN/m².

AESTHETICS

The effect of alloying additions on the appearance of gold has already been discussed. A range of yellow colours is available, depending on the composition, these being described as pinkish yellow, pale yellow, straw yellow, rich yellow, and so on.

CORROSION AND TARNISH-RESISTANCE

Similarly the effect of copper, silver, and platinum group metals on corrosion and tarnish-resistance has been covered earlier. In general a well produced casting in any of the gold alloys should not tarnish or corrode in the mouth. The one situation which does predispose to tarnishing is a heterogeneous or cored structure. This may arise in the higher platinum or palladium alloys but, of course, a homogenizing anneal should be used to obviate this problem.

It should also be noted that galvanic corrosion may arise if a gold alloy restoration comes into contact with a base metal alloy restoration, such as an amalgam filling. This, however, will result in accelerated corrosion of the base metal, which will become anodic with respect to the gold.

BIOCOMPATIBILITY

The extensive clinical experience with gold alloys in dentistry has shown that they have little or no harmful effect on the oral tissues. This arises largely from the nobility of the gold itself. The presence of copper, and to a lesser extent silver, could conceivably reduce the biocompatibility, but there is no evidence to suggest this is a problem. Very occasionally a patient may display a hypersensitivity response to the alloy, but such cases are extremely rare.

COST

The very high cost of gold is an important factor which may be considered a disadvantage. It has certainly provided motivation in the search for alternative alloys. Moreover, the high cost of the laboratory and additional clinical stages involved have to be added to that of the alloy, but the widespread use of precious metal alloys would suggest their cost is not yet prohibitive.

BONDING TO PORCELAIN

As discussed in Chapter 9, modifications may be readily made to these gold alloys to enable them to bond with porcelain with very effective results.

## White gold

A number of so-called 'white' gold alloys are used in dentistry which have compositions differing from those normally associated with Type I–IV alloys but which nevertheless can be produced with the same mechanical properties.

In these cases the manufacturer will describe the product as conforming to the mechanical property specifications of a particular type of gold alloy.

As the name implies, these alloys are pale in colour, this being due to the presence of substantial amounts of other elements, especially palladium and silver, at the expense of some of the gold. There are two types of white gold alloy. The first is similar in composition to the Type IV alloy, usually having just a little less gold and a little more platinum and especially palladium, and is still pale yellow. The second type is more common and contains much less gold. In fact, the two principal elements are silver and palladium and the total gold content may be less than 30 per cent. A usual composition range is 18–24 per cent palladium, 28–45 per cent silver, 16–29 per cent gold, and 14–20 per cent copper. They are silver in colour. These alloys are available in both the hardening and non-hardening varieties and tend to be relatively strong but less ductile than the normal gold alloys. They are particularly prone to the over-hardening mentioned earlier.

The advantage of these materials lies in the lower cost, although it is also claimed that some patients prefer the white colour to that of gold. One disadvantage is that they tend to have higher melting-points due to the palladium content.

### Applications of gold alloys

Obviously the use to which any gold alloy is put depends on its mechanical properties.

Generally Type I alloys are used for inlays, especially those which are subjected to low stresses. Manufacturers often provide a range of Type I alloys from which one of the appropriate strength can be chosen. Because they are soft, these alloys can be readily burnished in the mouth in order to improve marginal adaptation.

Type II alloys are harder and stronger and can be used for most inlays except those that have thin sections. In this situation Type III alloys are preferred since they have higher strengths to resist the stresses that are encountered. Type III alloys are also used for the full and partial veneer crowns that are often used in bridgework and occasionally for saddles, connectors, and clasps in partial dentures.

While Type IV gold alloys, with the highest strength, may be used for restorations of thin section exposed to high stresses, Type III alloys are generally adequate and are easier to finish and burnish accurately. However, the construction of cast cores and posts may be undertaken most reliably with the former. The properties of these alloys make them suitable for partial denture construction but, as explained in Chapter 10, alternative materials are generally used.

### Gold alloy solders

It is technically difficult to cast an entire bridge in one piece with sufficient accuracy to give a precise fit. It may be advisable to cast a complex bridge in a number of sections, which may then be accurately soldered together. Soldering is a process used to join metals in which a filler metal, known as the solder, fuses and bonds to the parts to be joined. The requirements of a gold solder, therefore, are the same as those of the gold alloy used in the casting, with the additional characteristics associated with low-temperature fusion.

Among the most important of these extra requirements is that the fusion temperature should be lower than that of the casting alloy. Usually a solder will fuse at a temperature about 50–100 °C below the melting-point of the casting alloy. Clearly it would be undesirable to use a solder that fused very close to the melting-point of the castings as the latter might start to melt and distort. Equally important, the molten solder must be free flowing. That is, it should have a high fluidity and a surface tension which will allow efficient wetting of the surfaces to be joined, just as discussed for general adhesion phenomena in Chapter 2.

The strength of a soldered joint depends to a large extent on its soundness, especially at the interface between the solder and the casting. This is controlled not only by the wetting ability but also by the behaviour of the solder subsequent to melting. For example, overheating of a solder rich in base metals may result in void formation at the interface due to volatilization of these metals. Ideally, of course, the strength of the soldered joint should be at least the same as that of the casting alloy itself.

It is obviously desirable that the solder should have the same colour and tarnish-resistance as the casting alloy. In practice it is difficult to obtain an exact colour match, but slight differences should not be noticed after polishing. While all gold alloys have good tarnish-resistance, problems could theoretically arise if quite different compositions were used for the solder and the casting alloy because of the formation of a galvanic cell. Thus the manufacturer's recommendations concerning the type of solder to use with any alloy must be followed.

Understandably the composition of gold solder is basically similar to that of the casting alloys, with slight variations to optimize the fusion temperature, fluidity, and surface tension. In addition, therefore, to the normal gold, copper, and silver, zinc and tin are present in the proportions shown in Table 8.4.

**Table 8.4** Composition of typical gold solder (melting range, 750–800 °C)

|    | %  |
|----|----|
| Au | 65 |
| Ag | 16 |
| Cu | 13 |
| Zn | 4  |
| Sn | 2  |

The fusion temperature range will typically be 750–800 °C. Solders of higher gold content but lower tin and zinc will give high fusion ranges.

An outline of the soldering technique is given in Chapter 10.

## BASE METAL CASTING ALLOYS

There are two types of base metal casting alloy in common use. Cobalt–chromium alloys are widely used for partial denture construction and are discussed in Chapter 10. However, nickel–chromium casting alloys have gained acceptance as alternatives to gold alloys for crown and bridgework.

### Composition of nickel–chromium alloys

Many nickel-based alloys have been made available by manufacturers and it is difficult to specify a range of composition which will cover all these products. Typically, however, the true nickel–chromium alloys will contain 70–80 per cent nickel and 12–20 per cent chromium. In addition there are usually small quantities of molybdenum (1–5 per cent) to refine grain size, aluminium (about 3 per cent), which allows precipitation hardening by the formation of a $NiAl_3$ phase, and traces of iron and silicon. Some of the alloys also contain beryllium in amounts up to 2 per cent both to refine the grain size and lower the fusion temperature, Beryllium may affect the bio-compatibility as noted below. A few commercially available base metal alloys deviate from this generalized formulation. One alloy, for example, has 24 per cent palladium and 10 per cent cobalt replacing some of the nickel while another could be more correctly called an iron–chromium alloy.

### Properties of nickel–chromium alloys

*Ease of casting.* The major disadvantages of these alloys are associated with the casting process. First, the melting range of 1200–1400 °C is higher than that of the gold alloys, with a larger gap between solidus and liquidus. Melting is therefore more difficult and cannot be achieved with conventional torches. This also necessitates the use of different investment materials for the moulds, as described later. Furthermore, the higher temperatures involved also lead to a higher solidifcation and thermal contraction and it is generally agreed that castings cannot be made with the same degree of precision as with gold alloys. The higher fusion temperature does have one significant advantage in the context of bonded porcelain (Chapter 9). In this sytem the cast metal substructure has to withstand the firing temperature of porcelain without melting or distorting. The higher the fusion temperature of the alloy over the firing temperature of the porcelain, the less risk there is of distortion.

*Mechanical properties.* A very wide range of mechanical properties has been reported. Alloys at the mid-point of the compositional range have a tensile strength in the region of 600–900 $MN/m^2$ but with a ductility of less than 10 per cent and usually around 5 per cent. They can therefore be compared to a hardened Type IV gold alloy with perhaps a little less ductility, but other compositions within the broad range can give lower strengths with slightly greater ductility, to correspond with other gold alloy types. These nickel–chromium alloys, however, are generally harder than the gold alloys, a typical Vickers Hardness Number of 300 being considerably greater than the 210–230 for a hardened Type IV gold alloy. This has some practical significance, for although it is useful to have restorations that are hard from the functional point of view, this does make them difficult to polish and adjust. High-speed equipment has to be used and the procedures take longer. Similarly, should fixed restorations need to be removed from the mouth at some subsequent stage, sectioning and removal is more difficult if these alloys have been used.

One further point is that the elastic modulus for these alloys is in the region of 200–210 $GN/m^2$, which is more than twice the value for gold alloys.

*Aesthetics.* These alloys display a normal silvery-grey metallic lustre and are, therefore, quite different in colour from gold. Also, as noted below, they do tend to tarnish a little more, which could adversely affect the surface appearance.

*Corrosion and tarnish-resistance.* The relatively short period of clinical use with these alloys has not allowed long-term assessments of their corrosion-resistance to be made. However, since they contain up to 20 per cent chromium, and therefore display passivity, these alloys should have very good resistance. This will depend on the composition and microstructure to a certain extent and there is some evidence that the alloys containing beryllium are a little more susceptible to corrosion. Generally these alloys, not possessing the nobility of gold, must be considered slightly inferior in respect of tarnish-resistance.

*Biocompatibility.* Both nickel and chromium can be regarded as potentially toxic metals, but cytotoxicity in oral tissues following the use of the nickel–chromium alloys does not appear to be a problem, because of the low levels of the elements that actually gain access to the cells. There are, however, two aspects of the biocompatibility of these alloys which deserve attention.

The first concerns the possibility of hypersensitivity responses to the alloy. A number of metals are sensitizers, and nickel is one of the most important. If nickel-based alloys are used in patients who are known to be sensitive to nickel there is a high probability that a hypersensitivity response will occur. These alloys are, therefore, contra-indicated in this type of patient.

Secondly, some of these alloys contain small quantities of beryllium, which is a highly toxic metal. The amounts involved are very small and unlikely to be of much danger to the patient, but concern has been expressed over the hazards in the dental laboratory. Here melting and grinding operations may cause a release of beryllium-bearing substances into the atmosphere where they may be inhaled by the technician.

*Cost.* These alloys are certainly cheaper than the gold alloys, although in many cases the cost of a restoration made from a nickel–chromium alloy may not be very much less than one made from a gold alloy, for reasons mentioned in Chapter 9.

*Bonding to porcelain.* It is possible to produce a bond between these alloys and porcelain, although this is not as easily or effectively achieved as it is with gold alloys (Chapter 9).

## COHESIVE GOLD

As explained at the beginning of this chapter, pure gold is not used to prepare cast restorations, in view of its low strength. However, it may be used in a number of forms as a direct filling material, and for convenience it is described briefly here.

Pure gold is able to weld to itself at room temperature. Unlike soldering, welding is the union of two metals without the presence of an intervening low-fusing material. Usually high temperatures are involved, but with some materials pressure alone at room temperature is sufficient. Gold may be presented in three forms for use as a direct filling material which are, nevertheless, handled clinically in much the same way. These forms are cohesive, mat, and powdered gold.

### Gold foil

Cohesive gold is produced from pure gold rolled into sheets about 0·001 mm in thickness. These are cut into small strips of varying size and loosely rolled into cylinders. Provided the surface is free from impurities and adsorbed gases, pressure will unite separate pieces. Although adhesion phenomena are involved, the nature of the bond can be compared to the cohesion within any individual piece of gold. This accounts for the name of the presentation.

During preparation of gold-foil sheet, work-hardening occurs and manufacturers undertake a stress-relieving anneal. Contamination with gases, such as oxygen and sulphur dioxide from the atmosphere, reduces the reactivity of the surface after annealing. Degassing of the product must be carried out by the dentist before it is used. Some gold foils are treated with ammonia following the anneal to prevent union between pieces during storage. This is then called non-cohesive gold, and may be easier to insert into the cavity during the initial stages of filling. Ammonia prevents contamination with other gases and is easily driven off by heat.

### Matt gold

Matt gold, produced by an electrolytic precipitation process, is presented as a powder. This is compressed into thin strips which are sintered by heating to a temperature just below the melting-point of the gold. While this material is presented as small cylinders, it contains more gold per unit volume and therefore requires less condensation than cohesive gold.

### Powdered gold

By chemical precipitation or atomization of molten metal a very fine powder of pure gold may be prepared. As this would be difficult to handle clinically the powder is generally encapsulated in a piece of gold foil to produce pellets of convenient dimensions. As the density is greater than that of cohesive gold foil, fewer pellets and less condensation are required to fill any given cavity.

### Manipulation of direct-filling gold

Cohesive, mat, and powdered gold are condensed into the prepared cavity in increments the size of which is determined by the dimensions of the pellets being used. Before this can be carried out, the gold is degassed by heating to 250–350 °C. This is easily carried out by placing the pellets on a heated mica tray for a few minutes immediately prior to use.

Condensation or compaction may be achieved in a number of ways. Hand condensers may be used in conjunction with a small mallet, but this is time-consuming and alarming to the patient. Automatic mallets are available which recoil when pressure is applied via the condenser nib. The fastest results are achieved with mechanical condensers which use a vibratory action. It is essential to condense the gold thoroughly to prevent small voids in the resulting filling, which reduce its strength. The condenser point should have a small surface area compared with that of those used to pack amalgam. Ideally its surface area should be about 0·4–1·0 mm². If it is too large inadequate pressure is achieved and if it is too small the point perforates the gold.

Absolute isolation of the cavity is important if the cohesive properties of the material are to be maintained. Rubber dam is mandatory and the cavity is slightly over-filled to allow for finishing.

### Properties

Although pure gold is relatively weak, especially following a stress-relieving anneal, it is work hardened during condensation. Despite the improvement achieved, direct-filling gold restorations should not be used in situations where considerable stress is anticipated. The strength is very much dependent on the efficiency of condensation, which determines the degree of work-hardening and the number of voids present. In a well-condensed filling the strength may approach that of Type I casting gold alloy.

Corrosion and tarnish-resistance are good and there is very little marginal leakage between these fillings and the cavity walls. Pure gold displays excellent biocompatibility. However, the technique is demanding, time consuming, and involves a certain amount of physical trauma to the tooth and its supporting tissues. In a small tooth this is an important consideration. The trauma from mechanical condensers is less than with the manual techniques which are also more distressing for the patient. In view of these factors direct-filling gold is not used extensively.

# 9
## Porcelain and bonded porcelain

It is apparent from Chapter 5 that many tooth-coloured materials are available for the restoration of anterior teeth. There are, however, situations where it is technically difficult to restore badly broken down teeth with conventional fillings and where the result would not necessarily produce an acceptable appearance. These problems may be overcome by using crowns that completely cover the remaining coronal tooth substance. Moreover, in carefully selected cases, missing teeth may be replaced by bridges which very often utilize crowns in their design.

Materials for the construction of these crowns and bridges require many of the attributes of the ideal tooth-coloured filling material (Chapter 5). An obvious consideration is that the appearance should closely simulate that of natural tooth substance in both shade and translucence. As these characteristics vary considerably from one patient to another, and even from one tooth to another, it is important that the system of crown construction is flexible enough to allow the simulation of the patient's natural teeth with great accuracy.

The materials should be strong enough to withstand the considerable forces associated with occlusion and articulation, as crowns made from them are not offered the same support and protection as a conventional filling. Similarly they must have high abrasion-resistance. Materials should be insoluble and not lose their colour or attract debris and stain. A crown is intended to be a durable restoration that will last the patient many years.

Very few materials possess adequate properties for the construction of tooth-coloured crowns, and dental porcelain is by far the most suitable in the majority of patients. This may be used alone or in combination with an alloy to which it is attached. Crowns made using the latter combination are usually called bonded porcelain crowns. Acrylic resin may be applied to crownwork but, as will be seen later, it offers so many disadvantages that it should only be considered for use on a temporary basis.

### DENTAL PORCELAIN

Dental porcelains are classified according to their fusion temperature and are graded as high, medium, or low fusing. The materials in the low range are used in the construction of crowns and bridges while the medium and high fusing varieties are used in the commercial preparation of artificial teeth for denture construction. The ranges of fusion temperature given for these three groups vary, but those below are typical.

| Low fusing | 850 – 1100 °C |
| Medium fusing | 1100 – 1300 °C |
| High fusing | 1300 – 1400 °C |

Variations in fusion temperature are the result of variations in composition, which are described in the next section.

Porcelains for dental use may also be described as vacuum-fired or air-fired, depending on the type of furnace employed during the construction of the restoration. This distinction, however, does not relate to specific differences in composition. The particle size of powders used for vacuum firing, while not uniform, tends to be smaller than in those fired in air, to allow a greater degree of compaction. This feature is explained more fully in a later section. Vacuum-fired porcelains tend to have fusion temperatures that fall into the medium range.

## Composition of dental porcelain

A complex variety of ingredients make up dental porcelains, and manufacturers are reluctant to reveal the precise formulation of their products. Porcelains are basically ceramic powders containing China clay, or kaolin, which is hydrated aluminium silicate, silica, usually in the form of quartz, and a low fusing flux. This flux binds the kaolin and silica together during maturation. The most commonly used flux is feldspar, which is a mixture of sodium, potassium, and aluminium silicates, the proportions of which determine the fusion temperature of the feldspar. The fusion temperature of the porcelain may also be lowered by adding other, low-fusing fluxes, such as carbonates and borax. China clay contributes strength and colour to the final porcelain while silica gives strength and translucence.

The composition of dental porcelain differs from that used for china, having a higher proportion of kaolin, and its formulation is varied to produce materials with different fusion temperatures.

### HIGH FUSING

High fusing porcelains generally contain less silica than those in the low and medium fusing range. Typically silica is present to about 15 per cent. The remaining 85 per cent may be almost entirely feldspar, but up to 4 per cent China clay may be included at its expense. Unlike the low and medium fusing porcelains these products are used directly by the manufacturers of denture teeth and bridge pontic facings without a frit stage being undertaken. Fritting is the fusion of the constituents at a high temperature followed by shock cooling and is outlined in the next section. During the production of denture teeth from high fusing porcelains a pyrochemical reaction occurs between the constituents.

### LOW AND MEDIUM FUSING

These depart from the basic formula by lacking clay and are typically made up of about 25 per cent silica and 60 per cent feldspar. The addition of other low fusing fluxes, making up the remaining 15 per cent, contribute the low fusing characteristic of this group. In addition there are small quantities of metal oxides to produce the desired shade and translucence. The basic porcelain is translucent, and oxides, such as those of tin, titanium, and zirconium, act as opacifiers. Pigments of this kind are, of course, present in high fusing products.

The method of preparation of low fusing porcelains is different from that of high fusing ones. Proportioned ingredients are heated to the fusion temperature of the fluxes, where a chemical reaction takes place between the components, the silica effectively dissolving in the feldspar. The fused mass is cooled rapidly by quenching. This leaves the product crazed, which facilitates the subsequent grinding into powder. This process, as mentioned earlier is referred to as fritting. It is very important to avoid contamination of the porcelain at any stage, especially with iron, as impurities affect the shade of the product. Thorough removal of iron from the ingredients is undertaken by the manufacturer, and the frit is ground in a ball mill to maintain the high level of purity. The powder particle size is carefully regulated and ranges from 7–70 $\mu$m. A range of particle sizes helps to minimize the production of voids, as the smaller particles occupy spaces between the larger ones.

The particles of the frit are all of the same composition, representing the overall composition of the porcelain. When the dental technician fires the porcelain powder during crown construction he is merely reuniting the particles by fusion rather than inducing a chemical reaction between them.

GLAZES

Porcelain is a porous material that will allow the permeation of oral fluids and bacteria. The rough nature of its surface thus facilitates the rapid accumulation of dental plaque. To avoid these problems the surface of a porcelain crown is glazed to produce a smooth, shiny, impervious outer layer. This may be achieved in two ways. Glazes are transparent, low fusing glasses that are available separately from the crown porcelain, and are applied to the crown after its construction. A brief period in the furnace at a relatively low temperature is sufficient to fuse the glaze. Usually, however, an equally effective result may be achieved by carefully controlling the duration of the final firing of the crown. By extending the period slightly, the superficial material fuses more confluently to glaze the surface. If the crown is left in the furnace too long, however, the surface features and contour are lost and the surface is excessively shiny.

It is important that glazes painted on to the constructed crown should have a coefficient of expansion the same as, or closely similar to, that of the underlying porcelain. If not, differential contraction on removal from the furnace will result in crazing of the glaze, which may subsequently peel off. If absolute matching of coefficients cannot be achieved, it is better for the glaze to have the lower value as this will result in compressive stresses rather than tensile stresses under which it would be more likely to fracture.

STAINS

It is often impossible to simulate a patient's teeth without reproducing additional artefacts such as staining, cracks, and even fillings. Stains are added during the fabrication of the crown or just prior to glazing. They are presented in powder form and are low fusing glasses with a high pigment content. Colours vary and are dependent on the particular metal oxides used. On fusion of the superficial layer of the crown during glazing the stains are incorporated in the restoration.

Alterations, in the form of stains, may be made to a completed crown prior to its cementation if it is found to be unsatisfactory. The glaze of the crown is lightly broken with a diamond stone and the powder, suspended in distilled glycerine, is painted on to the surface. Some permeation occurs and the crown is fired at a low temperature. Stains actually built into the crown during its construction usually produce a more pleasing result.

BINDERS

As discussed in detail later, the dental technician builds up the crown with a number of porcelain powders. These powders are mixed with distilled water to produce the paste which has the consistency of wet sand. It is necessary for the manufacturer to add binders to the powder to prevent disintegration of the paste crown by giving it some cohesion. Starch and sugar are used for this purpose and they burn away when the crown is fired.

## Firing

The process of firing displays certain recognizable stages. Initially the built-up crown should be heated slowly to prevent the formation of steam, which would lead to its disintegration. This drying-out phase is generally achieved in the open entrance to the furnace. As the crown is placed inside the furnace any binders present are burnt out and the surface of the crown becomes blackened. During this early stage some contraction occurs.

As the porcelain begins to fuse, continuity is only achieved at points of contact between adjacent particles. The surface and the mass of the material are still porous and little contraction occurs. This stage is sometimes referred to as the low bisque or biscuit. Continued firing brings about more cohesion of the mass as the fused fluxes flow between the particles drawing them closer together and filling in voids. These changes contribute the greatest amount of contraction and the resultant surface is glazed and non-porous, although the main mass remains so. This is the high biscuit stage. Sometimes a medium biscuit stage is described when cohesion has been achieved but contraction has not been identified. If the crown remains in the furnace for an excessive period it loses its form and becomes highly glazed. With modern porcelains a contraction of 30–35 per cent occurs on firing. To avoid cracking and crazing in the newly formed crown it should be allowed to cool gradually. Improved porcelains are less vulnerable to damage on rapid cooling.

FURNACES FOR FIRING PORCELAIN

There are many different varieties of furnace available for this purpose. They are broadly classified as air firing or vacuum firing, although the latter may be used for firing porcelain in air. In addition there are models that offer varying degrees of automation. These allow predetermined time intervals for the various stages of drying out and firing, and also move the restoration in and out of the furnace.

Vacuum firing produces a denser porcelain as air is withdrawn during the process. As fewer voids and areas of porosity are present the resultant crown is stronger and the shade can be more predictably reproduced. Areas of porosity in air fired crowns alter the translucence of the porcelain and may be exposed during grinding of the superficial layers. While voids may be present in the centre of vacuum fired porcelain they are not encountered during grinding.

Infrared furnaces have also been developed for use with dental porcelains. It is claimed that very accurate control over firing temperatures is achieved and the high temperatures are reached rapidly and uniformly throughout the entire mass of porcelain.

## Properties of porcelain

Porcelain was developed for dental use because of its superb aesthetic qualities which, in the well-made crown, are unparalleled. However, to achieve the best results the material must be used in reasonable bulk. If the available space is less than 1 mm there is a tendency for the opaque core material, on which the crown is based, to show through the overlying porcelain. It is obviously necessary for the clinician to reduce the tooth by an equivalent amount if over-contouring of the restoration is to be avoided. For a small tooth, such as a lower incisor, this may be a significant loss of tissue, and in this respect tooth preparation may be relatively traumatic to the dental pulp.

The aesthetic qualities of porcelain do not deteriorate with time, as it displays excellent colour stability and has an exceedingly high abrasion-resistance. Indeed, it is not uncommon for a porcelain crown to induce wear in the opposing natural teeth, and crowns may be observed that have failed to wear to the same extent as their natural neighbours. Porcelain is completely insoluble in oral fluids.

Despite techniques for crown construction which are designed to compensate for the large firing shrinkage, it is difficult to achieve the same quality of marginal fit as that associated with cast gold inlays or crowns. This is aggravated by the need to use a thick butt joint at the margin, as explained later. Fortunately the coefficient of thermal expansion of porcelain is similar to that of tooth substance, ranging from $6{-}8 \times 10^{-6}/°C$, and marginal percolation is not a problem.

Porcelain is extremely well tolerated by tissues, and in this respect can be considered inert. However, in the clinical situation, unglazed porcelain, with its rough, porous surface, allows the rapid accumulation of dental plaque with its attendant dental and periodontal problems. It is important to ensure, therefore, that the surface of the crown is adequately glazed before cementation.

The cements most frequently employed are zinc phosphate and poly-carboxylate cements. Neither offers specific adhesion to porcelain. Poly-carboxylate cement does display adhesion to tooth substance and induces a milder pulpal response. Modifications to the method of construction of porcelain crowns, to be described later, result in specific adhesion between the crown and polycarboxylate cement.

Clearly strength is important in a material used to crown teeth. Porcelain displays a reasonably high compressive strength ranging from 350 to 550 $MN/m^2$ but a low tensile strength of 20–40 $MN/m^2$. The inner surface of a porcelain crown is covered with microcracks induced during firing. These contribute, and are associated with, surface imperfections, which on propagation lead to instantaneous and complete fracture of the restoration. This is particularly important under tensile stresses for under these circumstances the microcracks tend to open and propagate (Fig. 9.1). The outer surface does not demonstrate microcracks as the glaze eliminates them, so most crown fractures are initiated on the inner surface. Porcelain crowns, therefore, exhibit poor tensile and impact strength. Being brittle, the material must be used in fairly thick section, preferably at least 1 mm. While in some

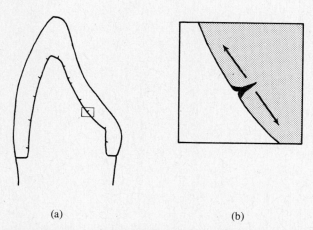

(a)                                    (b)

**Fig. 9.1** (a) Section through porcelain crown showing site of microcrack formation; (b) magnified microcrack. Tensile stresses (arrows) tend to open microcracks leading to their propagation.

situations a slightly reduced thickness gives adequate strength, the aesthetics suffer when the opaque core is visible through the superficial porcelain. Importantly, the gingival margin of the crown must not taper to a feather edge, as in a cast metal restoration, but must finish with a butt joint. Fine edges would fracture away to leave an undesirable marginal defect.

The manipulation of porcelain can alter the strength of the resultant crown. Best results are achieved when the recommended technique and firing cycle have been used. Loss of the glaze reduces the strength of the crown. The glaze appears to exert a 'skin' effect, which is lost if it is breached. The superficial layer or 'skin' cools and solidifies more rapidly than the central mass when the crown is removed from the furnace. Subsequently this layer resists the contraction of the main bulk of porcelain. The outer layer therefore exists in a state of compression and is able to resist the propagation of cracks to the surface. In this respect a glaze produced by controlled fusion of the superficial layer of the crown gives greater strength than glazes added as a separate veneer. With older dental porcelains the problem of fracture limited their usefulness, but more recently a number of ways of reducing this problem have been developed. These are all directed at preventing or limiting the propagation of microcracks and are discussed later.

## Technique of crown construction

The crown is constructed from a combination of three or more powders of varying shades and translucence. Thus, the incisal edge and proximal parts of the restoration are made more translucent in order to simulate the appearance produced by the natural enamel in these regions. The exact shade is selected using a guide which is compared with the natural teeth in the patient's mouth. A chart indicates to the technician which combination of powders should be used to achieve the chosen shade. Three basic layers are built up to construct the crown (Fig. 9.2). The central core is made up of an opaque porcelain to mask any discoloration of the underlying tooth preparation. This is particularly important when crowns are being constructed on a metal post cemented in the root canal of a non-vital tooth. The bulk of the crown is made up of a body or dentine shade, which is relatively opaque and contributes to the colour of the restoration. Finally, a more translucent material is placed incisally and proximally to achieve the effect described above.

All these powders are handled in an essentially similar way, being made into a paste with distilled water. Surface tension aids in the condensation of the powder by drawing the particles closer together. It is important, therefore, that the powder is not allowed to dry out. The porcelain is built up on a platinum foil matrix which is closely adapted to the die of the patient's prepared tooth. This allows the delicate unfired porcelain to be handled and supported prior to, and during, firing. Clearly such a matrix must have a higher melting-point than the fusion temperature of porcelain.

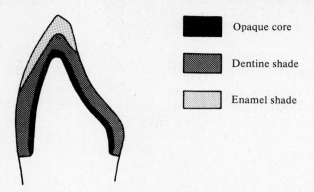

**Fig. 9.2** Section through porcelain crown showing distribution of opaque, dentine, and enamel shades.

Platinum is ideally suited to this purpose. When the core porcelain powder has been applied to the matrix, as much water as possible is withdrawn by vibrating the die to bring moisture to the surface, where it can be absorbed by a tissue. The removal of water by this and other techniques aids the compaction or condensation of the powder particles, minimizing the incorporation of voids and reducing firing shrinkage. If too much water is removed too quickly as it is heated, the crown may disintegrate. Porcelain pastes may be handled in a variety of ways to build up the crown and to achieve good condensation. These include the use of a brush or spatula. Where effective condensation has been carried out, the resulting crown is stronger. Poor condensation may also adversely effect the shade of the final product.

The opaque core of the crown is built up as a separate stage. Often some cracks form as this is fired, and these are filled in with more core material and the core is refired. As the core contracts there is a danger of the platinum foil covering the shoulder of the preparation being lifted, and following the initial firing the technician should confirm the close fit of the matrix against the die before continuing.

The main body of the crown, including dentine and enamel shades, are built up and intrinsic stains are added. In view of the large contraction during firing it is necessary to overbuild the crown quite substantially to achieve the correct final proportions. In order to distinguish between the dentine and enamel powders they are lightly pigmented, often pale pink and blue. These colours are, of course, lost when the crown is fired.

Contraction cannot be accurately assessed, and it is necessary to grind the fired crown to its final shape using diamond stones before it can be glazed. The foil matrix remains in place throughout and should only be removed when it is established that no adjustments requiring a refiring are necessary. If a crown is refired without the matrix there is a risk of distortion due to pyroplastic flow. While the foil may be quite difficult to remove, there is no specific adhesion between it and the porcelain.

## ALUMINOUS PORCELAIN

Most modern crowns involve the use of aluminous porcelain. The principle of composite structures discussed in Chapters 1 and 5 is used here to increase the strength of the porcelain by incorporating into it a dispersion of fine alumina. The difference in behaviour during fracture between porcelain with alumina, porcelain with another additive, and unfilled porcelain is shown in Figure 9.3. With unfilled porcelain there are no specific factors preventing the rapid propagation of microcracks, and the result is gross fracture. If a filler is present, the microcrack progresses through the porcelain until a filler particle is encountered. In the case of a material other than alumina the crack is redirected at each interface and eventually propagates throughout the porcelain to result in gross fracture. With alumina, redirection does not take place but the crack passes through the alumina particles. As alumina is a very hard material each particle encountered offers considerable resistance to propagation, and as the concentration of alumina particles increases so does the strength of the porcelain. The interface between the alumina particles and the main mass of porcelain is relatively stress-free as the coefficients of expansion of both phases are the same. With other fillers, with differing coefficients of expansion, the interfaces are stressed and break down more easily.

Unfortunately the addition of alumina to dental porcelain increases its opacity, detracting from its aesthetic qualities. Its use is therefore limited to the core of the crown where a degree of opacity is desirable. Aluminous porcelain carries about 40–50 per cent alumina in the core powder, which

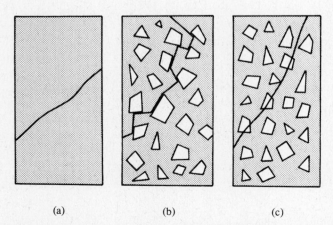

(a)　　　　　　　　(b)　　　　　　　　(c)

**Fig. 9.3** Propagation of crack through (a) unfilled porcelain; (b) porcelain filled with a substance other than alumina; (c) porcelain filled with alumina.

doubles the strength of the resultant crown. Some body shade porcelains contain up to 5 per cent alumina. For a given concentration of alumina the effect on strength will vary depending on the particle size. Thus, the use of small particles, by offering more interfaces, gives greater strength. However, the smaller the particle size, the greater the opacity, and a compromise is generally used. Alumina particles from 10 to 15 $\mu$m are generally employed.

It is an interesting observation that the glaze on an aluminous porcelain crown does not contribute the same increase in strength as the older porcelains. Presumably the strong inner layer of the crown, the core, offers all the resistance to fracture that was previously attributed to the glaze.

### ALUMINA INSERTS

A further increase in the strength of porcelain crowns may be achieved using inserts of pure alumina. In the conventional jacket crown these may be in the form of small flat or curved sheets of alumina placed palatally (Fig. 9.4).

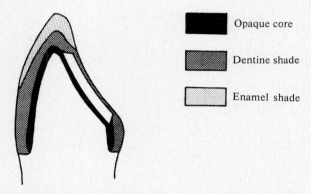

Opaque core

Dentine shade

Enamel shade

**Fig. 9.4** Section through porcelain crown incorporating a palatal insert of pure alumina.

Clearly these cannot be placed labially for aesthetic reasons and if they are too extensive palatally the overall translucence of the crown may be reduced. Because they are relatively bulky additions, alumina inserts of this type can only be placed where there is adequate clearance between the preparation and the opposing teeth. Moreover, when such space is present, a conventional crown with an aluminous porcelain core usually gives adequate strength. The use of pure alumina inserts can give a fivefold increase in the strength of a crown.

Porcelain post-crowns may be constructed around an alumina tube that fits over a cast metal spigot prepared specifically to fit its internal dimensions (Fig. 9.5). While these crowns have great strength, the resistance and retention form of the spigot is poor compared to a well-designed preparation or cast core and post. Alumina rods may be used in the production of a basic substructure on which a simple porcelain bridge is constructed.

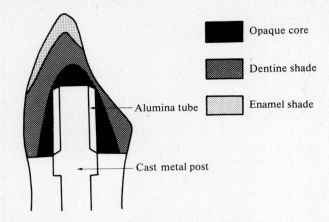

Opaque core

Dentine shade

Enamel shade

Alumina tube

Cast metal post

**Fig. 9.5** Porcelain post-crown constructed over pure alumina tube.

APPLICATIONS OF ALUMINOUS PORCELAIN

The majority of porcelain crowns are built on an opaque core of aluminous porcelain, and this is the widest application. However, the increased strength of aluminous porcelain tempted clinicians to use it for bridge construction. A great many fracture failures followed, despite the use of pure alumina rods across connectors and in pontics. These fractures occurred most frequently through the porcelain jacket crown retainers. As indicated earlier, porcelain will withstand relatively high compressive forces, but is weak in tension. During occlusion and articulation the abutment teeth, on which the bridge is supported, tend to move independently in their sockets. This results in complex stresses, including tensile stresses, within the porcelain bridge, which fractures as a result.

Interestingly, small bridges supported on a single tooth were successful as this conflict of abutment tooth movement was not present. These two unit bridges are the only ones that may be undertaken with a reasonable degree of confidence. Further developments in crown construction, to be decribed later, may, by offering improved strength, allow porcelain to be used in slightly larger bridges. This, however, must await the results of clinical experiments.

## BONDED PORCELAIN

The mechanism of fracture of porcelain crowns has been described in an earlier section. While aluminous porcelain employs a system that impedes micro-crack propagation, it does not reduce the presence of microcracks or prevent their initial propagation. Fusion of the porcelain onto a metal substructure, giving a bonded porcelain system, can effectively eliminate the formation of microcracks on the fitting surface of the crown. Porcelain used in this way will therefore withstand considerably greater forces. The physical properties and chemical composition of alloys used in bonded porcelain systems must be carefully controlled if a durable bond is to be achieved.

### SPECIAL REQUIREMENTS OF ALLOYS FOR BONDED PORCELAIN

Bonded porcelain restorations are produced by fusing the porcelain on to an already prepared alloy substructure (Fig. 9.6). Clearly the alloy must have a high melting-point if it is to withstand the high temperatures associated with firing porcelain. At high temperatures alloys tend to creep. The slight distortion in the substructure that may result can seriously prejudice the fit of the completed restoration. By carefully controlling the composition of the alloy, manufacturers can minimize this problem. With a high quality alloy a second phase is precipitated at the fusion temperature of the porcelain, which leads to a dispersion strengthening effect. As bonded porcelain alloys have a high melting-point it is necessary to use silica or phosphate-bonded investments during casting (Chapter 10).

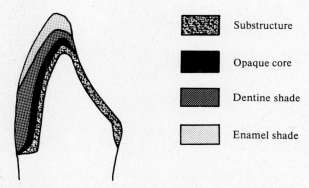

**Fig. 9.6** Section through bonded porcelain crown showing extent of substructure and distribution of porcelain.

For the bond to be effective and durable it is important to minimize residual stresses at the interface between the porcelain and the metal. To achieve this it is necessary to match the coefficient of expansion of the alloy closely to that of the porcelain. The compositions of alloy and porcelain are specifically adjusted to produce this match. If it is not achieved, stresses may be established at the interface and the porcelain veneer may even be displaced from the substructure during the construction of the restoration in the dental laboratory. The greatest temperature change the completed crown undergoes is, of course, on removal from the furnace when it cools from about 960 °C to room temperature. If the incorrect porcelain has been used the facing is lost at this stage.

Bonded porcelain alloys must be rigid. Any flexion occurring in the substructure will be transmitted to the porcelain which will fracture, as the latter is unable to withstand tensile stress. If the bond between the facing and the substructure is strong the tendency to fracture is reduced.

The nature of the bond between the porcelain and alloy is discussed in a subsequent section. It is important, however, that the chemical composition of the alloy permits the formation of oxides in small quantities. Reaction between oxides in the alloy and oxides in the porcelain is the basis of the bond between the two. Bonding alloys therefore contain small quantities of certain metals, in particular tin, that readily form oxides.

### Composition of alloys for bonded porcelain

A variety of alloys may be used for this purpose and it is difficult to find a reasonable basis for classification. However, as with the casting alloys discussed in the previous chapter, they may be divided broadly into those made up substantially of base metals and those of precious metals. Difficulty arises in classifying some products which contain a combination of both.

Alloys containing a large proportion of precious metals may be based either on a combination of gold, platinum, and palladium or of silver, platinum, and palladium. The former has a yellow colour while the latter has a silver appearance. Gold and silver contribute a resistance to tarnish and corrosion while platinum and palladium increase the hardness and raise the melting-point. Other metals are added to produce the desired physical properties, especially the carefully controlled coefficient of expansion. Indium, iridium, tin, and zinc may be present in small amounts to achieve this. Silver-based alloys have a melting-point between 1150 °C and 1250 °C while gold-based alloys have a lower melting-point of 1125–1150 °C. Bonding alloys should not contain copper as the interface between the substructure and the porcelain is discoloured green.

Many attempts have been made to develop a bonding alloy of base metals to reduce the otherwise high cost of the technique. These have not met with the same degree of success as the precious metals. The most common alloy in this category is one of nickel and chromium. These two metals are present in proportions that produce the appropriate coefficient of expansion, and chromium oxide is the important agent in achieving the bond.

In order to match the coefficients of expansion of the bonding alloys and the porcelain the latter may have modifications to the basic formulation given earlier. Alteration to the proportion of metal oxides present are used to achieve this and tin oxide may be added specifically to improve the bond between the porcelain and the precious metal alloys. If an exact match of expansion coefficients is not achieved it is desirable that the coefficient of the alloy is slightly greater than that of the porcelain. In this way compressive stresses develop in the porcelain as it cools rather than tensile stresses that would tend to result in fracture.

NATURE OF THE BOND

Many different factors have been implicated in the bonding of porcelain to the alloy substructure. These include mechanical adhesion, compressive forces, and specific adhesion (Chapter 2). It is now accepted that, while all these may contribute, specific adhesion is the principal mechanism.

When the porcelain and substructure are heated to the firing temperature of the former (about 980 °C), oxides from the superficial layer of the alloy migrate into, and combine with, the porcelain. There is chemical union between the two, giving strong adhesion. Should a fracture occur it is usually within the porcelain rather than as a result of bond failure. In the precious metal alloys tin oxide, and possibly iridium oxide, is responsible for the bond whereas in the base metals chromium oxide fulfils this role.

To aid good adhesion it is important to wet the alloy surface well. With most of the precious alloys available there is good wetting with a low contact angle between the porcelain and the metal, provided the surface has been prepared properly. An interface with less residual stress, and therefore better adhesion, is produced if the substructure surface is as smooth as possible. Despite technical steps directed at achieving this there are still microscopic irregularities on the alloy surface. Only with efficient wetting will such irregularities be completely filled with porcelain.

Clinical experience has shown that the bond with base metal alloys is not as good as that with the precious metals. This is probably because more residual stress is present. As explained earlier it is important to match the coefficients of expansion to minimize this. However, when chromium oxide migrates to the alloy surface and into the porcelain during firing it significantly alters the coefficient of expansion of the latter. Thus the originally close match is destroyed and the interface is unavoidably stressed.

## Technical considerations with bonded porcelain

### SUBSTRUCTURE DESIGN

A labio-palatal section through a bonded porcelain crown is shown in Figure 9.6. While a very thin section of metal would be effective in preventing microcrack formation and propagation in the overlying porcelain, it is not possible to cast these alloys in less than 0·5 mm thickness. The palatal metal is also difficult to manage below this thickness. As the porcelain contracts considerably on firing, there is a danger that the thin metal substructure will become distorted at the high temperatures involved. If this happened the resultant crown would display a deficiency at the gingival margin on the labial aspect. It is helpful, therefore, to leave a slightly thickened band of metal adjacent to the labial shoulder of the preparation to resist this tendency.

There is a potential problem with the aesthetics of bonded porcelain crowns that in many cases is difficult to overcome. The dark, opaque metal substructure tends to reduce the aesthetic benefit of the translucent porcelain placed over it. This results in a rather lifeless appearance. By reducing the bulk of the substructure and paying careful attention to its design it is often possible to overcome this to some extent. For a good apppearance the overlying porcelain must be used in a thickness of at least 1 mm. Part of this is made up of an opaque layer used to mask the dark metal backing and the remainder is built up in body and enamel shades, as with a conventional porcelain crown. This means that the total thickness of metal and porcelain on the labial surface of the crown is 1·5 mm.

In order to minimize residual stress in the porcelain the substructure should have no sharp features. The contour should be gently rounded.

### MELTING AND CASTING BONDING ALLOYS

Bonded porcelain crown substructures are produced by the lost-wax casting method, just as for gold inlays. The melting-points of these alloys, however, are higher, especially those of the base metal alloys. Precious metal alloys can be melted with a gas–oxygen torch. Insufficient heat is produced by these to melt the base metal alloys and a plasma flame must be used. This instrument is not as easy to control as the conventional flame, and it is possible to overheat the alloy, which results in its oxidation. The casting produced is pitted and porous. Moreover, the entire casting procedure for base metal alloys must be carried out with precision if a satisfactory casting is to be produced. Sprues must be relatively bulky to allow rapid progress of the molten metal. Unfortunately these alloys do not share to the same extent the capacity of the precious metals to be reused in future castings. There is therefore a large amount of wastage, which makes the use of the base metal alloy more expensive than its unit cost would suggest.

### SURFACE PREPARATION

Prior to fusing porcelain to the alloy substructure great care must be taken if a durable bond is to be achieved. The surface must be smooth, as explained earlier, and free from contamination. A process of degreasing and degassing is therefore undertaken. The surface is cleaned with fine abrasives and may be sandblasted with alumina dust. A final cleaning may be carried out ultrasonically prior to washing in water and drying. From this point on, the surface which has to bear the porcelain must not be contaminated by contact with the fingers. By heating the substructure in the furnace for 5 minutes at 1000 °C the surface is degassed and oxidized. With precious metal alloys the opaque porcelain may now be applied. With base metals, however, it is wiser to repeat the sandblasting and oxidation to ensure a uniform layer of chromium oxide. This is another stage where management of the base alloys is more critical than that of the precious ones. Opaque porcelain is then applied in the form of a paste in the same way as a porcelain crown is constructed.

By using solders of the appropriate melting-point it is possible to solder substructure components together before the fusion of the porcelain facings or after these have been applied. The latter technique, however, may lead to some discoloration of the porcelain and is best avoided.

### Clinical considerations for bonded porcelain

There are two major clinical drawbacks to the use of bonded porcelain crowns and bridges. As both metal and porcelain must be placed labially a total reduction of 1·5 mm has to be undertaken in this region. Even for an anatomically large tooth, such as an upper canine, this involves destruction of considerable proportions. On a small tooth it may be difficult to execute such a preparation without risking exposure of the pulp. Additional pulpal irritation may follow the cementation of the crown if an irritant cement is used. Furthermore, a small tooth may be considerably weakened by such a preparation.

The second problem relates to the first, and concerns aesthetics. If the 1·5 mm reduction, referred to above, is not achieved the opaque core can be seen through the dentine and enamel shades. A reduction in available space also minimizes the translucence achieved, which may even be limited in an optimal preparation.

By using a cast metal substructure it is possible to produce a minimal reduction in tooth tissue palatally, of about 0·5 mm. This has obvious conservative advantages over the porcelain crown and the margin may be finished to a feather edge, which favours a good fit. With casting gold alloys for inlays it is generally possible to burnish the metal at feather edge margins. In the case of bonded crowns this is not possible to a practical degree as the alloys are so hard, and only the smallest of errors may be effectively corrected.

APPLICATIONS OF BONDED PORCELAIN

It is clear from the foregoing pages that bonded porcelain is a system used primarily for crown construction. Because of the improved strength of such restorations over porcelain and aluminous porcelain they are used in situations were considerable occlusal stress is anticipated. Often this occurs in patients with a 'close bite' where contact between the opposing teeth is extensive and it would be difficult to guarantee an overall clearance of at least 1 mm during preparation. Where it is at all possible to construct an aluminous porcelain jacket crown this is generally preferable for aesthetic reasons.

Because of the superior strength of bonded porcelain crowns and the great rigidity of these restorations they are used extensively in bridgework as retainers and pontics. Using the same materials for all the components of a bridge produces aesthetic harmony. Pontics of bonded porcelain are more convenient to construct than those based on proprietary porcelain facings, and they can be shaped individually for the particular patient. However, the clinical drawbacks outlined in the previous section still apply.

### Porcelain bonded to foil

The improvement in the strength of porcelain for crown construction by bonding the inner surface to metal has been described. The main limitations of bonded porcelain crowns are the need for an extensive preparation to allow for both metal and porcelain labially and the possible loss of translucence accompanying the presence of the metal substructure. In order to take advantage of the bonded porcelain system without the above problems, a method of bonding porcelain to a platinum foil matrix has been developed. Although the foil matrix is of relatively small dimensions and is not in itself mechanically robust, the propagation of microcracks present on the inner surface of the crown is effectively prevented.

Following the construction of a conventional platinum foil matrix a second foil is placed on the die over the first, as illustrated in Figure 9.7. The second matrix, however, only covers the axial, incisal, and palatal surfaces, leaving the shoulder exposed. It is this second layer of platinum foil that becomes incorporated permanently in the crown. Both matrices are made from 0·025 mm platinum foil.

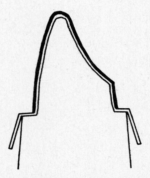

**Fig. 9.7** Twin platinum foil matrices on die. Superficial matrix (shaded) is incorporated permanently in porcelain crown.

The outer foil is tin plated in a solution of stannous sulphate to a thickness of 0·2–2·0 $\mu$m. The thickness of tin deposited is determined by the current applied. With a plating time of one minute, 50 mA is used for anterior teeth and premolars while 100 mA is used to plate the matrices for molar teeth which require a greater thickness of tin for optimal results. Prior to this the foil should be lightly sandblasted with alumina to increase the surface area available for bonding. A period of electrolytic degreasing is carried out in caustic soda and the foil is washed. Any caustic soda remaining is neutralized in citric acid and a final wash in water completes the preparation for tin plating. A commercially available degreasing and plating bath makes the whole process easy to execute.

To make bonding between the foil and porcelain possible it is necessary to oxidize the surface, as with the conventional bonded porcelain technique.

Initially the foil is placed in the furnace in vacuum at 800 °C and the temperature is raised 50° per minute for 4 minutes, by which time the temperature will have reached 1000 °C. This allows the tin and the platinum to alloy. Air is admitted to the furnace and the temperature maintained at 1000 °C for a further 2 minutes to allow oxidation of the tin to occur. It should be appreciated that both the inner and outer surfaces of the matrix are tin plated and oxidized during the process.

Construction of the porcelain crown over the twin foil matrix is essentially similar to that of a conventional restoration. A new range of porcelains has been developed for use with this system. The opaque core powders have an improved capacity to mask the underlying foil, which is quite dark following oxidation.

The superior strength of these crowns is derived from the prevention of microcrack propagation and by the use of an aluminous porcelain core. It is possible, therefore, that more complex bridges will be more successful than with conventional aluminous porcelain. As the completed crown is effectively lined with a layer of tin oxide, zinc polycarboxylate cement and glass ionomer cement offer specific adhesion to the inner surface. Therefore systems now exist that allow specific adhesion of cements to both the restoration and the tooth, with obvious advantages.

## MATERIALS FOR TEMPORARY CROWNS AND BRIDGES

Following tooth preparation for crowns and bridges it is necessary to restore the teeth temporarily while the permanent restorations are constructed. This protects the exposed tooth tissue from thermal and chemical irritation and maintains the anatomical relationship between the prepared teeth and those opposed and adjacent to them. Anteriorly the appearance is restored and speech and mastication may be facilitated. The materials available for tooth-coloured temporary crowns and bridges are all polymers.

### Acrylic resin

The chemistry of polymethyl methacrylate is described in Chapter 11 and its contribution as a tooth-coloured filling material is discussed in Chapter 5. The presentations used to produce fillings may also be used to produce temporary crowns. A preformed cellulose acetate crown former acts as a matrix, and one of suitable size and shape is trimmed to fit the tooth as accurately as possible. Acrylic resin monomer and polymer powder of an appropriate shade are mixed to a runny consistency and placed in the matrix, which is positioned over the tooth. A separating medium, such as vaseline (petroleum jelly), prevents mechanical adhesion of the resin to the tooth. Following polymerization, which takes about 2 minutes, the restoration is removed and trimmed before being cemented to the tooth. The matrix is peeled off the acrylic resin crown. Other methods of temporary crown construction are outlined in the next section, and these may be applied to acrylic resin.

The disadvantages of acrylic resin as a restorative material are mentioned in Chapter 5. These all apply to the resin used as a temporary crown material. However, temporary crowns are hopefully only left in the mouth for a few weeks at the most, and often only for a few days. Over such a short period of time they do not produce lasting damage, provided they are well fitting. The greatest problem is the relatively rough and porous surface, which allows the excessive accumulation of dental plaque, particularly in gingival regions where trimming has usually been necessary.

### Epimine resin

This is based on a complex long-chain molecule bearing imine groups (Fig. 9.8), and is the ethylene imine derivative of bisphenol-A. The product is presented as a base paste, which also contains about 25 per cent powdered nylon as a filler, and liquid reactor. This contains an aromatic sulphonate ester which causes polymerization of the base paste producing a hard mass. The system is chemically similar to the polyether impression material discussed in Chapter 6.

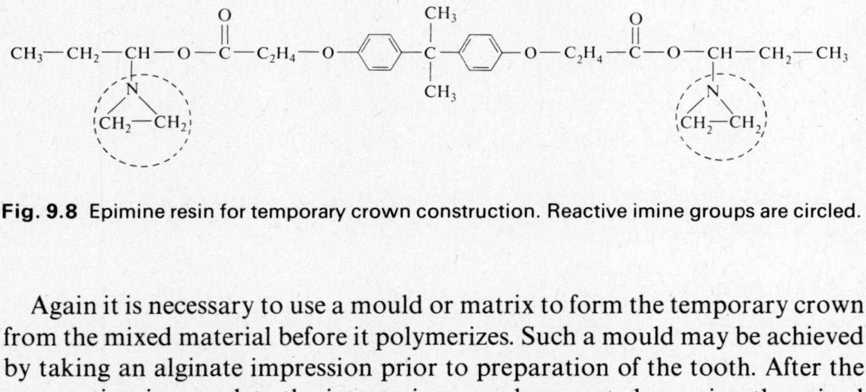

**Fig. 9.8** Epimine resin for temporary crown construction. Reactive imine groups are circled.

Again it is necessary to use a mould or matrix to form the temporary crown from the mixed material before it polymerizes. Such a mould may be achieved by taking an alginate impression prior to preparation of the tooth. After the preparation is complete the impression may be reseated carrying the mixed resin in the appropriate part. It will be appreciated that the resin will fill the space previously occupied by the tooth substance removed during preparation. Excess material is displaced to the periphery of the impression. After polymerization is complete, which takes 4–5 minutes, the temporary restoration may be trimmed and cemented. This technique has the advantage of accurately restoring the original shape of the tooth. A polythene matrix constructed on a model of the patient's teeth may be used in a similar way.

The mixed resin displays very good flow, and so excess material is easily displaced leaving a very thin film between the restoration and the periphery of the impression. It is non-irritant to the pulp and the exothermic heat produced during polymerization is slight compared to that from acrylic resin. However, the product is highly translucent, and offers only one shade, which leads to poor aesthetic qualities in many patients. The setting time is inconsistent, perhaps because of difficulty in standardizing the proportions of liquid to base paste. When the time comes to remove the restoration the resin is hard and brittle and it is often impossible to remove without fracturing, which would, of course, preclude its further use. The material may induce a hypersensitivity reaction in some individuals. This is not surprising as similar responses may be evoked by the polyether impression material, which has a fundamentally similar composition.

## Polycarbonates

The chemistry of polycarbonates is also described in Chapter 11. This material has been used to produce a wide range of tooth-coloured temporary crowns of different size and shape. After the gingival margin of an appropriate pattern has been trimmed, the crown, filled with acrylic resin, is placed over the prepared tooth. After polymerization of this resin the temporary crown is removed and final trimming undertaken before cementation. Although these polycarbonate crowns are difficult to separate from the underlying acrylic resin there is no chemical union between the two. The presentation offers only one shade but despite this a not unpleasing appearance may be produced in many patients.

## Cementation of temporary crowns

It is clearly important to achieve a seal at the margins of temporary crowns to prevent the ingress of fluid, and reasonable retention to prevent displacement of the restoration. However, it is also desirable to be able to remove the crown easily without resorting to its total destruction. For this reason relatively weak cements are used for this purpose.

Zinc oxide/eugenol has a wide application in this context and a relatively thin mix is used. There are a number of proprietary products specifically for the cementation of temporary restorations and for the temporary cementation of permanent restorations. One such material is a two-paste system based on zinc oxide/eugenol. It also provides a third paste, which reduces the hardness of the resulting cement without altering the setting time. By applying cements only to the gingival region of temporary crowns a seal is produced marginally but removal is far easier.

# 10

## Alloys used in denture construction: investments and casting techniques

Alloys are used in two different situations in denture construction. First, and of greatest significance, they are used in partial dentures where the strength and rigidity of metallic materials in the framework is essential. Type IV gold alloys, described in Chapter 8, are suitable, and at one time were used frequently in this situation. However, their high cost, especially in relation to the large volume required, is a severe limitation. The vast majority of castings for partial dentures are therefore made from base metal alloys, especially the cobalt–chromium casting alloys.

Secondly, alloys may be used for the base in full dentures. In practice, alloy bases are rarely indicated, as acrylic resin is the first choice, as described in Chapter 11, and alternatives are only considered when these are unsuitable. Even if this is the case, other polymeric materials, such as the modified acrylics, are usually preferred and alloys are rarely chosen. However, it is possible to either cast a full denture base in cobalt–chromium alloy, or form it in wrought stainless steel.

### COBALT–CHROMIUM ALLOYS

Cobalt–chromium alloys have been available industrially since the 1920s, their combination of high strength and excellent corrosion-resistance, especially at high temperatures, making them very useful for a number of applications. These alloys became known as the 'Stellites' because they maintained their shiny, star-like appearance under difficult conditions, and a range of compositions became available for a variety of purposes. An alloy based on 70 per cent cobalt and 30 per cent chromium, with minor additions of carbon, manganese, and silicon was first used in dentistry in 1929. The alloys used today vary a little from this original composition, small quantities of nickel and molybdenum replacing some of the cobalt. This is necessary because partial dentures require a little more ductility than is provided by the 70–30 alloy, but do not need the high-temperature strength that is associated with this level of cobalt. Replacement of some of the cobalt with other elements can increase the ductility at the expense of some of the strength.

#### Composition

Many cobalt–chromium dental casting alloys are available commercially and they display a wide spectrum of composition. It is not possible to define this precisely for these alloys, and indeed the only requirement of the ADA specification (No. 14) is that there should be a minimum of 55 per cent cobalt, chromium, and nickel together. The usual range of composition is given in Table 10.1, although it is possible that some alloys will be outside this range. Some other alloys, although basically of the cobalt–chromium type, have quite different compositions and are discussed at the end of this section.

**Table 10.1** Normal range of composition for cobalt–chromium dental casting alloys

|  | % |
|---|---|
| Co | 55–65 |
| Cr | 23–30 |
| Ni | 0–20 |
| Mo | 0–7 |
| Fe | 0–5 |
| C | up to 0·4 |
| W, Mn, Si, Pt | traces |

EFFECTS OF ALLOYING ELEMENTS

Cobalt is obviously the parent element and imparts the hardness, strength, and rigidity to the alloy. It also has a high melting-point.

Chromium forms a series of solid solutions with cobalt, the two elements having different crystal structures. The phase diagram is shown in Figure 10.1.

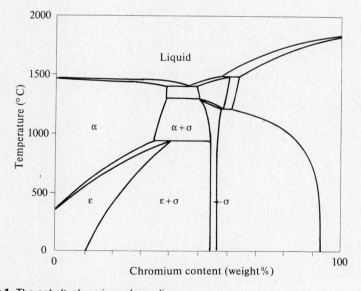

**Fig. 10.1** The cobalt–chromium phase diagram.

The limit of solubility in the binary cobalt–chromium system is about 34 per cent chromium at 1000 °C. Above this level the sigma phase is produced giving a two-phase structure. Unfortunately the sigma phase is very brittle and this type of two-phase structure is, therefore, undesirable. The actual limit of solid solubility is modified by the presence of other alloying elements, such as nickel, so that the chromium content will most likely be in the 20–25 per cent region in these alloys. The solid solution formed at high temperatures will be retained on casting because of the difficulty of diffusion as the alloy rapidly cools, so that alloys of this composition will tend to have the single solid solution structure.

The main role of the chromium is to impart corrosion and tarnish-resistance to the alloy. It will be recalled from Chapter 1 that chromium is one of the few elements that passivates readily and effectively and fortunately it carries this ability with it when alloyed. Cobalt also passivates to a certain extent and so the alloy is particularly good in this respect. Generally the higher the chromium content the better the corrosion-resistance, so that manufacturers usually aim for the maximum chromium content that is possible without risking the formation of a sigma phase.

It will also be noted from Figure 10.1 that chromium, in these proportions, reduces the melting-point.

The addition of nickel increases the ductility as noted above. It is usually added at the expense of the cobalt, the nickel going into solid solution in the cobalt and chromium. In effect, the nickel is interchangeable with the cobalt over a wide range of composition. The increase in ductility produced by nickel is, of course, achieved at the expense of a reduction in strength and hardness.

Molybdenum refines the grain size. It does this by providing more nuclei for solidification during casting, as discussed in Chapter 1. This is very important in partial dentures as the cobalt–chromium alloys tend to develop large grain sizes, which could result in the presence of very few grains in a cross-section of, say, a clasp or connector. A much finer grain size will increase the strength of such thin sections. Molybdenum also produces a significant solid solution hardening effect in the alloy and is normally present in proportions from 2·5 to 5 per cent.

Other elements are also present in small quantities. Some, like iron and beryllium, give solid solution hardening; others, like gallium and iridium, may refine the grain size, whilst others, such as manganese and silicon, act as deoxidizers.

The final element, which is of great significance, is carbon, which has a considerable influence on the mechanical properties. The carbon forms a very limited interstitial solid solution with the major elements, which gives some strengthening, but it also readily forms carbides, notably with chromium. A small quantity of carbides increases the strength considerably, the ideal situation being an array of discrete carbides distributed through the solid solution, as indicated in Figure 10.2a. This type of structure is produced

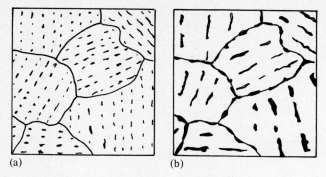

**Fig. 10.2** (a) Discrete carbides; and (b) continuous carbides in cobalt–chromium alloy microstructure.

because the carbides are associated with the last liquid to freeze and are therefore precipitated in the interdendritic spaces (Chapter 1). It is most important, however, that the carbides do not become continuous, either within the grain or at the grain boundaries (Fig. 10.2b) as this leads to excessive brittleness.

The control of carbide formation is, therefore, of great importance, although it is not easy to achieve. The basic carbon content is controlled by the manufacturer, but the final carbide structure is also affected by the pick-up of carbon during the melting and casting process and by the rate of cooling. Since the melting-point of these alloys is too high for a gas–air torch, an oxy-acetylene flame is sometimes used for the melting. With this method it is possible for carbon to be picked up from the flame, upsetting the carbon balance. This could also happen with the electric-arc method of melting involving carbon electrodes, so that induction heating is usually preferred. The precipitation of the carbide depends to some extent on the rate of cooling and the diffusion of atoms in the molten alloy immediately prior to its solidification. The faster the rate of cooling through the fusion range, the less chance there is for diffusion of the carbon and chromium to form carbides.

**Properties of cobalt–chromium alloys**

These will be discussed in the context of the requirements of casting alloys outlined in Chapter 8.

EASE OF CASTING

Although these alloys are described as casting alloys, since, in the compositions given, they are too brittle to be wrought, dental castings are not achieved without some difficulty, and certainly not so easily as with gold alloys. The important points to note are as follows.

**a** The liquidus may range from 1250 °C to 1480 °C. This is clearly higher than that for the gold alloys and, as discussed later, this means that all but those at the lower end of the range require different methods of melting than the gas–air torch used with most gold alloys, and the use of different mould materials.

**b** In relation to the reactivity of the molten alloy, the use of deoxidizers to minimize the effect of oxidation and the tendency to pick up carbon have already been mentioned. No undue difficulty should be encountered, provided the usual care is taken during casting, but it is important to remember that overheating is undesirable. This may lead to gas inclusions and a poor surface texture due to a reaction between the molten metal and the mould.

**c** The temperature difference between the liquidus and solidus is also relatively large and a cored, dendritic structure is usually recognizable after casting.

**d** The casting shrinkage of the cobalt–chromium alloys is greater than with the gold alloys. Typical figures for the total contraction on casting are 2–2·5 per cent for the former and 1·25 per cent for the latter. The significance of this is discussed later, but it is of relevance to note that in the partial denture framework for which the cobalt–chromium alloys are used, the accuracy required is slightly less critical than with the gold alloy restorations, so that clinically this difference may not be too important.

**e** These alloys are very hard, and finishing of the surface is considerably more difficult than with the softer gold alloys.

**Table 10.2** Mechanical properties of cast cobalt–chromium alloys

| Modulus of elasticity GN/m² | 0·1% proof strength MN/m² | U.T.S. MN/m² | Elongation % | Vickers Hardness Number |
|---|---|---|---|---|
| 250 | 500–580 | 725–860 | 1–4 | 370–400 |

MECHANICAL PROPERTIES

The range of mechanical properties obtained with these alloys is given in Table 10.2. Comparison with Table 8.3 shows that their proof and ultimate tensile strengths are very similar to those of the Type IV heat-hardened gold alloys. Three important differences do exist, however.

**a** The modulus of elasticity of the cobalt–chromium alloys is approximately twice the modulus of the gold alloys. This means they are stiffer, and, while this may not be of any great significance in inlays and crowns, it is important in connectors of partial dentures. On the other hand it is not always desirable for the clasps of the dentures to be too rigid, as more flexible clasps can be located in greater undercuts.

**b** The ductility of the cobalt–chromium alloys is generally lower than with the gold alloys. The former are very brittle, and work-harden so rapidly that even minor adjustments of clasps can result in fracture within a short period of use.

**c** The Vickers Hardness Number for a cobalt–chromium alloy is typically 370 and may even exceed 400, while that for a gold alloy is in the region of 210–230. This makes the finishing much more difficult.

AESTHETICS AND CORROSION-RESISTANCE

Clearly no base metal alloy can compete with gold alloys if the colour of gold is required in a denture. With this one reservation, however, cobalt–chromium alloys must be considered very suitable for intra-oral use. Although finishing is more difficult than with gold, a very good polish can ultimately be obtained. Moreover, this good surface finish is retained because of the excellent corrosion-resistance of the alloy in the oral environment. The suitability of these alloys for intra-oral use from the corrosion point of view can be judged from their general use for surgically implanted prostheses.

In spite of good corrosion-resistance in the oral environment, the alloys are attacked by chlorine-containing denture cleansers, such as hypochlorite solutions, which must be avoided.

BIOCOMPATIBILITY

The successful use for implants is proof of the good biocompatibility of these alloys. As with the nickel–chromium alloys described in Chapter 8, it is possible for some patients to display a sensitivity to these alloys, usually due to the cobalt content, although this is very rare. Hypersensitivity to cobalt has been implicated in the failure of some orthopaedic implants.

DENSITY

Although of no great significance in inlays, crowns, and bridges, the density of the casting alloy may be important in a denture framework which is larger than a simple restoration and which is not permanently fixed to the oral tissues. The density of a gold alloy is in the region of 15 $g/cm^3$ while that of a cobalt–chromium alloy is 8 $g/cm^3$. This provides a further reason for choosing the base metal alloy for the denture framework.

COST

This point has already been discussed in the context of the choice between gold and nickel–chromium alloys in Chapter 8. With partial dentures, the volume of material used brings this question into far greater prominence and the cobalt–chromium alloys are preferred largely for this reason.

### Possible alternative casting alloys

The poor ductility of the cobalt–chromium alloys has provided a stimulus for the search for alternative casting alloys for partial dentures.

Some of these alloys represent variations on the basic cobalt–chromium composition. Further replacement of the cobalt, either by greater amounts of nickel or possibly other elements may give some improvement. A 35 per cent cobalt, 26 per cent chromium, 26 per cent nickel, 13 per cent tantalum alloy, for example, gives much better ductility, although, as usual, at the expense of strength. One commercially available alloy contains up to 10 per cent titanium in addition to 5–15 per cent nickel, 5–15 per cent chromium, 3 per cent molybdenum, and traces of other elements in the parent cobalt. This alloy can give over 10 per cent ductility whilst retaining a high strength. A criticism has been the poor castability, due to the excessive oxidation and high viscosity, which leads to a high percentage of faulty castings.

Other commercially available alloys are based on the iron–chromium system. These, for example, could consist of about 50 per cent iron, 25 per cent chromium, and less than 10 per cent each of cobalt, nickel, and molybdenum. Since they are effectively the same as cobalt–chromium alloys, but with a very substantial amount of the cobalt replaced by iron, the strength is about the same, but the hardness slightly lower and the ductility somewhat greater than the cobalt–chromium alloys.

Some other alloys have attempted to reproduce a gold appearance through the use of copper. For example an aluminium bronze, basically of 80 per cent copper, 10 per cent aluminium, 5 per cent nickel, and 5 per cent iron composition, is commercially available. Although these have reasonable mechanical properties their long term corrosion-resistance is not very good.

A type of brass, based on copper and zinc with small amounts of nickel, cobalt, and iridium, has also been used. This has mechanical properties similar to a Type III gold alloy but has a high casting shrinkage.

## TECHNIQUES IN CASTING DENTAL ALLOYS

The stages in the casting of a dental restoration or appliance are illustrated diagrammatically in Figure 10.3. The same principles apply whether a small inlay or a large denture-base are involved, but for convenience the casting of an inlay will be discussed here. Also the techniques will be described in general terms in relation to gold, and the modifications necessary when other metals are involved will be indicated at the appropriate place.

The first stage is the preparation of the wax pattern as described in Chapter 7. This sprued pattern is then invested, or surrounded, by a slurry of a refractory material which sets and forms a mould for the casting (Fig. 10.3a). The material used for this is called an investment material. After the investment has set the wax is eliminated by heat, giving a hollow mould (Fig. 10.3b), which is then heated further to a temperature not far below the melting-point of the alloy. The molten metal is cast into this mould, generally

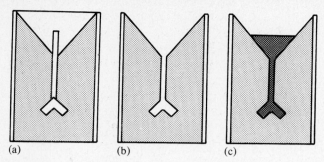

**Fig. 10.3** Stages in the casting process, showing (a) sprued wax pattern surrounded by investment; (b) mould after elimination of wax; (c) final casting.

in a casting machine, and allowed to cool (Fig. 10.3c). After removal from the investment, the casting is cleaned and finished.

## INVESTMENT MATERIALS

### Dimensional changes in the casting process

In a process involving numerous stages, there is ample opportunity for errors to arise which could result in the loss of dimensional accuracy of the restoration. It is, of course, absolutely essential for the restoration to fit the prepared tooth exactly. Great care is taken during the technical procedures, therefore, to minimize, or make allowances for, dimensional changes that take place. In this context it is very important to recall the point made earlier that metals contract when they solidify. This is an inherent characteristic of this type of phase transformation and, although the amount of contraction can be minimized by careful choice of the alloy, it cannot be eliminated. Therefore, if a molten metal is poured into a mould which is of exactly the right dimensions, it will contract on solidifying, so that the casting will be smaller than the mould. Methods have to be used to compensate for this shrinkage by making the original mould larger than the required casting.

In addition to shrinking on solidification, the metal will also contract as it cools to room temperature from the melting-point by an amount determined by its coefficient of expansion. This adds to the difficulty but is more readily overcome since the mould is heated to a point close to the casting temperature resulting in its expansion. It is the additional casting shrinkage that is the main problem. The situation is illustrated in Figure 10.4 where the contraction that takes place in the metal is shown alongside the dimensional change that is required in the mould.

So far it has been assumed that the wax pattern used to produce the investment mould is itself of the correct dimensions. However, as will be recalled from Chapter 7, wax contracts to a considerable degree on cooling, and patterns produced by the direct technique undergo a reduction in size

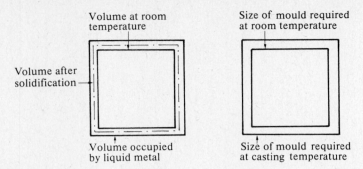

**Fig. 10.4** Casting shrinkage of the alloy and the corresponding dimensional change required in the mould.

from mouth to room temperature. Compensation must also be made for this contraction.

In practice the dimensional changes in the investment after its application to the wax pattern are controlled by the nature of the investment material itself. It is therefore appropriate to discuss these materials at this point.

### Requirements of an investment material

**a** The first and most important requirement of an investment material is the ability to compensate for the contraction from the sources described above.

**b** The material, when mixed, must have a consistency suitable for adaptation to the wax pattern, having a fine particle size to allow accurate and smooth reproduction of the surface.

**c** It must have a suitable setting time.

**d** The investment material must be able to withstand the temperatures associated with the casting process without undergoing any distortion or decomposition and without reacting with the metal.

**e** During casting, molten metal is forced into the mould under pressure and the investment must have adequate strength to prevent disintegration or fragmentation under this force.

**f** As explained below, it is important that the air within the mould should be allowed to escape as the molten metal is forced into the mould. The investment material should preferably be porous to allow the escape of air through the mould wall.

**g** The investment should be easily removed from the casting after it has cooled.

Based on these requirements, three types of investment material currently used in dental practice may be distinguished. They all have the same basic structure consisting of a refractory substance, the particles of which are held together by a suitable binder. A refractory material is a substance that can withstand high temperatures without decomposing. All three classes of investment materials utilize silica ($SiO_2$) as the refractory material, although it may be present in different forms. It is the nature of the binder that differs in these three materials.

The most common type utilizes gypsum as the binding agent. Such gypsum-bonded investment materials are widely used in the casting of gold restorations. There is a limitation on the maximum temperature at which they can be used, however, and there are two alternatives if high temperatures are involved. These are the phosphate and silica-bonded materials.

## Gypsum-bonded investment materials

COMPOSITION

These investments usually contain 60–65 per cent silica in one of its crystalline forms. In most cases this is either quartz or crystobalite or possibly a combination of the two, the significance of the choice being described later. A further 30–35 per cent of the material consists of gypsum. This is in the form of the autoclaved calcium sulphate hemihydrate (Chapter 7) and is preferred to the calcined hemihydrate because of its greater strength. The remainder of the material (about 5 per cent) consists of additives that are used to control properties, such as the expansion and strength, or substances, such as graphite, that help to produce a reducing atmosphere within the mould when it is heated. All these components are mixed together in the form of a powder which is mixed with water by the technician to form the slurry. The mixing is achieved in much the same way as the mixing of dental stone discussed in Chapter 7.

DIMENSIONAL CHANGES IN THE MOULD

Three factors may contribute to expansion of the gypsum-bonded investment material once it has been applied to the wax pattern.

**a** *Setting expansion.* The expansion that is associated with the setting of gypsum products has already been discussed in detail in Chapter 7. The presence of the silica in the gypsum, if anything, increases the amount of expansion observed, possibly by interfering with the inward growth of the dihydrate crystals. The total amount of setting expansion is of the order of 0·4–0·5 per cent, although this may be modified by the presence of accelerators and retarders, exactly as for dental stone.

**b** *Hygroscopic expansion.* The description of the setting process of gypsum products and their associated expansion has assumed that the reaction takes place in air. In the presence of excess water, the same reaction occurs, but there is a tendency for the observed expansion to be even greater, because the water facilitates the outward growth of the crystals. This additional expansion is termed hygroscopic expansion. Generally the same features that increase the setting expansion give greater amounts of hygroscopic expansion. It has long been a practice to enhance the contribution from hygroscopic expansion by immersing the invested wax pattern in water during setting. It is, however, very difficult to control the amount of additional expansion that occurs in this way and the technique is no longer common. Nevertheless, hygroscopic expansion must make a small contribution to the overall expansion since, as noted below in the discussion of techniques, wet asbestos is generally used to line the casting ring, in contact with the investment.

c *Thermal expansion.* After it has set, the investment will have expanded for the above reasons, but this will still be insufficient to compensate completely for the metal shrinkage. One further factor, related to the thermal behaviour of silica, is instrumental in providing this extra expansion.

Nearly all materials expand when heated, the amount being determined by the coefficient of expansion. Usually this coefficient is a constant over a wide range of temperature so that a graph of expansion against temperature should be a straight line. The dotted line in Figure 10.5 illustrates this behaviour. However, when certain types of silica are heated they show quite different characteristics and specifically display a far more rapid increase in expansion than the normal expansion coefficient would predict. This is due to a slight change in the arrangement of atoms in the crystalline lattice of the silica, which takes place because different types of crystal structure

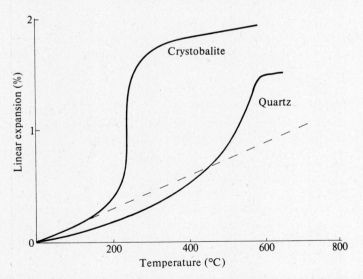

**Fig. 10.5** Thermal expansion. Dotted line shows expansion in normal material as the temperature is increased. The curves for crystobalite and quartz show increased expansion due to inversion.

are stable at high and low temperatures. This change in the crystal structure on heating is called inversion.

Silica exists in many different forms and the inversion phenomenon takes place at different temperatures, and is associated with different amounts of expansion, in each of the various forms. The two most commonly used forms of crystalline silica are quartz and crystobalite, the thermal expansion curves for these being illustrated in Figure 10.5. Clearly the crystobalite gives the greater amount of expansion, and this also takes place at a lower temperature than quartz.

Although the investment shows an overall expansion on heating, there is also a tendency to contract a little because of the effect of heat on the calcium sulphate dihydrate. The loss of water of crystallization from the dihydrate on heating to produce the anhydrite has already been described in Chapter 7. This loss is accompanied by a shrinkage and takes place as the investment is heated in the 100–200 °C range. Thus, the thermal expansion curve for a gypsum-bonded investment material will just show a slight thermal expansion up to about 100 °C, then a period of no change, or slight contraction, as the further thermal expansion of silica competes with the contraction due to this loss of water from the binder, followed by a further expansion as the temperature rises and the inversion phenomenon occurs. Generally the total expansion is adequate to compensate for the shrinkage encountered with gold alloys.

OTHER PROPERTIES OF GYPSUM-BONDED INVESTMENTS

Although they cannot be considered perfect, the gypsum-bonded investment materials are very satisfactory and meet most of the requirements. They are sufficiently thermally stable to be used with virtually all the gold alloys. The consistency is good and the particle size adequate for reproduction of surface detail. The material is generally of sufficient strength to withstand the casting process, but may be removed easily from the casting following quenching. Since gypsum is slightly porous, so is the set investment material which allows the escape of some air during casting.

The one problem with these materials is their inability to be used at very high temperatures, which precludes their use for the casting of nickel-based or cobalt-based alloys. This is because the calcium sulphate and the silica react at about 1200 °C:

$$CaSO_4 + SiO_2 \longrightarrow CaSiO_3 + SO_3$$

This results in the breakdown of the surface and, as the equation implies, the release of sulphur trioxide, which is a gas. Although the mould will not normally be preheated to these temperatures, the reaction would take place as molten metal impinged on the investment surface. The sulphur trioxide produced would then become trapped in the metal, giving porosity, and the contamination of the surface might decrease the corrosion-resistance.

### Phosphate-bonded investments

In these materials the binder is magnesium ammonium phosphate. They differ from the gypsum-based products in two respects. First, the setting reaction is not a simple hydration phenomenon and secondly the phosphate can react with the silica refractory to give superior strength.

The powder consists of three components. First, there is the silica, which acts as the refractory and constitutes about 80 per cent of the powder. Secondly, there is a source of phosphate ions, usually as the ammonium phosphate $NH_4H_2PO_4$. The third substance is magnesium oxide, which reacts with the phosphate in solution to give magnesium ammonium phosphate. This reaction may be represented by the equation

$$NH_4H_2PO_4 + MgO \longrightarrow NH_4MgPO_4 + H_2O,$$

although a number of different hydrated or non-hydrated magnesium ammonium phosphates may be produced. When set, this phosphate has a moderate strength, which is usually improved by the addition of alkaline colloidal silica to the liquid that is mixed with the powder.

On heating, a reaction takes place between the silica and the phosphate to produce a layer of silicophosphates around the silica particles, giving even greater strength. The material is then thermally stable, allowing its use at the casting temperatures of the base-metal alloys.

The setting expansion of this type of material is similar to that of the gypsum-bonded product. If colloidal silica is used in its preparation, there is also a significant contribution from hygroscopic expansion. Again the thermal expansion is similar as it is largely controlled by the silica content.

### Silica-bonded investments

There are a number of ways in which silica can be·used as a binder in investment materials. Most frequently in dental investments the setting reaction involves the use of sodium silicate, colloidal silica, or ethyl silicate. In the latter case, the ethyl silicate in polymer form is hydrolyzed to give a sol, silicic acid

$$Si(OC_2H_5)_4 + 4H_2O \longrightarrow Si(OH)_4 + 4C_2H_5OH,$$

which, when mixed with the quartz or crystobalite under alkaline conditions, gels to give the silica-based binder. Since this process is relatively slow, an amine can be added to the ethyl silicate which accelerates the process so that hydrolysis and gelation occur simultaneously.

In contrast to the other two investments the silica-bonded material shrinks on setting because of the loss of alcohol $(C_2H_5OH)$ and water. However, the far greater amount of silica in the material, by giving a much greater contribution to the thermal expansion, compensates for this and again good dimensional accuracy may be achieved. These investments tend to be more refractory than the phosphate-bonded products.

One disadvantage with this material is the lack of porosity which arises from the decrease in the volume of the binder. In order to avoid the problems of back pressure exerted by trapped air, venting of the investment is essential. Venting is, in fact, now common with all products as better investing processes result in denser, less porous moulds. Vents are usually produced by attaching one end of a wax sprue to the top of the casting ring and placing the other end close to, but not touching, the pattern. It is also essential with the denser investments to restrict the thickness of investment between the end of the pattern and the top of the casting ring to 6 mm to facilitate the escape of gases.

### Investment of wax patterns

The investment of the wax pattern is a very critical stage in the casting process. One of the first points to note is that there must be a suitable channel through the investment material for the molten metal to enter the mould. This channel is produced by attaching a rod of either wax or metal to the pattern. These are called 'sprues' or 'sprue formers'. Wax sprues are eliminated from the mould in the same way as the wax pattern itself, while metal sprues are removed after the investment has set.

Several features of sprue design will influence the success of the casting.

**a** It is necessary to place the sprue in the most suitable position where it will allow easy flow of the molten metal, without creating turbulence, to give rapid and complete filling of the mould.

**b** The sprue should be of sufficient diameter to facilitate the rapid passage of the molten alloy into the mould. For a small inlay this need only be about 1·5 mm, but for larger restorations a sprue approximately 2·5 mm in diameter may be needed. With large castings, such as partial dentures and bridges, several sprues may be required. Bridges based on nickel–chromium alloys should have a broad sprue to each unit.

**c** On casting, more alloy is drawn into the mould as it contracts, but this is only achieved if the sprue is sufficiently short. Under these circumstances additional alloy is taken from the excess at the mouth of the sprue channel. If the sprue is too long the alloy in the channel tends to draw material back from the mould, leaving the casting porous. This may be overcome by placing a wax reservoir on the sprue close to the pattern. This wax is lost to create a space in the investment adjacent to the mould. Provided the cross-section of the reservoir exceeds that of the pattern, any additional alloy required to compensate for the contraction is taken from the reservoir by the casting. Normally a sprue length of 9 mm is recommended. Patterns with and without reservoirs are illustrated in Figure 10.6.

**d** Finally, the length of the sprue and the height of the casting ring should be designed to leave the pattern, and thus the mould, reasonably close to

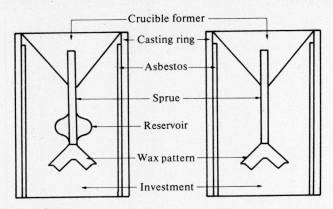

**Fig. 10.6** Patterns (a) with; and (b) without reservoirs, showing casting ring, pattern and former.

the end of the investment block. This, in conjunction with the porosity of the investment, allows the escape of air and gases during casting.

At the end of the sprue-former is the crucible-former. This is cone-shaped piece of metal or wax which allows a funnel to be formed in the investment which acts as a crucible for the melting of the gold in some techniques and guides the molten metal into the mould.

The wax pattern, with attached sprue and crucible former, is placed inside a casting ring, which has an inner lining of asbestos. The latter is used to allow the setting and thermal expansion to take place without the direct constraining influence of the casting ring. The asbestos is soaked in water and this may contribute a certain amount of hygroscopic expansion, as already mentioned. The arrangement of lined ring, pattern, and formers is shown in Figure 10.6. The pattern should be cleaned and painted with a wetting or degreasing agent before investing.

Investing can either be performed in air or under vacuum. In the former case the investment is mixed carefully, according to the manufacturer's instructions, and is placed on a vibrator to eliminate air. The method of applying the investment varies but a commonly used technique involves coating the wax pattern by brush first and then immersing it into the casting ring filled with investment. Alternatively the pattern may be placed in the ring and the investment poured around it. It is usual to continue careful vibrating of the investment during these stages.

Air inclusions are best avoided by the use of a vacuum. Either a vacuum pump or water aspirator may be used to obtain a partial vacuum over the investment. Several different types of commercially available apparatus are suitable for this purpose. The resulting investment has less porosity and greater mechanical strength.

MELTING AND CASTING

About 30–45 minutes are allowed for the investment to set before the next stage is carried out. The crucible former and sprue are carefully removed, the wax being eliminated by heating the investment. This may be done as a separate process or as a part of preheating prior to casting. A temperature of 150 °C is sufficient to remove most of the wax from the inverted casting ring, the last traces being burnt out at a higher temperature.

The ring may then be heated to about 700 °C, either gradually or by placing in a preheated furnace, and held at this temperature to allow uniform heat distribution in the mould. This is called heat-soaking and 25–30 minutes is usually sufficient.

There are several different kinds of casting machine but all provide some mechanism for forcing the metal into the mould under pressure. In some systems, compressed air, gas, steam, or a vacuum is used, whilst centrifugal force is used in others. The preheated casting ring is placed into the casting machine. The alloy may be contained in either the funnel provided by the crucible former in the investment, or in a separate crucible that is located adjacent to the mouth of the ring.

Melting may be achieved by a gas–air or gas–oxygen torch, by an electric arc, or by an induction coil. The former two methods are generally used with gold alloys, the gas (natural gas)–air mixture being sufficient for alloys with a melting range below 1000 °C. A gas–oxygen mixture is needed for higher melting gold alloys. The reducing part of the flame is used for melting. Once the metal has started to melt, flux is added to increase the fluidity of the metal and prevent contamination by oxidation. When the alloy is completely fluid the flame is removed and the casting machine activated to force the molten metal into the mould.

The casting ring and contents are left standing until they have lost all traces of redness, which may take 5 minutes, after which quenching is carried out by complete immersion in cold water. The investment disintegrates on quenching and is easily removed from the casting. Removal of investment from the casting ring is facilitated by the asbestos liner.

CLEANING AND FINISHING THE CASTING

Gold castings may appear dull because the surface has slightly oxidized. The surface layer can be removed by a process known as 'pickling', which involves heating the casting in an acid. Sulphuric, hydrochloric, and nitric acids have all been used, the former two usually being preferred. Dilutions in the range of 10–50 per cent are employed and the pickling may be achieved by placing the casting in the acid solution and warming it to 70–80 °C or alternatively heating the casting in a flame and dropping it into acid. The former technique is usually recommended because of the possibility of the flame melting thin edges. Oxides may also be removed by ultrasonic cleaners.

Sprues and excess metal may be removed with a piercing saw, and gross irregularities by an appropriate stone or bur. The surface can be smoothed with a hard rubber wheel and polished with an abrasive compound on a felt wheel. The final polish may be achieved with a wool mop, following which the casting is thoroughly cleaned. With inlays prepared by the indirect technique, finishing should be carried out on the die to protect the fine feather edges of the restoration.

### HEAT TREATMENT

As discussed earlier, gold alloys may require heat treatment. This may be either an homogenizing or stress-relieving anneal, or a heat-hardening treatment. In the former case the casting is placed in a preheated furnace at 700 °C for 3–4 minutes, quenched, and then pickled. The heat-hardening process, details of which have already been given, may be achieved either in air or in a salt bath. In the latter case, the casting is placed in a mixture of molten sodium and potassium nitrates. This is a better method of heating, preventing oxidation of the surface.

### REUSE OF GOLD

Excess gold remaining from a casting may be reused. It has to be thoroughly cleaned, preferably by sand blasting, to remove all traces of oxide and investment adhering to the surface which would otherwise contaminate subsequent castings. It is good practice to add at least one-third of new alloy to this reclaimed alloy, but the new and used parts must be of the same alloy type.

### VARIATIONS IN CASTING WITH BASE METAL ALLOYS

The technique of casting the nickel–chromium and cobalt–chromium alloys is basically similar to that for the gold alloys, but there are a few important differences, which are related to the melting range. First, the higher temperatures involved necessitate the use of either phosphate or silica-bonded investments because of the instability of the gypsum-bonded material. Secondly, alternative sources of heat for melting may be required for these higher temperatures. The gas–air torch can only be used for alloys with a melting range below 1000 °C. Other types of torch can be used to melt alloys above this temperature. The oxy-acetylene torch has been used for cobalt–chromium alloys and the problem of carbon pick-up from the acetylene has already been mentioned. Gas–oxygen torches may be used but the maximum temperature attained is around 1300 °C and suitable for only a few of the base metal alloys.

Electrical heating methods are therefore usually preferred. In the electric-arc technique, a high current is passed between two carbon electrodes, which are held about 12 mm away from the alloy to be melted. A uniformly molten mass is produced within about 30 seconds. Great care must be taken in this technique to avoid damage to the eyes by the arc. The other electrical methods are induction heating where the alloy is contained within a coil and heated by induction as a current is passed through the coil, and resistance heating, where the current is passed through the metal itself.

## Soldering techniques

The need, under certain circumstances, to solder together separate sections of bridges was mentioned in Chapter 8 in relation to the composition of gold solders.

Before soldering, the surfaces to be joined should be thoroughly smoothed and cleaned to allow the solder to flow easily over them. It is sometimes helpful to prevent solder flowing too far by applying colloidal graphite to nearby areas where the solder is not required. Clearly the components must be located in the correct relationship to one another, and this may be achieved in the mouth or on a model. In the mouth a plaster locating impression or cold-cure resin may be used for this, while sticky wax serves the same purpose in the laboratory.

The located bridge is surrounded with investment, so that only the area of the proposed joint is exposed. After an initial drying-out period the invested bridge is heated slowly in a furnace to a temperature close to the melting-point of the solder to be used. To maintain heat, soldering may be carried out on a preheated soldering block and sufficient solder is added to adequately fill the joint. Gold solders are easily melted for this process with a gas–air torch.

Components of bonded procelain may be soldered before or after the construction of the porcelain facing. Clearly if soldering is undertaken before-hand, the melting-point of the solder must be higher than the fusion temperature of the porcelain, and the converse is also true. When investing a bridge carrying porcelain facings it is wise to protect them from the abrasive action of the investment by applying a thin film of wax. In view of the higher temperatures involved in soldering bonded porcelain, a phosphate-bonded investment should be used.

## Casting defects

An error at any stage of the casting process may result in a defect. These defects may be considered in four categories:

**a** incomplete castings;

**b** inaccurate castings;

**c** porous castings;

**d** rough casting surfaces.

INCOMPLETE CASTINGS

These occur when alloy fails to reach all parts of the mould. This may arise from:

**a** use of insufficient alloy;

**b** inadequate heating of the alloy so that it is not completely molten;

**c** premature solidification of the metal as it enters the mould, usually due to inadequate heating of the latter;

**d** the inability of the alloy to reach all parts of the mould because sections are too thin;

**e** use of a casting force that is too low;

**f** sprues that are too narrow or blocked by investment or flux, limiting the flow of the alloy;

**g** the inability of gas to escape from the mould, leading to back pressure which resists the force of the molten metal. This may be due to an investment that is not sufficiently porous, a lack of vents, or a mould space that is too far from the end of the ring.

Clearly all these errors are very elementary and should be easily avoided.

INACCURATE CASTINGS

A casting may not accurately fit the prepared teeth, either because it is distorted or the wrong size. In practice it is often difficult to distinguish between these sources of inaccuracy. Distortion, when present, is almost invariably produced at the wax stage. Residual stresses in a wax pattern are gradually relieved over a period of time, resulting in distortion. Investing soon after the pattern has been made minimizes this problem. Distortion may arise during any stage in the handling of a wax pattern, especially when it is being removed from the tooth or die, and during investment.

The factors which influence the dimensional accuracy of the casting have already been discussed in some detail. The use of the wrong investment will result in an inaccurate casting if its expansion is not balanced with the contraction of the alloy. Also if the mould is heated above the recommended temperature, excessive expansion of the mould will occur, leading to an oversize casting. The opposite result is achieved with under-heating.

POROUS CASTINGS

The types of porosity observed in castings are illustrated in Figure 10.7. Some of these are almost inevitable to a certain extent whilst others are more easily avoided.

The first type is really a minor version of the incomplete casting and involves the fine margins which may be rounded, pitted, or even absent. All the reasons for incomplete castings may apply in this case, the back pressure of the gases in the mould probably being the most important.

Casting shrinkage may result in porosity, especially near the sprue attachment. Here the metal in contact with the mould walls solidifies first and

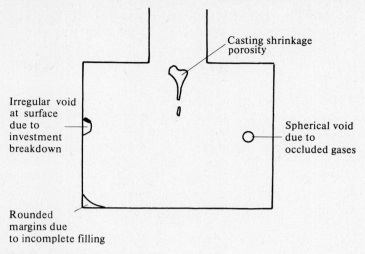

**Fig. 10.7** Types of casting porosity.

contracts. If there is insufficient molten metal available, via the sprue, voids form in this region. They may be minimized by using thick sprues or appropriately placed reservoirs and by ensuring that the sprues are attached to the thickest sections of the pattern.

Some irregular voids may be produced at the surface of a casting if the investment breaks down, the fragments preventing the molten alloy reaching all parts of the mould.

Finally, spherical voids may be found throughout the casting. These are due to gases that dissolve in the alloy at high temperatures but which come out of solution as it solidifies. The use of too high a temperature or prolonged heating of the alloy will aggravate this situation. Gases coming out of solution in this way are called occluded gases.

ROUGH CASTING SURFACES

A rough surface on a casting may be produced for a variety of reasons, many of which have already been discussed. Occluded gases may produce small surface defects as well as internal porosity. An air bubble trapped on the surface of the investment will produce surface nodules on the casting as these bubbles fill with molten metal. This may be obviated by careful technique and vacuum investing. If the casting ring is disturbed before the investment has set, a series of ridges may be produced. Sharp fins can arise if the set investment cracks, thus allowing the molten metal to enter the cracks on casting. This is usually associated with overheating of the mould or heating it too rapidly. The breakdown of the investment may also lead to a rough surface. Improper investment technique and the use of too high a casting force can contribute to this effect. As noted earlier in this chapter, sulphur trioxide formed when gypsum-bonded investments are overheated may contaminate the surface. Further contamination may arise through oxidation of the alloy.

## STAINLESS STEEL

For reasons discussed in Chapter 11, it is sometimes desirable to construct a full denture base from a metal. This may be done by using a casting process with a cobalt–chromium alloy, although it is difficult to cast the very thin sections often required in the base. A more suitable alloy is stainless steel which, unlike the cobalt–chromium alloy, can be wrought. Unfortunately the process involved in fabricating the stainless steel denture base does need equipment which is not normally available in small dental laboratories, and the use of this material is probably restricted by this limitation.

As mentioned in Chapter 1, stainless steels comprise one of many categories of steel, their main attribute being a very good resistance to corrosion. Since they also have good mechanical properties, can be wrought, and are relatively cheap, these steels enjoy widespread use and are employed in dentistry for orthodontic appliances and denture bases, and indeed for internal prostheses in orthopaedics. The metallurgy of stainless steel is covered here in relation to their use in prosthetics, while the orthodontic applications are discussed in Chapter 13.

### Composition and structure of stainless steel

Steels, by definition, are alloys of iron and carbon, with or without the addition of other elements. Steels that contain a minimum of about 12 per cent chromium will possess good corrosion-resistance because of the passivating effect of this element, and are generally known as stainless steels.

There are three different forms of stainless steel each with a different crystal structure that is largely determined by the composition. First, there are the ferritic stainless steels, with a body-centred cubic structure similar to that found in many simpler types of steel. The chromium content is in the range 12–28 per cent, but no other major alloying element is present. Martensitic stainless steels contain 12–17 per cent chromium, a small amount of nickel, and a relatively large amount of carbon. They have a body-centred tetragonal structure and are the hardest of the stainless steels, being used for surgical instruments including scalpel blades. Thirdly, and most important in the context of dental materials, there are the austenitic stainless steels which contain 16–25 per cent chromium and at least 8 per cent nickel (the 18–8 steel) and are widely used for domestic products. These steels have a face-centred cubic crystal structure.

Because corrosion-resistance is very important in any intra-oral appliance, the austenitic stainless steel is used in the construction of orthodontic appliances and dentures. The composition may vary, but will usually lie in the range of 17–19 per cent chromium and 8–19 per cent nickel with less than 0·15 per cent carbon.

## Properties of austenitic stainless steel

### EASE OF FABRICATION

Steels are not easily cast, because of their high melting range and are generally used in the wrought state. These particular austenitic stainless steels possess a reasonable degree of ductility and can be processed by many techniques, but they work harden very readily, as discussed below, so that great care has to be taken during deformation.

### MECHANICAL PROPERTIES

The elastic modulus for an 18–8 stainless steel is about 200 $GN/m^2$, which is just less than that of cobalt–chromium alloys.

Because of the work-hardening effect, the strength and ductility depend on the extent of prior deformation. In the so-called 'soft' state, where there has been little or no deformation, the alloy is relatively weak, with a yield strength of less than 300 $MN/m^2$ and an ultimate tensile strength of about 600 $MN/m^2$, but with an exceptionally high ductility of 50 per cent. However, as stress is applied and the steel deforms, the face-centred cubic, austenitic structure transforms to a martensitic type of structure and the material work-hardens rapidly. The yield strength of a 'hard' steel may then approach 1500 $MN/m^2$ and the ultimate tensile strength 1700 $MN/m^2$. The ductility is, of course, reduced at the same time, and in a fully work-hardened steel will be less than 5 per cent.

These characteristics have a number of important consequences. First, a wide range of mechanical properties is available for one composition of alloy, which provides considerable versatility. This is especially important in orthodontic appliances as the wires can be provided in soft, half-hard, or hard condition, the selection being dependent on the work to be performed, as discussed in Chapter 13. Secondly, the rapid loss of ductility during work hardening may result in cracking as deformation proceeds. This can be avoided in some circumstances by the use of annealing heat treatments (Chapter 1), which soften the material and allow further deformation to take place.

### CORROSION-RESISTANCE

As already mentioned, the austenitic stainless steels are the most corrosion-resistant steels available and generally they are very suitable for use in the oral environment. Their corrosion-resistance is not as good as that of gold, nickel–chromium, or cobalt–chromium alloys, the latter two generally containing more chromium. In particular, great care has to be taken if the steel is heated to the region of 650–1000 °C during any part of the process, since chromium carbides may be precipitated. The large amount of chromium that is tied up in such carbides means that there is insufficient in the remainder of the material to afford complete corrosion-resistance. A steel in this condition is said to be sensitized and the problem most frequently arises if welding has been performed.

### Fabrication of stainless steel denture bases

As noted earlier, stainless steel denture bases are not easily fabricated. Swaging was the most commonly used method for many years, a method in which a stainless steel sheet was pressed between a die and a counter-die in a hydraulic press. A large number of stages were involved in the preparation of dies and counter-dies, so that dimensional inaccuracy and loss of fine detail were significant problems.

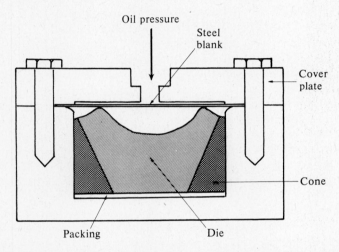

**Fig. 10.8** Apparatus used for the hydraulic forming of stainless steel denture bases.

A far better slow-rate hydraulic forming technique is now used where only one die is involved and pressure is applied directly to the steel by the oil. The forming chamber, illustrated in Figure 10.8, consists of two halves that are securely bolted together. A circular stainless steel blank is clamped between these two halves. The die, usually made from a hard dental stone, is supported by a brass cone and fluid pressure is applied to the top surface of the blank by a suitable pump. The plate may vary in thickness from 0·25–0·35 mm and the oil pressure needed to deform the plate will naturally vary with this thickness.

The forming process is carried out in a number of stages which involve progressively increasing pressures. In simple cases three forming operations may be involved, but deeply vaulted palates may require more. The final pressure may be of the order of 50 MN/m$^2$. The plastic strain induced in the steel during this process may be considerable, and, as work hardening takes place, there is a risk of cracking in some parts of the plate. The annealing treatments referred to above may be used to soften the steel between the forming operations to reduce this risk. Beading wire and wire gauze to retain the pink acrylic resin bearing the denture teeth may be attached to the periphery of the trimmed base by spot welding (Chapter 13).

# 11
## Denture base resins

A full denture consists of two parts, the artificial teeth and the denture base which rests on the oral soft tissues. Artificial teeth are made from either acrylic resin or porcelain and are described briefly at the end of this chapter. The properties of the denture base are generally more important to the performance of the denture for it is the base that controls the retention, mechanical properties, and biocompatibility. As usual, a large number of requirements can be listed.

### Requirements of a denture base resin

Virtually all denture bases are constructed from polymeric materials. Very occasionally these will be unsuitable and a metal has to be used, as discussed in the previous chapter, but the properties of a polymer are far more appropriate to this application and the following list of requirements refer specifically to them. The clinical use of alternative materials is discussed later. It should be noted that the terms denture base polymers and denture base resins are generally used interchangeably.

#### EASE OF FABRICATION

A prime consideration in the selection of a material is the ease of fabrication, as dentures have to be prepared to fit individual patients. In terms of plastics technology the shapes are complex and the moulding of polymers to the desired form is not easily achieved. As noted later, the prevailing use of acrylic resin for denture bases is largely based on its exceptional ease of fabrication.

Two other factors are important. First, the artificial teeth have to be incorporated into the base and the moulding process has to allow for their accurate placement and permanent retention in the resin. Secondly, as dentures may break, it is highly desirable for them to be capable of easy but effective repair. This is largely controlled by the nature of the denture base resin.

#### ACCURACY

It is, of course, essential that a denture adapts well to the oral tissues, implying good dimensional accuracy and surface reproducibility. All resins undergo some contraction on polymerization and this has to be kept to a minimum.

#### MECHANICAL PROPERTIES

Dentures are subjected to reasonably high stresses during use, and fracture of the base is still quite common. Good mechanical properties are therefore required, the more important ones being listed below.

**a** *A high proportional limit:* this ensures that plastic deformation does not take place under normal use.

**b** *A high ultimate tensile strength:* fracture owing to overloading is thus avoided.

**c** *A high fatigue limit:* this minimizes the risk of fatigue failures. It will be readily appreciated that denture bases are flexed many times during use so that fatigue, which is the failure of the material under repetitive stresses (Chapter 1), is likely to be more of a problem than simple overloading.

**d** *A good impact strength.* A common cause of failure with removable dentures is their accidental dropping by the patient, often during cleaning. Ideally the base should have a high impact strength to resist this abuse. An important factor here is the effect that notches have on impact strength since cracks are more easily nucleated at any irregular feature.

**e** *Resistance to viscoelastic deformation.* Loads applied to a polymeric material may, over a period of time, produce permanent deformation even though the elastic limit, as determined by a simple tensile test, has not been exceeded. This phenomenon of time-dependent deformation under low loads, sometimes referred to as 'creep', has been discussed in Chapter 1. It is obviously desirable that such deformation is restricted. It is important to bear in mind that such deformation is very sensitive to temperature and there is a close relationship between viscoelastic behaviour and the thermal behaviour described below.

**f** *A reasonably high elastic modulus.* Although the ideal elastic modulus for a denture base has not been determined, it would seem desirable to avoid the great flexibility associated with very low modulus materials.

It should be remembered that the mechanical behaviour of a denture is dependent on the design of the denture as well as the materials. The relationship between impact strength and notches mentioned earlier is a good example of this.

AESTHETICS

Ideally the denture base should have a natural appearance, which implies that the polymer chosen should be easily pigmented and be either transparent or translucent. Moreover, the appearance should not change with time, either by loss of substance or by surface contamination.

STABILITY IN THE ORAL ENVIRONMENT

As with any material used for an intra-oral restoration or appliance, the denture base resin should be chemically stable. That is it should not dissolve or be otherwise affected by either the oral fluids or other substances taken into the mouth, nor should it absorb any fluids to such an extent that its properties change. It should also be resistant to the types of chemical used for cleaning the dentures.

BIOCOMPATIBILITY

Similarly, the material must not have any adverse effect on the oral tissues. Clearly it must be non-toxic, but, probably of more importance, it should be non-irritant. Hypersensitivity to denture base resins is possible, especially as they may still contain a significant amount of irritant monomer after processing. High molecular weight polymers themselves are inert in this respect but low molecular weight substances are often highly irritant.

In addition to a lack of irritation of the tissues, the denture base material must not have an unpleasant taste or in any way be objectionable to the patient.

The question of contamination must also be considered in this context. Both the presence of porosity in the resin and the susceptibility to water absorption leads to a risk of microbial contamination within the mouth, especially by yeasts, which can lead to denture stomatitis. Materials that minimize this risk are preferable.

THERMAL PROPERTIES

Since polymers frequently melt or undergo structural transitions at relatively low temperatures, it is essential that any critical transition temperature should be above the maximum that will be encountered. Thus the thermal behaviour of the materials should be such that no softening or warpage results from normal use, either in respect of hot fluids taken into the mouth or hot cleaning solutions. For the same reason care must be taken to avoid excessive heating of the denture base during the polishing and finishing processes that follow moulding.

The coefficient of expansion of the resin should ideally be the same as that of the oral soft tissues and should also be similar to that of the material used for the artificial teeth. Also it is desirable for the denture base to have a reasonably high thermal conductivity so that the sensation associated with hot and cold fluids in the mouth is still experienced by the denture-wearer.

MISCELLANEOUS PROPERTIES

a It is usually considered desirable for the denture base resin to be radiopaque so that any fragment that is inhaled or ingested can be readily detected radiographically.

b The cost of the material and the equipment necessary for its processing should be low.

c The density should be low in order to facilitate the retention of upper dentures.

## Choice of resins

Since the 1940s acrylic resins have been the materials of choice for denture bases. They possess many, although not all, of the ideal properties listed above. Various modifications have been made over the years, and several versions of acrylic resin are available, although all are based on the same polymerization process.

There are some alternatives, which are used either when acrylic resin is contra-indicated for some reason or because they offer a very specific advantage in a specific situation. One of these, vulcanite, was in use long before the acrylics were developed, but now its use is rarely considered. Several polymers, including polycarbonate and some styrene co-polymers, offer improved impact strength but have yet to displace acrylic as the most popular material.

## ACRYLIC RESINS

Acrylic resins have been widely used in dentistry, not only for denture bases but also as a restorative material (Chapter 5), and for artificial teeth, splints, and other appliances. Strictly speaking the term 'acrylic resin' is used to describe a resin that is structurally derived from ethylene and is based on a vinyl monomer that contains a double carbon–carbon bond. Acrylic acid, $CH_2$=CHCOOH, and methacrylic acid, $CH_2$=CCH$_3$COOH, form the basis of two series of acrylic polymers. These polyacids are not widely used as structural materials because of their tendency to soften in water, but their esters are far more stable. The general form of the esters of polymethacrylic acid is shown in Figure 11.1a. If the ester radical R is a methyl group, then the polymethyl methacrylate structure of Figure 11.1b is produced. It is this polymer that is widely referred to as 'acrylic resin'.

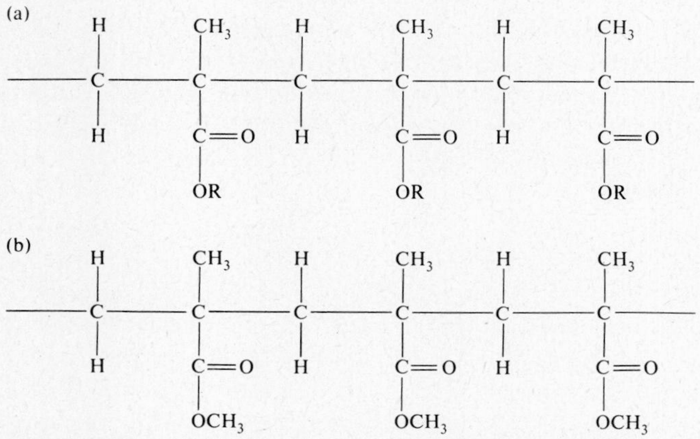

**Fig. 11.1** (a) Esters of polymethacrylic acid; (b) polymethyl methacrylate.

### Chemistry of methyl methacrylate polymerization

Polymethyl methacrylate is prepared by the addition polymerization of methyl methacrylate. One of the most significant features of dental acrylic is that this can be achieved quite readily and without resorting to the difficult conditions and expensive equipment associated with most polymerization processes.

Methyl methacrylate is a liquid that has the structure shown in Figure 11.2a. The addition polymerization of a vinyl compound of this type takes place in a number of stages. The first requires the presence of free radicals. These are molecules which have unpaired electrons and are, therefore, highly reactive. Free radicals are usually produced by heating a large molecule which splits into small fragments which may be free radicals. By convention they are generally denoted R˙. A free radical may react with a molecule of methyl methacrylate, as shown in Figure 11.2b, the unpaired electron combining with one of the extra electrons in the double bond. This leaves the other electron free and turns the monomer itself into another free radical.

The process propagates by the reaction between the newly activated molecule and another methyl methacrylate molecule (Figure 11.2c) and continues until a polymer chain is formed. It is easy to see from this why these are called 'addition polymers'.

The process may terminate in a number of ways. The growing chain itself may react with a free radical, should they collide, giving a stable molecule, as in Figure 11.2d. Alternatively the active state may be transferred from the chain to another species present, as indicated in Figure 11.2e. This leads to termination in that particular chain but also the generation of a new, more mobile, radical.

Further polymerization can obviously continue as long as there are free radicals and unterminated chains left. As the chains get longer, however, the probability of collision between free radicals and double bonds in a monomer becomes smaller so the process slows down very considerably. Eventually diffusion of the active species becomes very difficult and it is likely that the reaction will effectively cease before reaching completion; that is, while some monomer is still available. The presence of this residual monomer, which may vary from 0·2–5·0 per cent of the original monomer depending on the conditions, has a significant effect on the properties of the resin, as discussed later.

GENERATION OF FREE RADICALS: ACTIVATION, INITIATION, INHIBITION

Free radicals may be generated in many ways, but with denture acrylic they are invariably produced from benzoyl peroxide. This is an unstable substance which readily decomposes to give two free radicals per molecule as shown in Figure 11.3a. The initial reaction between the free radicals and the monomer (Figure 11.2a) is called the initiation process. Before this can take place,

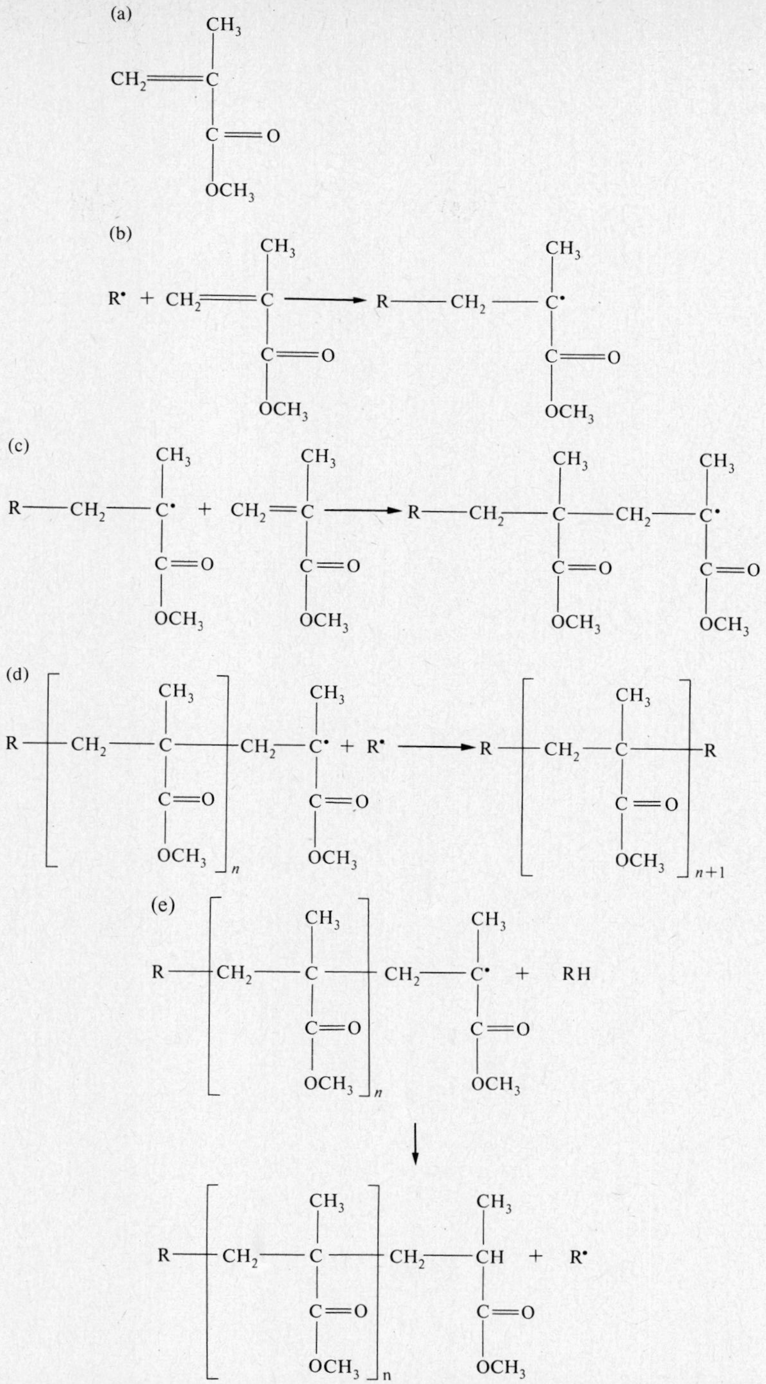

**Fig. 11.2** (a) Methyl methacrylate; (b) reaction between free radical and methyl methacrylate; (c) propagation of polymerization; (d) termination of polymerization by interaction between growing chain and free radical; (e) termination by transfer of active state to another species.

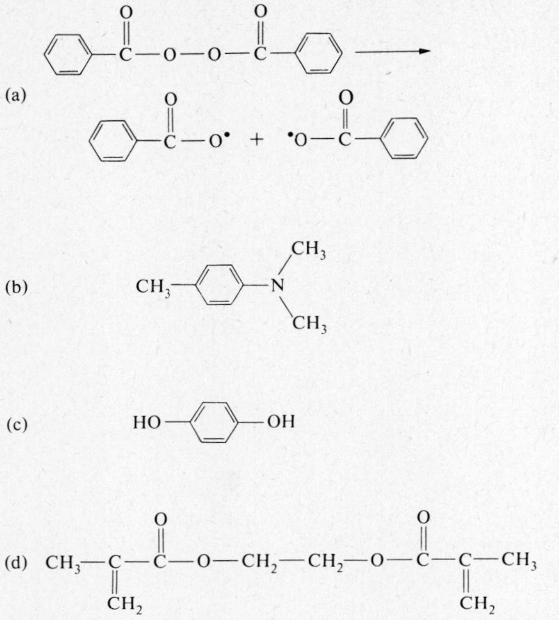

**Fig. 11.3** (a) Breakdown of benzoyl peroxide to give free radicals; (b) dimethyl-p-toluidene; (c) hydroquinone; (d) ethylene glycol dimethacrylate.

however, the benzoyl peroxide has to decompose. This generation of the free radicals is called the activation stage and may be achieved by:

**a** ultraviolet light (or other radiations);

**b** a chemical reaction;

**c** heat.

Ultraviolet light is sometimes used in the curing, or polymerization, of restorative materials and fissure sealants where the structure also contains vinyl groups (Chapters 5 and 13), but the latter two methods are used for denture construction. The most commonly used chemical activators are dimethyl-p-toluidine, a tertiary amine the structure of which is shown in Figure 11.3b, and various sulphinic acids and their derivatives. It is important to note that no heat is required for the reaction between activator and initiator to take place, and simple mixing of the two will produce the free radicals. For this reason, these acrylics are usually referred to as 'cold-cure' or 'self-cure' resins.

A high temperature will also decompose the peroxide. Generally about 60 °C is needed to initiate the polymerization and 75 °C gives a reasonable rate of reaction, although 100 °C may be used to give a quicker cure. These resins are called heat-cured acrylics.

If pure methyl methacrylate is left standing, it may polymerize very slowly without the aid of intentionally added activators and initiators. This occurs because of chance collisions between the molecules of methyl methacrylate and the few free radicals that will inevitably be present. To give stability on storage and prevent this premature polymerization, an inhibitor is added. Hydroquinone, shown in Figure 11.3c, is a very effective inhibitor, reacting with any active species present, either free radicals or activated methyl methacrylate, using up the unpaired electrons and producing a stable molecule.

## Heat-cured acrylic resin

### PRESENTATION

It is generally agreed that the heat-cured acrylics provide better properties than the cold-cured resins, and they are therefore used in the majority of denture bases. It is impractical and unnecessary, however, to use methyl methacrylate as the sole starting material for the denture construction. Instead, a large amount of previously polymerized material is presented, in powder form, and this is mixed with a smaller amount of monomer. This monomer is then polymerized in such a way that it binds the original powder, as shown in Figure 11.4.

There are numerous advantages of this technique. First, it is far more convenient, because, soon after mixing, a dough is formed which can be moulded very readily. Secondly, since the powder can be prepared under more controlled conditions by the manufacturer, materials with better mechanical properties are produced. Thirdly, there is less polymerization shrinkage since a much smaller volume of monomer is employed.

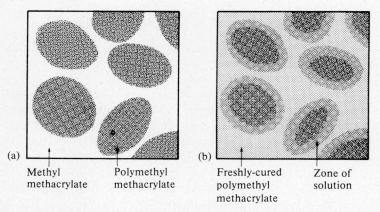

(a) Methyl methacrylate / Polymethyl methacrylate  (b) Freshly-cured polymethyl methacrylate / Zone of solution

**Fig. 11.4** Binding of polymer powder during polymerization of methyl methacrylate.

The material for preparing a denture base is therefore presented as a powder and a liquid, the powder consisting largely of the polymethyl methacrylate and the liquid of methyl methacrylate monomer. Other substances are also present as indicated in Table 11.1. The monomer and initiator have to be kept apart to minimize spontaneous polymerization on storage so that the benzoyl peroxide is included in the powder. This will also contain any pigments, dyes, fibres, and opacifiers that give the desired appearance. In some presentations, a quantity of a radiopaque substance, usually a glass, is also added to the powder.

**Table 11.1** Composition of denture acrylic resin: powder and liquid

POWDER
       Polymer (polymethyl methacrylate)
       Initiator (benzoyl peroxide)
       Pigments
       Radiopaque filler
LIQUID
       Monomer (methyl methacrylate and possibly others such as ethyl acrylate)
       Inhibitor (hydroquinone)
       Cross-linking agent (ethylene glycol dimethacrylate)

In many materials, the polymerization process is not quite as simple as that described above. Cross-linking agents are usually present in amounts up to 2 per cent. These are molecules with a $C\!\!=\!\!C$ group at each end, which can link two growing polymer molecules together. Ethylene glycol dimethacrylate (Fig. 11.3d) is frequently used for this purpose. A cross-linked polymer is more resistant to surface crazing, as discussed later. Sometimes co-monomers are used in addition to the methyl methacrylate. These are usually acrylic monomers of very similar structure that modify the properties slightly. They are also widely used along with some plasticizers in the preparation of soft linings for dentures and are discussed under this heading later in the chapter.

LABORATORY TECHNIQUES

It is not necessary to explain here the details of preparation of a denture mould. Briefly, a master stone cast is made from the impression and a wax denture containing the artificial teeth is prepared on this model. The waxed denture and cast are placed in the lower half of a metal flask filled with freshly mixed plaster (Figure 11.5a). When set, the exposed surface of the plaster is coated with a suitable separating medium, such as vaseline. The inverted upper half of the flask is filled with plaster and the lower section containing the wax denture is lowered into place. The complete flask is illustrated in Figure 11.5b. After the plaster has set, the flask is heated to soften the wax and the halves separated. The artificial teeth remain in the plaster of the upper half of the flask. The wax is removed, final traces being eliminated by boiling water.

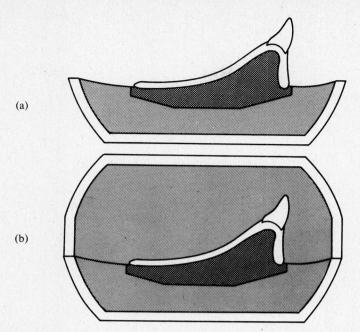

(a)

(b)

**Fig. 11.5** (a) Waxed denture and cast invested in lower half of flask; (b) complete flask.

*Separating medium.* After removal of the wax, a space, corresponding to the dimensions of the required denture, is left in the flask, which has to be filled with acrylic. It is very important, however, that the resin is protected from the gypsum, since water released from the latter would affect both the polymerization process and the properties of the cured resin. Monomer would also soak into the mould, again affecting the resulting resin, but also joining the gypsum in the two halves of the flask, preventing them from being separated easily. Therefore a separating medium, sometimes referred to as a cold mould seal, has to be used as a barrier. Usually this is a solution of sodium alginate which is brushed onto the investment surface.

Tin foil was, at one time, used extensively as a separating medium, being burnished on to the surface. This process was very time consuming, and is no longer used routinely. However, since the alginate film is not completely water-resistant, the surface of the cured acrylic may be slightly opaque as a result of the interaction with water. Therefore, if perfect clarity is absolutely essential, this tin foil technique may still be used.

*Dough preparation.* The powder/liquid ratio used is dependent upon the character of the powder, including particle size and shape. It is always quoted by the manufacturer for a specific product and the instructions should be carefully followed. The critical factor is the ability of the liquid to wet all the powder completely, and this is usually achieved with a liquid volume/

powder volume ratio of $1:3.3$ or $1:3.5$ which corresponds roughly to $1:2.5$ by weight. Excess liquid is undesirable as this gives a greater amount of polymerization shrinkage.

Measuring devices are usually provided by the manufacturer and the powder is added to the liquid. The mix is spatulated for a short time, typically 45 seconds, and then allowed to stand, in a closed container to prevent evaporation of the volatile monomer, for a length of time determined by the manufacturer. This is usually for about 18–20 minutes, during which time the powder and liquid interact. The monomer first wets the powder and produces a coarse-textured material with a consistency similar to that of wet sand. As the monomer starts to dissolve the surface of the polymer particles, the mixture becomes tacky and then, as it becomes saturated with more and more polymer in solution, it looses its tackiness and forms a dough. At this dough stage it is ready to be packed into the mould.

The material should not be left longer than the dough stage before packing, since it becomes too rubbery and eventually quite stiff. However, the dough condition is usually maintained for quite a length of time so that the timing is not too critical.

The dough time is influenced by a number of factors. If a high powder/ liquid ratio is used, it is reduced. Small powder particles and lower molecular weights of the polymer also aid rapid dissolution and give shorter dough times. The same effect is produced by raising the temperature and, conversely, refrigeration will slow the process down. This latter fact may be utilized to extend the dough stage, although there is a risk of moisture contamination arising from condensation when the resin is brought back to room temperature.

*Packing.* The dough is shaped by hand into a horseshoe form and placed in the upper half of the flask, over the teeth. Sufficient resin should be used to ensure complete filling of the mould space. A polyethylene or similar sheet is then placed over the resin to prevent its adhesion to the lower half of the mould during trial closure. This is achieved by pressing the two halves slowly together, so that the dough spreads out to fill the mould space. Any excess resin will flow out between the two halves of the flask, producing a flash. This is removed and additional trial closures made until no appreciable flash is produced. The model is then repainted with cold mould seal and the protective sheet removed. The flask is reassembled and placed in a flask clamp so that curing may be achieved under pressure. The presence of excessive flash leading to incomplete closure of the flask results in an increased vertical dimension in the denture and a corresponding reduction in the freeway space. Some denture base resins flow readily at the dough stage and a trial closure may not be necessary.

*Curing.* As mentioned previously, 60 °C is required to decompose the benzoyl peroxide, but at this temperature the polymerization process would take a very long time. A temperature of about 75 °C is sufficient to bring the time down to a practical value, while higher temperatures still, up to 100 °C, will produce very short curing times. In practice, curing cycles involving temperatures between 60 and 100 °C are used.

There are both advantages and disadvantages in reducing the time needed for curing by increasing the temperature. The obvious advantage is that the total processing time is much shorter, and with curing cycles that may last about an hour, the technician is able to provide a same-day service. On the other hand, it has always been thought advisable to use longer curing times for better quality dentures. The main reason for this is the greater risk of porosity with the rapid cure. This arises because the polymerization process is exothermic and the temperature of the resin will exceed the water temperature at some stage of the process, the surrounding gypsum being a very poor conductor of heat. The boiling-point of methyl methacrylate monomer is 100·3 °C. If the resin is heated rapidly, the exotherm occurs early at a time when there is still a large amount of monomer. The vaporization of this monomer causes the porosity, which may reduce the strength of the denture and increase the risk of microbial contamination. With a slower rise in temperature, and hence a slower rate of reaction, the maximum temperature of the resin is reached later when there is less monomer available for vaporization. In addition to this problem, a rapid cure may result in warpage of the denture after removal from the flask.

For many years the orthodox curing cycle involved heating the flask, in water, to about 72–75 °C and leaving it at this temperature for at least 9 hours, usually overnight. Not only was this thought to give best results, but it was also a convenient method and was suited to the routine of a dental laboratory.

The problems associated with the fast cure can be largely avoided if the rate of increase in temperature is kept reasonably low, even if the final temperature is much greater than 75 °C. This allows sufficient time for most of the monomer to be used up before the temperature reaches its boiling-point. This is usually achieved by heating the flask, either in air or water, to about 75 °C for 1–2 hours before raising the temperature to 100 °C for about an hour. There are many time and temperature variations and it is emphasized that the manufacturer's instructions should be followed carefully in each case.

Many denture base resins are now supplied in a form suitable for even quicker setting. For example, the curing cycle for one commercially available resin involves immersing the flask in boiling water, with the heat source removed, and leaving for 20 minutes, then reapplying the heat to bring the temperature back up to 70 °C for a further 20 minutes and then boiling for a final 20 minutes.

*Deflasking and finishing.* It is important that the flask is cooled in a controlled manner and that it reaches room temperature before it is opened. Rapid cooling and premature removal from the flask can lead to residual stresses in the denture, which, in turn, may result in distortion. Therefore, the flask is generally allowed to cool slowly in air. Deflasking is also performed carefully to avoid damaging the denture, the plaster being removed with a saw. Polishing is usually carried out wet for the same reason of avoiding a rise in temperature and subsequent warpage. Polishing procedures are not carried out on the fitting surface of the denture.

### Properties of heat-cured acrylic resin

These properties will be discussed in relation to the requirements of a denture base given earlier in the chapter.

EASE OF FABRICATION

Although the method of fabrication just described involves numerous stages, each of which has to be carried out with care, the dough-moulding process is highly suited to denture preparation, and no other polymer is available that can be fabricated in the same way. This will become evident when alternatives are discussed. This unique property of acrylic resin is one of the main reasons why it is chosen for denture construction. Furthermore, it is relatively easy to repair and rebase and there may be good compatibility between base and teeth since the latter may also be made of acrylic. These two points are discussed more fully later.

ACCURACY

Polymerization shrinkage has already been covered in some detail in Chapters 1 and 5. Theoretically methyl methacrylate should display a considerable contraction on polymerization and a total volume shrinkage of 6–7 per cent can be calculated on the basis of a 3:1 powder/liquid ratio. In addition to this, the high coefficient of expansion of acrylic in relation to that of plaster, should result in a thermal contraction as the resin cools after curing. However, in practice, acrylic dentures do not show dimensional changes of these proportions, but appear to contract by only 0·2–0·5 per cent. This is an acceptable amount, while the value of 7 per cent or greater would result in very poorly fitting dentures. The discrepancy between theoretical and actual values is presumably due to the restraining influence of the mould. It must be emphasized that the good accuracy obtained will be lost if the denture is not handled with care during deflasking and finishing.

As far as surface detail is concerned, the dough-moulding technique is ideal as the viscosity of the resin at the packing stage allows the resin to flow very easily throughout the mould space.

MECHANICAL PROPERTIES

Polymethyl methacrylate does not possess properties typical of plastics. Whereas most plastics display high ductility, toughness, and low elastic moduli, polymethyl methacrylate is a brittle, relatively rigid material. This presents some problems with acrylic denture bases which are known to be susceptible to mechanical failure in service. Some typical mechanical properties are given in Table 11.2.

**Table 11.2** Mechanical properties of denture base acrylic

| | |
|---|---|
| Elastic modulus (GN/m²) | 1·8–2·6 |
| Proportional limit (MN/m²) | 25–30 |
| Compressive strength (MN/m²) | 75–80 |
| Tensile strength (MN/m²) | 45–65 |
| Elongation (%) | 1–3 |

The pattern of mechanical failure related to the length of time the denture is in use (Figure 11.6) indicates this susceptibility of acrylic to various failure mechanisms. There is a relatively high incidence of fracture during the first 12–18 months. These are largely due to deficiencies in design or processing which either place abnormally high loads on the denture or result in a very weak material, in both cases failure being due to simple overloading. The strength of acrylic is, in fact, comparable to many engineering plastics and these fractures cannot really be blamed on inadequacies in this class of material.

There is a further peak of failures at about three years. These are generally fatigue failures, the susceptibility to which is again dependent upon the stress level and the quality of processing. Clearly the number of load applications experienced in three years is sufficient to cause failures in a significant number of dentures. Presumably the stress level in those dentures that do not fail at this time is below the fatigue limit for those particular appliances.

Superimposed on the peaks of the graph which reflect overloading and

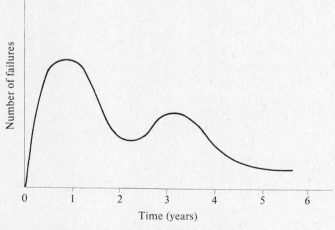

**Fig. 11.6** Pattern of mechanical failures in acrylic dentures.

fatigue is a general background rate of failure. These failures may arise in a number of ways, but fractures following the accidental dropping of the denture are of significance here, such events occurring at random. The low impact strength of acrylic is perhaps its biggest disadvantage, and since it is possible to prepare many plastics with ductilities several hundred times that of acrylic and with impact strengths more than ten times greater, this has been one reason for the search for alternatives.

Several factors related to the processing technique influence the fracture behaviour. The presence of porosity after curing, which has already been mentioned, can facilitate crack nucleation and propagation. Rapid deflasking and careless handling may result in internal stresses, which contribute to the early failure of a denture.

Generally, for a given processing time, the higher the maximum temperature reached, the greater the degree of polymerization and the greater the strength. This is of some relevance to the strength of thin sections, since the heat generated during polymerization is directly proportional to the mass of the resin. Since the investment and the acrylic itself are poor thermal conductors, this means that there is a variable temperature rise over the different sections of the base. The thicker sections become hotter and hence develop a greater inherent strength than the thin sections. The degree of polymerization is related to the strength by the molecular weight of the cured polymer. Generally, as was indicated in Chapter 1, a higher molecular weight implies a stronger, more rigid material, because of the greater resistance to deformation it manifests compared with a lower molecular weight resin. Although the molecular weight relates to the average length of the molecular chains, any residual monomer present can have an effect out of proportion to its quantity because it may act as a plasticizer and allow deformation to take place readily. In the same context, the intentional addition of plasicizers, or, conversely, cross-linking agents, will also have a pronounced effect on the properties of the resin.

AESTHETICS

The aesthetic properties of denture base acrylic are excellent. Polymethyl methacrylate itself is a clear plastic, a property derived from its amorphous nature, as described in Chapter 1. Most high-strength polymers are opaque in sections as thick as a denture base. Starting with a clear material, it is relatively easy to add the pigments necessary to produce the correct appearance, acrylic resin being particularly compatible with these additives. A small number of different shades which contain pigments and fibres to give a type of pink or veined pink appearance is available commercially, but, if necessary, localized pigmentation can be achieved with various tinting kits. The surface also takes a good polish, which is an advantage, although the appearance will be spoilt if there is any surface porosity.

Of equal importance is the fact that the colour stability is also good. Manufacturers are required to test each material under a high-intensity light-source for a period of time, and it has been found that all materials that do not show a change during this test will be satisfactory in service for many years.

It is possible for the surface of the denture to be slightly opaque. This may arise from water contamination during processing because of the lack of complete water-resistance of the separating medium. It is also possible that crazing in the polymer, mentioned below, will produce a hazy surface appearance and the polished finish may be lost over a period of time as a result of abrasion.

STABILITY IN THE ORAL ENVIRONMENT

Acrylic resins are virtually insoluble in the fluids they are likely to encounter in the mouth. They are, however, soluble in many organic solvents, so that, although they will not dissolve in normal use, care must be taken to avoid contact with such solvents during cleaning and storage.

These resins do, however, absorb water, up to an equilibrium content of between 1 and 2 per cent. It may take many days for this equilibrium to be reached as it relies on diffusion of the water molecules into the denture.

The presence of this quantity of water in the resin influences the properties of the denture. First, since the water molecules may act as plasticizers, the flexibility of the resin may increase. Secondly, and possibly of greater significance, the water absorption is associated with an expansion. A 1 per cent water absorption results in 0·23 per cent expansion. This may be desirable as it could compensate for the small contraction that occurs on curing. However, if the denture is alternately transferred between dry and wet conditions, the varying expansion and contraction would result in stresses which could lead to small cracks on the denture surface. This phenomenon is known as 'crazing' and is associated with a fine array of cracks on the surface. This will inevitably weaken the denture as cracks may open up to produce failure during use. This situation will be considerably exaggerated if the denture is exposed to solvents at any time. The presence of cross-linking agents considerably reduces the susceptibility to crazing.

To avoid any problems associated with water sorption, it is recommended practice to keep acrylic dentures under water whenever they are not in the mouth so that they do not dry out at any time.

BIOCOMPATIBILITY

In common with all high molecular weight synthetic polymers, polymethyl methacrylate has a low order of toxicity and is not known to produce any tissue irritation. Some problems of sensitivity to acrylic dentures may arise, although these are attributed to components other than the polymer itself. In particular, residual monomer is quite irritant so that improperly cured dentures are far more likely to induce sensitivity reactions. Other additives present may also be the cause of irritation, and sometimes a change from one product to another may resolve the problem.

A very common problem is denture sore mouth in which the mucous membrane under the denture becomes inflamed. It is a condition that is associated with a variety of factors, both local and systemic, an allergy to the denture base material sometimes being quoted in this context. It is, in fact, unlikely that allergies are responsible for denture sore mouth, the two most important features appearing to be the mechanical trauma from an ill-fitting denture and the presence of a large population of *Candida albicans*. The characteristics of the material do have some influence on the latter as candidiasis is more common and more difficult to eradicate where dentures have a porous surface.

THERMAL PROPERTIES

Acrylic resin does not normally soften below 75 °C and it is, therefore, unlikely that a denture will encounter any conditions during service that would result in softening. Repeated contact with some fluids, including alcohol, will lower the temperature at which some structural changes take place, but with the present formulations used this should not be clinically significant.

The coefficient of expansion of acrylic resin is high. It is unlikely that this affects the dimensional stability of the denture since variations in temperature within the mouth are only experienced transiently, the denture being a relatively large mass of poor thermal conductivity. Since porcelain has a low coefficient of expansion, thermal cycling of the denture could result in internal stresses and microcracks around the teeth, should they be made from this material. There is obviously an advantage here in using acrylic teeth. The low thermal conductivity does mean that there is reduced sensation in the underlying mucosa to temperature changes; however, the same problem would be encountered whatever the plastic used, since they all have low conductivity.

MISCELLANEOUS PROPERTIES

**a** *Radiopacity*. Acrylic itself is radiolucent. However, radiopaque fillers may be used to provide a certain amount of contrast on radiography. Barium sulphate has been used for this purpose, but, at the levels needed to give adequate radiopacity (10–20 per cent), the mechanical properties of the acrylic are reduced, including the impact strength, which is low, even in the unfilled material. Some acrylics are available with other fillers (details of which are not usually disclosed by the manufacturer) which may not have these problems.

**b** *Cost*. Acrylic resin is a reasonably inexpensive material.

**c** *Density*. There is little difference in the density of plastics, acrylic having a value of 1·18 g/cm$^3$.

## Cold-cured acrylic resin

These differ from the heat-cured material in the method of polymerization, a chemical activator being used to generate the free radicals rather than heat. The activator, which may be dimethyl-p-toluidine, a sulphinic acid derivative, or similar substance as discussed before, is present in the liquid and reacts with the initiator on mixing with the powder.

Once the polymerization has been initiated, the propagation and termination phases are exactly the same as in the heat-cured material. Again the reaction is exothermic, but since there is no externally applied heat, the maximum temperature reached is not as high. This means that the reaction does not go to completion and that the cured resin has a greater amount of residual free monomer. Since the process is initiated chemically when initiator and activator meet, polymerization starts as soon as the powder and liquid are mixed. The technique of packing is, therefore, slightly different since it has to be achieved more quickly.

### PROPERTIES OF COLD-CURED ACRYLIC RESIN

Generally the properties of heat and cold-cured acrylic are similar, with the following exceptions.

**a** The greater amount of residual monomer in the cold-cured materials results in a greater flexibility because of its plasticizing effect. The molecular weight of the cured resin is also lower and the strength of the cold-cured resin is only about 80 per cent of that of the heat-cured. Some of the strength and rigidity is regained over a period of time as the monomer slowly leaches out.

**b** There is also some evidence that there is a greater risk of sensitivity to the cold-cured resin because of the monomer content.

**c** The dimensional accuracy of dentures made from cold-cured resin tends to be better. This largely arises because of the lower temperature involved in processing, which results in both lower internal stresses and reduced thermal contraction.

**d** If a tertiary amine such as dimethyl-p-toluidine is used as the activator, the colour stability of the cold-cured resin may be poor because of oxidation of the amine. The sulphinic acid derivatives give better results in this respect.

### USES OF COLD-CURED ACRYLIC RESIN

With properties slightly inferior to those of heat-cured acrylic, the cold-cured material is not widely used as a denture base material. It is, however, popular for the repair of dentures and may be used for relining or rebasing processes as described later. Cold-cured acrylic is also used in a number of other dental applications, such as in the special trays for impressions and in removable orthodontic appliances.

### Pour-type acrylic resins

The cold-curing resins are also available in a slightly different form, which, it is claimed, gives good results with much shorter technical working times. These are usually called the 'pour-type', 'fluid', or simply 'pour' resins. They are similar to the cold-cured resin in composition, but are used with a significantly lower powder–liquid ratio. This ranges from $2:1$ up to $2·6:1$ compared with the conventional $3·5:1$.

The main differences with these materials lie in the methods of flasking and curing. Different investing materials are used, a reversible hydrocolloid being most common, although a soft gypsum stone is also available. Waxing the denture is performed in the usual way, and investing is carried out in a special flask. With the hydrocolloid, flasking is very easily achieved and it is here that most of the time is saved. After elimination of the wax and application of the separating medium, the cast is reseated in the mould and the flask reassembled.

When using the gypsum investment, curing is performed under pressure, typically from $140–300$ kN/m$^2$, depending on manufacturer's instructions. It is advisable to transfer the flask to pressure equipment before packing to minimize handling, which could result in tooth movement within the mould. The resin is poured into the mould and, after standing for a few minutes, the pressure is applied and the flask heated in warm water (35–60 °C, depending on the product). The curing time is usually 30 minutes, although some materials have a recommended time of 20 and some 45 minutes. Deflasking is easily and quickly performed.

The advantages claimed for the pour resins are greater accuracy in the denture base and a shorter processing time. Results obtained with different pour resins are, in fact, quite variable. Although a smaller amount of shrinkage is observed after processing, when compared to a heat-cured denture, the differences are usually small after the material has reached saturation with water.

The technician's working time can be considerably reduced by the use of these resins. However, the main disadvantage is that the technique is unreliable and a significant percentage of the dentures have faults which require repair. If the repair time is added to the normal processing time then the difference between heat-cured and pour resins is much smaller. The use of the soft stone investments with the pour resins give considerably inferior results in this respect.

There are a number of disadvantages associated with the pour resins, especially in relation to the mechanical properties.

**a** These materials usually have lower bend strengths than heat-cured resins.

**b** They also display a significantly lower fatigue strength.

**c** They are softer, abrade more easily, suffer slightly greater creep under constant load, and have a lower impact strength.

These poorer mechanical properties arise because of the low temperature used, which limits the degree of polymerization that is achieved. The amount of residual monomer present immediately after curing may be as much as 5 per cent in some cases.

In general, therefore, the advantages of pour resins are minimal, and there are some significant disadvantages. Since the cost of material in a denture base may be between 2 and 10 times that involved with a heat-cured resin, the use of pour resins is not very widespread.

## Denture repair, rebasing, and relining

It is desirable to be able to repair broken dentures or restore ill-fitting dentures to an appropriate shape without the necessity of making a completely new appliance. Acrylic resin is well suited to such processes.

*Repair*. Repair work may be achieved with either heat or cold-cured resin. The choice may be dependent upon the time available, but the heat-cured resin is preferable because of better properties. The disadvantages of the cold-cured resin already discussed in relation to the original denture construction apply equally well to repairs, the much lower strengths being particularly important. A residual monomer content of about 3 per cent is quite typical. The disadvantages of the heat-cured resin are the longer processing time and the tendency of the denture to warp as it is reheated to the curing temperature. It is generally found, in fact, that the cold-cured acrylic repairs give a slightly better fit.

When using cold-cured resin, the broken pieces of the denture are held together with sticky wax and wires and a model cast in plaster. The denture fragments are removed from the model when it has set and the fractured edges are trimmed and bevelled to allow a 3–5 mm separation. The parts are replaced on the cast after it has been treated with a separating medium, and the resin, mixed to a reasonably fluid consistency, is applied to the gap between the fracture surfaces. It is common practice to cure the resin under pressure and at slightly elevated temperatures in a manner previously described for the pour resins. When a heat-cured resin is used, the denture has to be completely invested in a flask and cured at no more than 75–77 °C for at least 8 hours.

*Rebasing*. The contour of the soft tissues under a denture may change gradually and the underlying bone may resorb. Thus a denture that fits the patient well originally may become ill-fitting over a period of time. In some circumstances, it is desirable to retain the dimensional relationships of the teeth in the denture but to provide a new base. Such a technique is called rebasing. Any denture base polymer may be used for this process. The existing denture base is used as the impression tray, and a stone cast is made from the impression. Care is taken to ensure that the correct vertical and horizontal relationships between the teeth and the cast are maintained. The teeth may be removed from the denture and maintained in their correct positions for reuse. Heat-cured material is then used in the normal way for the preparation of the new base.

*Relining.* It is more usual to reline a denture, adding a thin film of resin to the base to accommodate the changes in contour of the tissues. There are a number of ways in which dentures may be relined. Sometimes special soft linings are added because the patient is unable to tolerate the irritation produced by a hard denture. The use of soft linings, which may be made from quite different materials from the conventional acrylic resin, is discussed in a later section. Relining to achieve a better fit where there are no clinical indications for a soft lining may be achieved with either heat-cured or cold-cured acrylic resin. Usually the relining process is carried out in the laboratory in a similar manner to that used in the preparation of the original denture, although some materials are available which allow relining to be performed directly in the mouth.

In the conventional process, an impression is taken of the mouth, again using the denture as the tray. The cast is made and invested as usual, and after the flask halves are separated, the impression material is removed. The new resin is added to the inside of the denture after the surface has been softened by painting with monomer. Generally, low curing temperatures are used to minimize warpage of the denture.

The so-called chairside reliners were introduced in order to reduce the time taken. These materials are cold-curing acrylics that usually contain plasticizers and solvents to increase their fluidity and enhance their wetting of the base to be relined. The denture surface is roughened to improve the bonding of the lining. The material is mixed, applied to the denture, and held in the correct position in the mouth during curing. The total time taken may be only 15 or 20 minutes. Because of the exotherm and the presence of monomer, the process may be a little unpleasant for the patient. The results obtained with this relining technique are not always very good, as there is a tendency towards discoloration and failure of the bond to the original base. It is widely accepted, however, that such processes are useful in some situations.

## Soft lining materials and tissue conditioners

As mentioned above, it is often desirable to reline a denture with a soft material in the case of patients whose tissues in the denture-bearing area show signs of irritation from the denture. This may be due to some specific short-term condition that will soon resolve and which therefore requires a soft lining as a temporary expedient, as an alternative to not wearing the dentures at all, or to a more chronic condition that requires a permanent soft denture base.

### PERMANENT SOFT LININGS

The requirements of a soft lining material are essentially the same as those for the denture base itself, with a few additional points.

**a** The lining must form a strong and durable bond to the denture base resin.

**b** While the lining should be soft and resilient it should also possess good abrasion-resistance.

**c** The mechanical properties must not alter over a period of time; in particular, the linings must retain their resilience in use.

Since the soft lining materials often contain plasticizers and other lower molecular weight components to give the resilience, they are far more susceptible to interactions with the oral fluids. The loss of these substances by their leaching out into the oral fluids is particularly important as this may radically alter the mechanical properties.

Although there are many different proprietary soft lining materials available, they can, with one or two exceptions, be divided into two groups, the soft acrylics and silicone rubbers. There are a few cold-curing soft linings available but the majority are of the heat-curing type. The powder is generally polyethyl methacrylate or an ethyl-butyl methacrylate co-polymer and the monomer a higher methacrylate such as a butyl, nonyl, or lauryl methacrylate. The materials produced are soft at room temperature when incorporated with a suitable plasticizer. This is usually a phthalate such as butyl phthalyl butyl glycolate and may be present in amounts up to 30 per cent.

The dough is produced in the normal way and processed at the same time as the denture. This gives very good adhesion to the base. However, in other respects these materials have some deficiencies. First, they are substantially less resilient than silicone rubbers. Secondly, some of the plasticizer is leached out and replaced by water, so that the lining gradually becomes even less resilient. The use of a plasticizer, such as di-2-ethyl hexyl maleate, which itself polymerizes to a certain extent, minimizes this effect by inhibiting the leaching phenomenon.

The silicone rubber soft linings are essentially similar to the conventional impression rubbers discussed in Chapter 6, but contain 10–35 per cent by weight of a filler such as an inorganic silicate. These materials are resilient but have relatively poor abrasion-resistance. Silicone rubber does not bond well to acrylic resin, so an adhesive has to be used. This is a silicone polymer in a volatile solvent, the molecules of this polymer diffusing into the denture base, cross-linking then taking place as the lining cures. The relatively low bond strength produced becomes even lower over a period of time as the silicone rubber absorbs water, mainly because of the filler that is present, which hydrolyses the cross-links that give the adhesion. Thus silicone soft linings tend to peel off the denture during use.

A further problem with these materials is that, being slightly porous, they have a tendency to encourage the growth of oral micro-organisms including *Candida albicans*. This is aggravated by the difficulty of cleaning the lining surface adequately because of its poor abrasion-resistance. Some silicones contain a fungicide to overcome this problem. Cleaning dentures with silicone soft linings is also made more difficult by the bleaching and hardening effects of hypochlorite or other denture cleansers.

TISSUE CONDITIONERS

As noted above, a soft lining on a denture may be required as a temporary expedient when there is inflammation of the oral mucosa. This lining is usually called a 'tissue conditioner'. It is desirable that the material should be soft and viscoelastic, for it will then be viscous under a constant force, allowing a uniform transfer of load from denture to tissues, but resilient under the higher and more rapid forces involved in mastication.

The materials most commonly used as tissue conditioners are, in fact, viscoelastic gels consisting of a plasticizer dissolved in a polymer. The polymer is usually polyethyl methacrylate. It is mixed with a liquid that contains the plasticizer, generally butyl phthalyl butyl glycolate, and ethanol, the latter constituting between 5 and 25 per cent of the volume. The ethanol is a solvent for the polymer and as it diffuses into and swells the polymer beads, it carries plasticizer with it so that the latter is distributed throughout the material. Initially a fairly sticky liquid is produced, and this is coated onto the denture, which is placed in the patient's mouth. The material flows into all the spaces between the denture and the tissues and gels completely in about 30 minutes.

As with the soft acrylic linings, these tissue conditioners may harden, in some cases quite rapidly, as the ethanol and plasticizer are leached out.

## ALTERNATIVE DENTURE BASE POLYMERS

Although acrylic resins cannot be considered ideal for the construction of dentures, they have many desirable features and have been the materials of choice for many years. There are some alternative materials available, but they are rarely used. There are, however, a few indications for using an alternative. First, some patients may be unable to wear acrylic dentures because of an apparent hypersensitivity to the material. Quite frequently a change from one proprietary type of acrylic to another is a sufficient remedy, but sometimes it is necessary to resort to a different material altogether. Secondly, the dentures of some patients suffer repeated mid-line fracture and it may be thought appropriate to use a different material. This is the usual indication for using an alloy denture base. Thirdly, when a soft lining is required, it may be necessary to remove a substantial thickness of the base to allow room for the lining. In such cases, the remaining section of the base may be too thin for adequate impact strength so that a tougher material may be selected.

If an alternative denture base material is indicated, there is a choice between alloys and plastics. The two alloys, stainless steel and cobalt–chromium alloy, have already been discussed in this context. The alternative plastics may be grouped into two main categories. The first are those miscellaneous materials that have been used in the past but which are not considered to have acceptable properties and are rarely, if ever, used. These include vulcanite, which is discussed very briefly. The second group consists of those materials that have been employed for their greater impact strength.

## Vulcanite

Before the introduction of acrylic resins, vulcanite was by far the most popular material for dentures. Vulcanite is made from natural rubber, or polyisoprene, where the polymer is highly cross-linked by the use of sulphur. This process has been described in Chapter 1, the vulcanite, which is up to 32 per cent sulphur, being a hard, relatively rigid polymer. The vulcanization process is carried out under steam pressure at about 168 °C. The main disadvantages are:

**a** The rubber is opaque and impossible to prepare with a fully natural appearance.

**b** The dimensional accuracy is not very good because of the changes which take place on vulcanization.

**c** It easily becomes contaminated because it absorbs saliva.

## Materials with improved impact strength

These again can be divided into two groups, those which are based on non-acrylic polymers and the modified acrylics. Included in the first group is polycarbonate whilst the most common example of the latter group is the acrylic-butadiene-styrene polymer.

### POLYCARBONATE

Polycarbonate is the name given to polymers with a structural formula of the type shown in Figure 11.7a, R being an organic group. Typically polycarbonates are derived from bisphenol-A and their structure will be similar to that given in Figure 11.7b. Usually the polymer contains about 10 per cent glass fibres for greater strength. These materials have about the same strength as heat-cured acrylic resin but have a ductility of 60 per cent compared to that of 2–3 per cent, and may have an impact strength nearly 10 times that of acrylic. They display much less water absorption and have a coefficient of expansion less than half that of acrylic.

The one major disadvantage with polycarbonate is the difficulty experienced with fabrication. The dentures have to be constructed by a special injection moulding process since the polymer cannot be dough moulded. Injection moulding involves heating the polymer until it flows readily, in this case to about 330 °C and injecting it under pressure into the mould. The machines necessary for this process are expensive and not readily available. Moreover, the moulding has to be performed very carefully, especially in relation to the temperature. Overheating can result in discoloration of the polymer, but it will be too viscous if underheated. One final

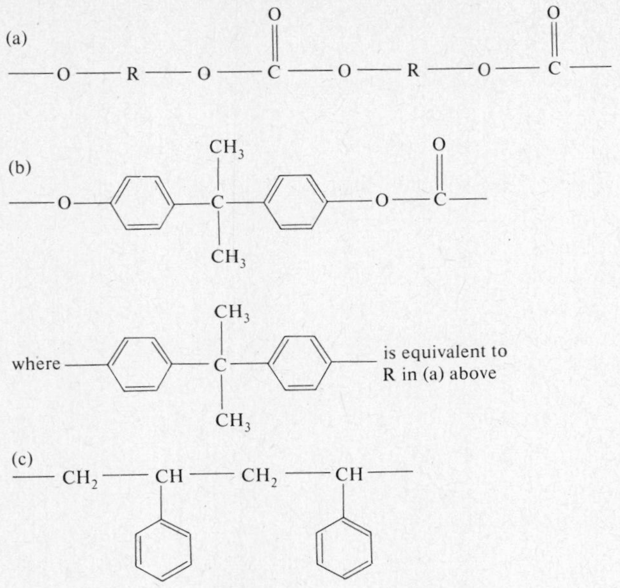

**Fig. 11.7** (a) Structural formula of polycarbonates; (b) polycarbonate derived from Bisphenol A; (c) polystyrene.

problem is that polycarbonate cannot be mechanically polished but requires a chemical polish, usually with methylene chloride, to give a good surface finish.

These processing difficulties have resulted in polycarbonates being used only rarely; very few laboratories possess the necessary equipment. This is unfortunate as it would be very desirable to have a polymer that was not based on acrylic, which had these mechanical properites and which could be used for patients in whom hypersensitivity to methyl methacrylate was suspected.

MODIFIED ACRYLICS

Some other polymers have also been used for injection moulded denture bases, but again the difficulties of processing have led to their very infrequent use. Some, however, may be co-polymerized with acrylic resins to give some improvement in mechanical properties whilst retaining the dough moulding capability. Polystyrene is one of these polymers, its structural formula being given in Figure 11.7c. As an engineering material styrene is often co-polymerized with either butadiene, acrylonitrile, or both of these, resulting in exceptionally tough plastics. Similar materials containing a high proportion of polymethyl methacrylate are suitable for denture bases. For example, a methyl methacrylate-styrene-butadiene terpolymer is commercially available.

Such materials possess many of the desirable features of the conventional heat-cured acrylic resin with the added advantage of increased toughness. Since the toughness may be obtained at the expense of rigidity, care has to be taken to ensure that the material is not too flexible. The major disadvantage of these so-called 'high-impact' acrylics is their greater expense, which precludes their use in routine denture production.

## ARTIFICIAL TEETH

Acrylic resin, very similar to the heat-cured denture base material, is most commonly used for denture teeth. Such teeth have good aesthetic qualities which are retained in most patients, they bond readily to acrylic denture bases, and are simply adjusted by grinding. Although porcelain denture teeth are still available, they are infrequently used. The porcelain is similar to that described in Chapter 9.

As no chemical bond occurs between this material and the denture base, mechanical methods of retention have to be employed and the great difference in thermal expansion between the base and the teeth leads to the localized production of stresses in the denture. Porcelain teeth tend to make a clicking noise during mastication and speech, which does not occur with acrylic resin teeth.

## DENTURE CLEANSERS

Food and plaque readily accumulate on dentures, and a wide variety of proprietary denture cleansers and general household cleansers are used for the routine removal of these deposits. One type of material used is simply an abrasive, supplied either as a powder or paste, which may be quite successful, but may abrade the base or teeth themselves. At least three types of solution are available. Hypochlorites, similar to those used in domestic bleaches, are common. They do not appear to affect the polymer in any way, but they can cause corrosion of chromium-containing alloys. Oxygenating solutions, such as perborates or percarbonates, usually supplied as a tablet to be dissolved in water, may also be used. These do not appear to be quite as powerful, but even so they may adversely affect the denture base, especially if soft lining materials have been used. Thirdly, some very dilute acids may be used.

Despite the availability of many such proprietary denture cleansers patients are often advised that appliances may be more easily maintained with soap and water, possibly applied with an ordinary toothbrush.

# 12

# Materials in root-canal therapy

There are many occasions when it is considered desirable to conserve a non-vital tooth by endodontic treatment. Indications range from the maintenance of an anterior tooth for optimal appearance and to avoid the need for a prosthesis, to the restoration of an isolated posterior tooth to be used as a partial denture abutment.

Treatment is carried out in a number of stages, each of which makes use of specific types of material. Following removal of necrotic pulp tissue the root canal is mechanically enlarged, and the adjacent dentine removed. This process may be termed biomechanical cleansing. The objective is to leave the canal clean, free from infected tissue and exudate, and prepared to receive the root filling. It is the hermetic sealing of the root canal, in particular the apical foramen, that is the most important factor in achieving a successful result. By eliminating the source of irritation from the root canal, periapical inflammation is prevented in the early case and allowed to resolve in the chronic established case.

Materials used in endodontic treatment are grouped below:

a  materials to aid sterilization of the canal;

b  preformed root-canal fillings;

c  root-canal sealers;

d  root-canal filling pastes;

e  others—absorbable pastes, mummifying pastes, chelating agents.

While some of the materials described may more aptly be termed medicaments they are included for completeness, as some, such as the polyantibiotic paste dressings, are handled in a similar way to many of the other materials and are left within the root-canal for an extended period.

## Materials to aid sterilization of the root canal

The mechanical enlargement of the root-canal by filing and reaming is made simpler and more effective by the use of intermittent irrigation. The irrigant lubricates the root-canal instruments and flushes dentine debris from the canal. While physiological saline or local anaesthetic solution will achieve these objectives, the use of a mild antiseptic has the additional advantage of reducing the number of living micro-organisms in the canal.

Sodium hypochlorite is widely used in this role and it produces its effect by releasing chlorine in the canal. Dilute solutions of 1–5 per cent dissolve organic debris while having a lesser effect on the adjacent viable tissues. Care should be exercised in its application, however, as sodium hypochlorite forced beyond the apical foramen may induce periapical inflammation. Although such a response is probably slight, it places an additional burden on the healing capacity of the periapical tissues. The effectiveness of sodium hypochlorite is rapidly reduced in the presence of excess organic debris and its use is therefore of little value unless augmented by thorough mechanical cleaning.

Sodium hypochlorite may be used in conjunction with 20 vol. hydrogen peroxide, as their combined action leads to the liberation of nascent oxygen and chlorine. The bubbles of gas produced tend to lift debris from the root-canal, leaving an environment unsuitable for the survival of many bacteria. Once again this technique should be used cautiously as gas may penetrate the apex, causing periapical inflammation or even surgical emphysema. For these reasons hydrogen peroxide should never be applied to the canal under pressure from a syringe and, following its use, irrigation with sodium hypochlorite should be carried out to ensure its complete removal. Indeed, it has been suggested that hydrogen peroxide should never be used.

In many cases it is desirable to medicate the canal for a limited period after biomechanical cleansing and before the placement of a root filling. Recently there has been a trend away from this practice, but two categories of material are still widely used, antiseptics and antibiotics.

Many, and often strongly caustic, antiseptics have been used, but the most popular compound in current use is parachlorophenol (PCP). Two preparations are available for clinical application, both in the form of solutions of PCP crystals, one aqueous and one in camphor. The former penetrates the dentinal tubules of the root for a considerable distance where it reaches bacteria that would otherwise be unaffected. Both forms of PCP are irritant to tissues even in the low concentration normally used (1–2 per cent). Higher concentrations bring about the coagulation of protein and tissue necrosis. Great care must therefore be taken in applying the medicament to avoid the penetration of the apical foramen. It is now generally agreed that the application of PCP on a paper point placed in the root canal is unnecessary and a pledget of cotton wool moistened with the solution and sealed into the coronal pulp chamber allows adequate medication of the dentine surface, enhanced by the low surface tension of the medicament. PCP is bactericidal to the vegetative organisms with which it comes into contact. Clearly every precaution should be taken to avoid the inadvertent spillage of PCP on the oral and facial tissues.

The specific antibacterial action of antibiotics has been used in polyantibiotic dressings, in the form of pastes topically applied to the canal. These medicaments are usually left in the root canal between visits prior to the placement of a root filling.

Many antibiotics have been employed in this way, and the use of some has been criticized. One of the claimed advantages of the antibiotics is that they are less irritant than the antiseptics, and this is certainly true of penicillin. However, the inclusion of antibiotics used widely in general medicine may run the risk of rendering the bacterial flora of a patient resistant to the drug, which may otherwise have been useful in the treatment of a serious systemic disease, particularly as low concentrations may leak slowly through the apical foramen into the tissues over an extended period. The risk of sensitizing patients to antibiotics is also recognized.

These problems have been overcome to a certain extent by the inclusion of antibiotics used only rarely in medical practice. However, the reason many of these antibiotics, for example bacitracin, are not generally popular is that they tend to be more irritant to tissues. Indeed, some preparations contain an anti-inflammatory agent, which suggests that they may cause periapical inflammation if used without. Resolution of a periapical lesion may also be impaired by the effect of anti-inflammatory drugs.

Most preparations include antibiotics which collectively are effective against a broad spectrum of micro-organisms. Penicillin, streptomycin, chloramphenicol, neomycin, and polymixin-B are among the antibiotics in use in various combinations, often in conjunction with an anti-fungal agent, such as sodium caprylate or nystatin. Modern materials are presented in the form of a paste, sometimes in a cartridge for easy placement in the root canal from a syringe. One disadvantage of the use of paste medications in root-canals is that they must be thoroughly removed before root fillings can be accurately placed and, as some are in a hydrophobic vehicle based on silicone, this can be difficult. The inclusion of a radiopaque substance, such as barium sulphate, renders preparations detectable radiologically.

## ROOT-FILLING MATERIALS

The obturation of the prepared and disinfected root-canal may be carried out using a variety of techniques and materials. The use of prefabricated root-filling points is probably still the most popular method, and these are placed with a sealer in an attempt to produce an apical seal that prevents the ingress of fluids to the canal. Many of the sealers used in this way have also been used alone to fill the root-canal space, and other materials have been developed specifically for use in this way. More recent developments in instrumentation have made dental amalgam practical and efficient as a root-filling material.

### Gutta percha points

Gutta percha occurs naturally as the coagulated exudate of mazer wood trees native to Malaysia, and is an isomer of natural rubber which has the same basic unit, isoprene (Chapter 1). At room temperature gutta percha is about 60 per cent crystalline and 40 per cent amorphous, the crystals of *trans*-polyisoprene occurring in two forms. The properties of the final material are partly dependent on the percentage of crystals present and the proportions of the two forms. Before the incorporation of additives, gutta percha is pliable at 25–30 °C, becomes soft at 60–65 °C, and melts and decomposes at 100 °C.

For dental use gutta percha contains up to 80 per cent additional material, the greatest bulk of which is an inert filler, usually zinc oxide. Other constituents include waxes as plasticizers, radiopacifiers, and colouring agents. To prevent the oxidation of the material in the presence of light and air some materials contain an antioxidant. Oxidation leads to the formation of a more brittle material that tends to fracture in the root-canal. This transformation can be seen in some varieties of gutta percha points that have been stored for long periods, and they are best discarded. The precise nature and proportions of ingredients of gutta percha for dental use are not generally made known by the manufacturers.

At mouth temperature gutta percha is, to a certain extent, mouldable, but retains sufficient rigidity to allow insertion of all but the smallest points into the root-canal. The material behaves viscoelastically and it is generally agreed that this allows closer adaptation to the root-canal wall if any irregularities are present. However, the use of a sealer in conjunction with the point is still essential if an adequate seal is to be achieved. The capacity of the material to mould against the canal wall may be enhanced by the use of a warmed condensation instrument.

The cytotoxicity of gutta percha is low even when tested by the more sensitive tissue-culture techniques. However, as more irritant sealers are always used with gutta percha and are more likely to come into contact with the periapical tissues it is these that determine the tissue response.

GUTTA PERCHA WITH SOLVENTS

Gutta percha is soluble in chloroform and other organic solvents, such as eucalyptol. This property has been used to produce a sealing paste of the material, either independently for use with a suitable point or by softening the surface of the selected point prior to its condensation. These pastes, often referred to as chloropercha and eucapercha, harden by the gradual volatilization of the solvent. In the environment of the sealed root-canal this is necessarily a slow procedure. It is, however, of more significance that the loss of the solvent is associated with contraction of the root filling, which clearly has a detrimental effect on the seal of the filling against the root-canal wall. For this reason, and because of the availability of suitable substitutes, the technique is becoming less popular.

**Silver points**

Silver is a more rigid, unyielding material than gutta percha, and this property is useful when root filling fine, curved canals, as greater control may be achieved over the final position of the apical end. However, the same property makes the filling of irregularities in the canal wall impossible, and it is necessary to rely on the sealer to fill such deficiencies. This is borne out by the fact that a poorer seal is achieved with silver than with gutta-percha points. Rigidity in the root-filling point is advantageous when a sectional root filling is to be placed in the apical third or fifth of the canal. The silver point may be notched, leaving the apical portion connected only by a narrow waist, which may be easily fractured following its cementation. Sealer is only applied to the apical fragment in such a technique, allowing the removal of the coronal portion of the point.

The bactericidal properties of silver were a major consideration in its selection as a root-filling material. Silver ions have an affinity for certain enzymes associated with the denaturation of protein. In contact with tissue fluids silver corrodes with the production of silver chloride, oxide, and carbonate. This is most likely to occur in the apical region, especially if the point penetrates the apical foramen, but despite this drawback silver is well tolerated by the tissues.

Silver used for root-filling points is over 99·8 per cent pure, containing only traces of nickel and copper. The shape and surface texture of the finished points are governed by the manufacturing technique and vary considerably. These factors will affect the adaptation of the point to the root canal, the adhesion of the sealer to the point, and the resistance of the filling to corrosion. While the adaptation of silver points to the root-canal walls may not be as good as with other materials, they are generally extremely difficult to remove from the canal, which is considered by some to be a disadvantage. If silver points that have a tight fit in the root canal are selected it appears likely that deformation of the dentine will allow close adaptation. In root-filled teeth subjected to apicectomy, silver points maintain their integrity and close adaptation to the root-canal wall, whereas gutta-percha points are grossly disrupted and the material smeared across the cut root surface.

## Silicone points

Encouraging results are being achieved with silicone rubber points (Silastic, Chapter 14). Various sealers have been investigated for use with this material, including polycarboxylate cement and silicone and cyanoacrylate adhesives. The last material was found to be highly irritant to periapical tissues, and in its present form is unsuitable for clinical use. A delay in the healing of periapical lesions also occurs if the silicone root filling is placed beyond the apical foramen, but the material is generally well tolerated. The great flexibility of root-filling points made from this material may make their placement difficult in narrow canals.

## Root-canal sealers

Root-canal filling points used alone do not produce an adequate apical seal, and a wide range of materials has been used between the points and the root-canal wall to overcome this problem. Indeed, the sealer may be con-sidered as the more important material, the root-filling point being used only to ensure its close adaptation to the root-canal wall and its placement in defects and accessory canals. While lining materials, such as zinc phosphate cement, zinc oxide/eugenol, calcium hydroxide, and zinc polycarboxylate cement are all in use as sealers, the most widely used materials are specifically modified zinc oxide/eugenols and resins.

## MODIFIED ZINC OXIDE/EUGENOL

An early product still in use (Rickert's formula) has a powder containing, in addition to zinc oxide, precipitated silver to give bactericidal properties and to increase the radiopacity, white rosin as a filler, and thymol iodide as an antiseptic. The liquid is oil of cloves with Canada balsam to increase the tackiness of the mixed cement. Discoloration of the dentine by the precipitated silver is a disadvantage, and care must be taken to avoid leaving material in the coronal access cavity where the overall appearance of the tooth may be affected.

A second formulation (Grossman's formula) later overcame this problem by replacing the silver radiopacifier with barium sulphate. The powder also contains zinc oxide as the principal reagent, staybelite resin, bismuth sub-carbonate, and anhydrous sodium borate. The last material, by removing water, reduces the rate of the setting reaction, giving an extended working time. The liquid is eugenol. Contraction on setting is small, which potentially improves the apical seal. However, if used in conjunction with well fitting root-filling points the thickness of material present is, in any event, small.

Both the above materials contain resins of fairly large particle size, which gives a gritty texture to the resultant mix unless thoroughly efficient spatulation is carried out. To overcome this, newer preparations are presented as two-paste systems. One such material, based on zinc oxide/eugenol, contains oleo resins, oils and waxes in the form of a paste together with bismuth trioxide, which gives a high degree of radiopacity, and thymol iodide as an antiseptic. The reactor is eugenol made into a paste by the incorporation of polymerized resins and annidalin. The material is convenient to mix and place in the root canal and its creamy consistency allows easy positioning of the root-filling point.

## RESINS

Two varieties of resinous root-canal sealers are in popular use. One is an epoxy resin system formed from bisphenol diglycidyl ether and a hardener, hexamethylene tetramine. The material also contains the oxides of bismuth, silver, and titanium. A degree of adhesion is claimed between the material and the dentine of the root-canal wall, and this, if it occurs, would improve the seal produced. A setting time of about 48 hours gives ample working time and the polymerized resin is chemically and biologically inert.

A second material is a polyvinyl resin in a polyketone vehicle and also contains hexachlorophane as an antiseptic. Polyketones are formed by the reaction of basic salts and metal oxides with the organic constituents. These in turn combine with metallic substances to produce the complex polyketone vehicle. Unlike the epoxy system the reaction is fast, giving a working time of only 5 minutes. The mix, produced from a viscous liquid and a fine powder, is sticky and more difficult to manipulate than other materials. Both these resins have the advantage of being insoluble in water and tissue fluid, although they may be dissolved in organic solvents.

A new hydrophilic acrylic resin is at present being investigated for use as a root-canal sealer, and early results are promising. It has been demonstrated that apical healing proceeds well even when the canal has been overfilled. The material adapts well to the root-canal wall.

The tissue reaction to root-canal sealers is important in view of the ease with which they may be forced into the periapical tissues. All the sealers mentioned are irritant to the tissues before they have set. Thereafter the response is largely determined by the degree of solubility, and in this respect the resins are superior. Free eugenol appears to evoke a relatively severe reaction and as all the zinc oxide materials contain free eugenol, even when set, they produce greater irritation. This is enhanced by the gradual dissolution of these materials, which leads to the liberation of more eugenol. However, an even more important factor influencing the periapical reaction is the quality of the apical seal, and it must be stressed that this is the most important factor governing success.

### Root-filling pastes

The use of root-canal sealers alone as permanent root-filling materials has been advocated. In general, however, their handling in the root canal is uncontrolled and it is difficult to know if the canal is adequately filled or if material has passed beyond the apex. As the zinc oxide/eugenol materials are all soluble to a certain extent in tissue fluid their use in any bulk must be suspect, particularly in view of the continued tissue irritation produced by liberated eugenol. Again the resins prove superior in this role. All the sealers contract on setting, and when used in greater bulk this prejudices the seal of the material with the dentine of the root-canal wall. Certain pastes have been developed specifically for use as root-filling materials, some claiming to offer therapeutic benefits.

One such popular material is available as a powder based on zinc oxide but also containing the anti-inflammatory agents hydrocortisone and dexamethasone and the antiseptics di-iodothymol and paraformaldehyde. The last material is highly irritant to periapical tissues, a fact that is probably masked by the presence of the anti-inflammatory drugs. Delayed symptoms associated with the use of this material as a root filling may occur because of the more rapid absorption of the steroids which leaves the irritant antiseptic in the tissues. The powder also contains bismuth subnitrate as a radiopacifier and the liquid is pure eugenol. It has been suggested by the manufacturers that any material passing beyond the apex is absorbed while that within the root canal is not, but it is difficult to appreciate how this distinction is achieved. While it is important to have a root filling that is not absorbed, it is undesirable to have such a material in the periapical tissues, particularly if it is irritant.

A second preparation with a fundamentally similar formulation suffers similar disadvantages. This material based on zinc oxide/eugenol has many constituents including anti-inflammatory drugs, antiseptics, radiopacifiers, and, importantly, paraformaldehyde, as well as being presented in a variety of forms. In addition to being advocated for the root filling of non-vital teeth the manufacturers recommend its value in vital pulpectomy where the apical portion of the pulp may be left in the canal and covered with the material. It has been found, however, that the remaining pulp tissue may become necrotic and periapical inflammation may follow.

## Dental amalgam

Dental amalgam has several properties that suggest it would be a satisfactory root-filling material, including good adaptation to the cavity and slight expansion on setting. Recently new instrumentation has made the use of amalgam a feasible proposition in practical terms. With the use of small amalgam carriers and matching condensers it is possible to deposit and condense small increments of amalgam in the apical third of most root canals. In large teeth the process may be time-consuming and it may be necessary to use more than one mix of amalgam. The filling of the small amalgam carriers may be facilitated by using a fine grain or spherical particle amalgam. When completely set, amalgam is well tolerated by the tissues. The material would be difficult, if not impossible, to remove and this would appear its only disadvantage. In this respect, however, it would be no worse than apical third fillings of silver and even gutta percha. Amalgam has been successfully used as a retrograde filling material at apicectomy for many years, where it has demonstrated a good apical seal and tissue tolerance.

## Absorbable pastes

Where it is anticipated that a root-filling sealer or paste could easily pass into the periapical tissues, some clinicians prefer to use a resorbable or, more aptly, absorbable paste. A commonly used material consists of parachloro-phenol, menthol, camphor, and iodoform. The resultant paste does not set. While material accidentally or deliberately passed into the periapical tissue is removed rapidly by phagocytosis, its presence is associated with a severe inflammatory reaction which may take some months to subside. Clearly a material that is absorbed readily will not achieve a lasting apical seal, and over a period of time it is removed, not only from the periapical region but from the root canal as well. For this reason such materials are not recommended as permanent root fillings or as a permanent sealer for a conventional root-filling point.

## Mummifying agents

In primary teeth it is not always feasible to carry out classical endodontic treatment, yet it may be desirable to conserve a tooth. Techniques employing mummifying pastes may help to overcome this dilemma. Formocresol is such an agent and is available in a preparation containing 19 per cent formaldehyde and 35 per cent cresol in a base of glycerine and water. A cotton wool pledget moistened with the material is applied to the exposed dental pulp for a five-minute period or may even be sealed into the tooth between visits. The mixture is bactericidal and brings about fixation of a superficial layer of tissue beneath which is normal pulp, a zone of inflamed pulp tissue being present between the two. A lining of zinc oxide/eugenol is used to replace the formocresol dressing before the tooth is permanently restored.

## Chelating agents

Narrow pulp canals or canals obstructed by calcific deposits may sometimes be filed and reamed more easily with a chelating agent to induce partial decalcification of the adjacent dentine. Ethylenediaminetetra-acetic acid (EDTA) is such a material and may be used in a 15 per cent solution buffered to pH 7·3. Its action begins immediately after introduction into the canal and conventional mechanical preparation is used. Any residual solution must be washed from the canal on completion of the preparation. Chelating agents used in similar fashion may also be helpful in the retrieval of broken instruments from the root canal.

# 13
## Materials in preventive dentistry and orthodontics

Dental caries is a very prevalent disease affecting nearly all people to a greater or lesser extent. Carious teeth may be restored using a variety of materials that have been discussed in earlier chapters. However, much attention has been directed towards the prevention of this disease. While it is unlikely that caries will be totally eliminated, it is possible that its incidence in the population may be reduced to a level that can be dealt with more effectively by restorative treatment.

Although the aetiology and spread of dental caries is not completely understood, certain essential conditions have been identified, without which carious lesions are not initiated. These are the presence of bacterial plaque adhering to the tooth surface, a suitable substrate, primarily from the diet, that may be metabolized within plaque to form acids, and finally a susceptible tooth surface. If any one of these is absent, caries is not initiated, and different preventive measures have been designed to influence each. For example, some progress has been made in the control of plaque by chemical as well as conventional mechanical means.

Techniques have been developed to alter the tooth surface, either totally or in part, to make it less susceptible to carious attack. This can be achieved by altering the solubility of enamel by the systemic or topical use of fluoride. Fluoride ions become incorporated into the calcium hydroxyapatite lattice partly converting it to calcium fluorapatite which is less soluble in dilute acid. Of practical importance to the clinician is the use of topical fluoride, and a number of methods of application are available. These have quite different degrees of effectiveness, and although they may have an effect on the entire enamel surface, some areas of the tooth appear to benefit more than others.

The morphology of many posterior teeth leads to the accumulation of plaque and food debris in areas that are not readily cleaned. Modification of this morphology may eliminate many stagnation areas and this provides the basis for fissure-sealing techniques.

### Topical fluorides

The beneficial effect of the ingestion of 1 ppm fluoride from the drinking water has long been recognized. Caries is markedly reduced in geographical areas where the drinking water contains fluoride at this concentration, either naturally or by the intentional addition of fluorides. Greatest benefit occurs if fluoride is ingested throughout the period of dental development from birth to the end of the first decade. In this situation all the enamel contains calcium fluorapatite so that it is uniformly rather than superficially resistant to caries.

While the use of topical fluoride applications may contribute some slight additional benefit to those derived from systemic sources, they are of greatest value to patients living in areas with low-fluoride water supplies. Topical fluoride does not confer the same degree of resistance to caries as systemic fluoride and its effect is clearly superficial. Therefore, as the surface of the tooth is gradually lost by abrasion, fresh enamel, with reduced resistance, is exposed. In addition, fluoride is gradually leached from the surface of the enamel. From this it becomes clear that in order to confer any long-term benefit, the procedure must be repeated at intervals. The frequency of treatment is determined by a number of factors, including the type and concentration of fluoride, its method of application and the caries suscepti- bility of the patient.

MODE OF ACTION

A number of factors may account for the action of topical fluoride. The situation is complex and incompletely understood, but the following may play a part.

**a** Crystallites of calcium fluorapatite tend to be larger than those of calcium hydroxyapatite and they therefore offer a smaller surface area in any given volume, and this reduces the rate at which dissolution occurs.

**b** Enamel contains carbonates which, being soluble, contribute towards the overall solubility of the tissue. Enamel rich in calcium fluorapatite contains less carbonate and is therefore less soluble.

**c** It is thought that the solubility of calcium fluorapatite and hydroxyapatite are initially similar. However, the secondary precipitation of substances, such as calcium fluoride, on the surface of the fluorapatite, reduces the diffusion of acids and free hydrogen ions into the latter.

**d** The presence of fluorides favours the crystallization of reprecipitated calcium phosphate as an apatite rather than as a more soluble form.

These factors are all concerned with the enamel. Other benefits may result from the effects of fluoride on the deposition and metabolism of dental plaque suggested below.

**a** A reduced surface energy for enamel treated with topical fluoride may inhibit the adsorption of salivary glycoprotein, which is the initial stage of plaque formation.

**b** Fluoride ions may inhibit the enzymes concerned with the metabolism of carbohydrates to acids.

**c** By reducing the amount of carbohydrate stored intracellularly in plaque, fluoride may inhibit acid production between meals.

**d** In high concentrations, fluorides have a toxic effect on plaque and will therefore lead to its short-term inhibition.

It is doubtful that this second group of factors plays a major part in reducing caries unless the application of fluoride is carried out on a regular basis.

MATERIALS

Sodium and stannous fluoride are the two most widely used substances, the former being popular in an acidulated form.

*Sodium fluoride.* This was the first widely used topical fluoride solution. The concentration used is dependent on the mode of application and the frequency of treatment. When applied by a clinician, a 2 per cent solution is used, generally with a 4-minute exposure. Unfortunately to give an appreciable benefit the application must be carried out four times at weekly intervals. This regime is recommended at ages that coincide with the eruption of new teeth, at for example, 3, 7, 11, and 13 years.

Sodium fluoride, unlike stannous fluoride, is stable and can be stored in plastic bottles. It does not stain the teeth or restorations and does not cause any apparent damage to the gingivae. The taste is acceptable.

*Stannous fluoride.* Solutions of 2 and 8 per cent stannous fluoride have been used, the latter being more common. It is claimed the treatment with these solutions produces better results than those achieved with sodium fluoride. In addition, only one application is required either every 6 months or annually, depending on the caries susceptibility of the patient.

Hydrolysis and oxidation soon lead to the deterioration of stannous fluoride solutions and fresh ones must be used for each treatment. Staining of the teeth occurs and this may make diagnosis of early caries confusing. The more concentrated solution has an unpleasant taste that cannot be masked by flavouring agents and some gingival irritation may also occur.

*Acidulated phosphate fluoride (APF).* It is generally agreed that the higher the concentration of fluoride, as calcium fluorapatite, in the superficial enamel the greater will be the resistance to caries. An increased absorption of topical fluoride may be achieved either by raising the concentration of fluoride applied to the tooth or by reducing the pH of the solution used. However, under the latter conditions the enamel dissolves, liberating phosphate ions. It is also important not to introduce too much fluoride as there is a tendency to form calcium fluoride and decomposition of the mineral phase occurs. This is also associated with the liberation of phosphate.

By the use of a low pH phosphate solution containing fluoride these side effects can be reduced, and this forms the basis of the APF solutions which are produced from sodium fluoride and phosphoric acid. They may be applied in solution or in the form of 'gels'. The addition of flavouring agents is possible and staining of the teeth does not occur. APF solutions are stable in plastic containers and are not appreciably irritant to the gingivae.

METHODS OF APPLYING TOPICAL FLUORIDES

*Solutions.* All three types of fluoride described above may be applied directly to the teeth by a clinician. Sodium fluoride is employed in a concentration of 2 per cent while 8 per cent stannous fluoride is used. APF is used with an effective fluoride-ion concentration of 1·2 per cent.

Prior to the application of topical fluoride as a solution, gel, or varnish the teeth to be treated are given a thorough prophylaxis, especially inter-proximally, and are isolated and dried. The use of a fluoride-containing prophylaxis paste has been recommended as a prelude to topical fluoride treatment, although additional benefit from this has not been clearly identified. A number of such pastes are available, including zirconium silicate–stannous fluoride and silicon dioxide–APF products.

Solutions of stannous fluoride are applied for about four minutes during which time the teeth are kept moist with the solution. It is possible to encourage the solutions between the teeth with unwaxed dental floss. The patient should not rinse or eat for at least 30 minutes following the applications. With sodium fluoride, a single application is allowed to dry on the teeth over a four-minute period.

*Gels.* Many of the APF gels available are not strictly gels but viscous liquids that flow fairly readily under the influence of gravity. Some products, however, do have thixotropic properties and are more jelly-like. This increase in viscosity is achieved by the inclusion of polymers, such as sodium carboxymethyl cellulose, up to about 5 per cent.

These materials are applied to the teeth using one of a number of different applicators, which generally contain an absorbent liner of paper or foam. With these techniques the entire dentition may be treated at one time, whereas solutions usually have to be applied to one quadrant at a time. It is also important, however, to ensure close adaptation of the applicator to all the available tooth surfaces. Again, exposure is about four minutes and the patient is discouraged from rinsing afterwards. With the more viscous products some of the gel is retained interproximally, increasing the amount of fluoride uptake in these areas.

Ingestion of some of the gel occurs during application, and this may result in nausea shortly afterwards. With well-designed applicators, however, this should not be a major problem.

*Mouth rinses.* Mouth rinses have the advantage of being self-administered and can therefore be used with much greater frequency than those treatments undertaken by a clinician. The solutions used are more dilute than those described above. Typically, 0·2 per cent sodium fluoride is used every two or four weeks while a 0·05 per cent solution may be used daily. APF solutions may also be used for mouth rinses.

*Toothpaste.* Toothpastes, used by a large proportion of the population, provide a convenient vehicle for topical fluoride. Sodium and stannous fluoride are both employed in addition to sodium monofluorophosphate ($Na_2PO_3F$). Clearly fluorides added to proprietary toothpastes must be compatible with their other constituents as any interaction would remove their beneficial effect. To ensure safety, a concentration of 0·8 per cent is typical.

*Varnishes.* Experiments have been carried out with varnishes containing fluorides. By remaining on the tooth surface for longer periods than with other techniques these might allow more exchange of fluoride to the tooth, which could result in a high concentration in the enamel immediately afterwards. Fluoride varnishes are not yet established as media for the application of topical fluoride.

EFFECTIVENESS OF TOPICAL FLUORIDE

Evaluation of the effectiveness of topical fluorides in their various forms is extremely difficult, and the literature is inconsistent in the methods of assessment employed. Variations occur in the method of patient selection and examination, treatments applied, the indices used, and the statistical methods applied to the results. Therefore it is often impossible to make direct comparisons between studies.

It is clear that topical fluorides increase the resistance of teeth to caries, and application by the clinician appears to produce the best results. The APF gels seem to be the most satisfactory, and indeed the most convenient to use. Their superiority may be due to the simpler handling technique, as incorrect or inadequate application is less likely.

The greatest benefit occurs on the smooth surfaces of the teeth, including the interproximal surfaces. However, topical fluorides do not result in any appreciable change in the incidence of fissure caries. More marked protection is imparted in non-fluoride areas, although evidence does suggest a small additional benefit in areas with an optimal amount of fluoride in the drinking water. In any event, topical methods are not as effective as systemic fluoride.

If topical fluoride applications are stopped, the benefit derived is gradually lost, in part due to the abrasion of the superficial enamel that was affected by the treatment. It is important, therefore, to continue a topical fluoride regime to maintain the benefits, although it may be possible to reduce the frequency of treatments as the patient becomes older, and presumably less caries-susceptible.

## Fissure sealants

The pits and fissures of the occlusal surfaces of the posterior teeth are the most common site for carious attack. In these regions the enamel is chemically the same as elsewhere, but the morphology allows plaque and food debris to accumulate readily, and their removal is difficult by conventional means. In addition, fissures are often extremely deep and narrow, reaching close to the amelo-dentinal junction (Fig. 13.1). As pointed out in the previous section,

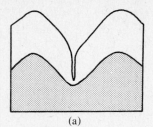 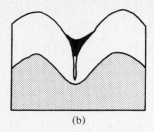

(a)                                    (b)

**Fig. 13.1** Cross-section through (a) deep enamel fissure; (b) fissure following sealing.

topical fluoride applications do not impart the same benefit to pits and fissures as to smooth surfaces. Therefore, a need exists for a preventive measure for these particularly susceptible areas.

By sealing the mouths of pits and fissures, and ideally filling the entire system, the accumulation of cariogenic material can be reduced (Fig. 13.1). The technique is referred to as fissure sealing and the materials used are fissure sealants. As carious lesions are often initiated in fissures soon after the eruption of the teeth, and, as progress is frequently rapid, fissure sealants should be applied early. The longer the time-interval following eruption, the greater will be the chance of placing the fissure sealant over an active carious lesion. This must be considered undesirable in all but the very earliest of lesions. Indeed, if early caries is detected clinically it is wiser to treat the tooth with a conventional restoration.

It should be stressed that fissure sealing alone does not constitute a comprehensive preventive dentistry regime, as only a limited area of the tooth is treated. However, used in conjunction with topical fluoride and plaque control techniques, it offers a useful contribution to the overall management of caries prevention.

REQUIREMENTS OF FISSURE SEALANTS

Fissure sealants require many of the attributes of any dental restorative material, and these are outlined below.

**a** As fissure sealants are applied to a surface that has not undergone mechanical preparation it is important that adhesion should exist between the sealant and enamel. Contributions from specific and mechanical adhesion may be utilized and thermal cycling should not reduce the bond strength or permit leakage.

**b** Contamination with moisture should not unduly affect the setting reaction or final properties.

**c** The sealant should flow readily into the depths of the fissure, this being a prelude to good adhesion.

**d** Strength and hardness are required to prevent fracture and abrasion, since fissure sealants are used in a vulnerable situation where damage may occur from occlusion and articulation.

**e** They should be insoluble in oral fluids in order to give good durability.

**f** The coefficient of thermal expansion should be close to that of enamel and dimensional change on setting should be minimal to reduce stress at the enamel–sealant interface.

**g** There should be a convenient and cheap method of application.

MATERIALS

A number of materials have been used for fissure sealing. Most of these are polymers, but the glass ionomer cement ASPA has been modified for this application.

*Cyanoacrylates.* Substances such as methyl-2-cyanoacrylate have been used with and without fillers. The fillers, such as polymethyl methacrylate powder and various metal powders, were added in an attempt to improve the durability of the product. Dissolution and loss when exposed to the oral fluids was the main problem, six-monthly replacement being necessary. Little success has been reported with this presentation, despite the claimed advantage that it could be applied to the tooth with good adhesion, even under slightly moist conditions.

*BIS–GMA resins.* These have been described in detail in Chapter 5 but are generally used in this context in the unfilled state. Presentations may be activated by chemicals or ultraviolet light. The latter systems have the advantage of an indefinite working time. However, the light source is expensive and, as explained in Chapter 5, it may not be consistent in emission of the appropriate wavelength. With this system once the initiator has been added to a capsule of resin the shelf-life is limited, even though activation with ultraviolet light has not been undertaken. This leads to a certain amount of wastage.

*Glass ionomer cement.* The product ASPA has also been discussed as a tooth-coloured filling material in Chapter 5, but has also been tested as a fissure sealant. Clearly the specific adhesion of ASPA to tooth substance is a potential advantage, and early results are promising in this role.

TECHNIQUE OF FISSURE SEALING

Teeth to be treated are given a thorough prophylaxis, washed, and dried. Pastes used for this purpose should not have a glycerine base, as a thin film remains on the surface and interferes with the effectiveness of the subsequent stages. It is also suggested that fluoride pastes should be avoided as they reduce the solubility of the enamel in the acid used to condition the surface prior to the application of the sealant.

While a certain amount of mechanical retention of the sealant in the fissure may occur, this cannot be guaranteed, and, in any event, it would not be adequate. Therefore, specific and microscopic mechanical adhesion must be employed. The glass ionomer cement offers specific adhesion but most fissure sealants rely on mechanical adhesion for their retention, and the acid-etch technique is used for this purpose. Chapter 5 deals with this in detail and the materials, methods, and mechanisms are essentially similar when they are applied to fissure sealing.

A number of etchant solutions have been tried, including 30 per cent unbuffered phosphoric acid and 50 per cent phosphoric acid buffered by the addition of 7 per cent zinc oxide. The former is claimed to be the more effective. Following prophylaxis the teeth are isolated and dried and the etchant is applied to the fissure for one minute (or longer in a high fluoride area), a fine brush being the most effective instrument for this purpose. The excess acid is washed away and the tooth dried again before the sealant is painted into the fissures, where it sets. As explained earlier, this is achieved in some products by exposure to ultraviolet light.

EFFECTIVENESS OF FISSURE SEALANTS

As with topical fluoride, it is difficult to evaluate the success achieved with this treatment, but a significant reduction in fissure caries has been reported.

Success is dependent upon a number of factors. Early treatment, prior to the initiation of carious lesions in the depths of the fissures, is clearly advantageous. Very early lesions are probably arrested by the elimination of the nutrient supply to the bacteria, which occurs with treatment. However, it is not always possible to be sure of this outcome, and the enamel barrier at the base of the fissure is often extremely thin. Retention of the sealant in the fissure is of obvious importance, and this is related to the materials and techniques used. The most common cause of retention failure is thought to be incorrect technique, in particular failure to clean, dry, and isolate the teeth adequately before and after etching.

While fissure sealing may not eliminate all fissure and pit caries, it will have a delaying effect, and restorative treatment, although ultimately necessary in some cases, may be carried out at an age when patient co-operation should be more favourable. Fissure sealing has been criticized as a preventive measure, since it is only directed at one part of the problem. As stated earlier, this should be recognized and the technique integrated into an overall preventive dentistry regime.

## MATERIALS IN ORTHODONTICS

Orthodontics is the study of growth and development of the occlusion and the prevention and treatment of abnormalities of this development. The treatment of malocclusion is most frequently undertaken with the use of appliances that produce tooth movement. When a force is applied to a tooth, the bone at the side of the tooth where there is a compressive stress tends to resorb, while there is bone deposition on the side of tension, allowing movement of the tooth in the direction of the force. This force can be applied by a suitable orthodontic appliance. The pressure exerted on the tooth must, of course, be large enough to produce the required movement, but should ideally be less than intra-capillary blood pressure, which is about $2-2 \cdot 5 \, kN/m^2$. Higher pressures may compress capillaries and lead to undesirable changes in the periodontal tissues. It is therefore important that the force exerted is relatively small and well controlled.

Several different types of appliance are available. These may be either removable by the patient, or fixed, in which case they are attached to the teeth and only removable by the dentist. In some cases, the forces are exerted intermittently by the use of screws, which are periodically adjusted, while in other cases they are applied continuously by the use of metal wires or elastic bands, from which stored elastic energy is released to the teeth over a period of time.

Removable orthodontic appliances generally consist of a plastic base, which is located around certain teeth, from which the force is applied to those teeth requiring movement by means of the active component. With fixed appliances, some type of bow wire, lying lingually or labially to the teeth, exerts force to the relevant teeth via brackets. These are either fixed to a band that is placed around the tooth or directly bonded to the enamel. For a long time bands were in universal use, but the advent of dental adhesives radically changed the situation, giving a far greater preference for direct bonding.

Within this array of appliances, several different types of material are used. These may be considered in the following groups:

**a** the plastic used for the base of removable appliances;

**b** the metals used for the wires in fixed and removable appliances;

**c** the materials used for elastic bands;

**d** the materials used for brackets, bands, and screws; and

**e** the adhesives used in the direct bonding of appliances to teeth.

### BASES FOR REMOVABLE APPLIANCES

Cold-cured acrylic resin, identical to that discussed in Chapter 11 in relation to denture bases, is used for the preparation of the bases of removable appliances. After the appropriate wires, such as springs, clasps, and bows have been formed, they are secured to a cast with sticky wax. The cast may then be coated with a separating medium to allow easy removal of the base, and the resin, prepared from a powder and liquid, is applied to the surface of the cast. Although the resin will cure by itself, best results are obtained when the acrylic is cured under pressure at an elevated temperature. After removal from the cast, the appliance can be trimmed and polished.

## Orthodontic wires

The most important requirements of an orthodontic wire relate to the mechanics of producing tooth movement and the methods of fabrication of the appliance. It is also desirable that the material should have good corrosion-resistance in the mouth, although this must be considered a secondary requirement since the appliances are used for only two years or less.

MECHANICS OF ORTHODONTIC APPLIANCES

It is not necessary to consider the mechanics of these appliances in great detail, but merely to discuss their influences on the selection of materials. An orthodontic appliance can be considered as having active and reactive components. The active component is that which delivers the force to the tooth requiring movement, while the reactive component fixes the appliance firmly to other teeth that do not have to be moved.

In the reactive member, a material of high elastic limit and high rigidity is required, for ideally it has to deform as little as possible, either elastically or plastically, during use of the appliance. On the other hand, if an active component has to deliver a force to a tooth, it must have the ability to absorb and release elastic energy readily. Since this is achieved through the use of large elastic deformations, this requirement is incompatible with that of the reactive component, assuming the same material is used in both cases.

There are several factors which need to be considered in more detail in relation to the active member. It is important to appreciate that the tooth movement is produced by inducing elastic deformation in the active member and then allowing the energy absorbed to be released to the tooth over a period of time. In an efficient appliance, the force exerted on the tooth by this member must be constant and must be maintained over a wide range of tooth movement. It would be of little use if the active member imparted a force to a tooth initially, if that force decreased to zero after the tooth had been moved just a little way.

There are two mechanical properties of the wire which control this efficiency. The first is flexibility. Ideally the wire must be sufficiently flexible so that it applies a small force to the tooth but over a wide range of deflection. If a very rigid wire is used, then either only a small degree of elastic strain could be induced (producing a correspondingly small movement) if the force to be applied is kept within the desired limits, or, alternatively, the force on the tooth would be too large if a more realistic strain were induced. This situation is illustrated in Figure 13.2. It will be recalled from Chapter 1 that the rigidity of a material is controlled by the elastic modulus. In considering the bending of a wire, the term flexural rigidity is used to denote the ease with which this elastic deformation will take place. This is controlled by both

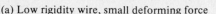

(a) Low rigidity wire, small deforming force

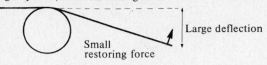

Large deflection

Small
restoring force

(b) High rigidity wire

(i) Small deforming force

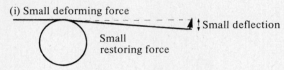

Small deflection

Small
restoring force

(ii) Large deforming force

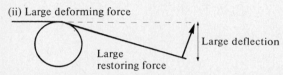

Large deflection

Large
restoring force

**Fig. 13.2** Forces and deflections in a palatal spring: (a) low rigidity wire. A large deflection is produced with a small deforming force. (b) High rigidity wire, where either (i) a small deforming force gives a small deflection resulting in a small restoring force but over a small distance; or (ii) a large deforming force gives a large deflection, which exerts a force over a large distance but where this force is high.

the elastic modulus $E$ and the geometry of the wire, measured in terms of the second moment of area $I$. Thus

$$\text{flexural rigidity} = E \times I.$$

For a single round wire, $I = \pi R^4/4$, where $R$ is the radius of the wire, so that

$$\text{flexural rigidity} = \frac{E\pi R^4}{4}.$$

From this it can be seen that it is much easier to alter the flexural rigidity by changing the wire radius than by choosing a material with a different elastic modulus. For example, an increase in the wire radius from 0·2 mm to 0·25 mm increases the flexural rigidity by more than 2·5 times.

The second property is the amount of energy that can be stored in the wire after it has been deformed. This is the resilience discussed in Chapter 1. For a given force, this is directly proportional to the distance over which that force can be moved. Since the above reasoning has shown that the most efficient appliance will allow the greatest degree of tooth movement on the application of a small force, a high value of maximum stored energy is required. In the stress–strain curve shown in Figure 13.3 the stored energy is measured by the area under the curve up to the elastic limit. It can be seen

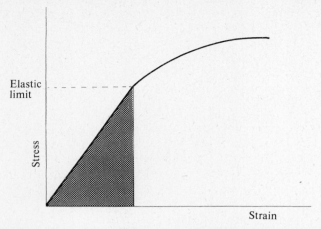

**Fig. 13.3** Stress–strain curve. The shaded area represents the stored elastic energy.

that the combination of a high elastic limit with a large elastic strain at this limit, implying a low elastic modulus, gives a high value of the stored energy. If two materials have the same elastic moduli, then that with the higher elastic limit will give the greater maximum stored energy. If two materials have the same elastic limit, this situation will be achieved in that material with the lower modulus. In practice, most metals have moduli within a narrow range (100–250 GN/m$^2$) so that variations in the elastic limit are more significant. Moreover, a material with a low elastic modulus will also be susceptible to deformation by extraneous forces in the mouth, so that a compromise of a relatively high elastic modulus and a high elastic limit is considered desirable.

EASE OF FABRICATION

For the greatest ease of fabrication of an orthodontic appliance, the wire should have a low elastic limit, high ductility, and low resilience. These properties are generally contradictory to those required for good function, as discussed above. Since the ability to produce tooth movements is obviously the more important, the high elastic limit remains as a most desirable feature. One significant factor, however, is that, if the material is susceptible to work hardening, the ductility and strength must be balanced, both during the formation of the appliance and during use, as discussed below in relation to stainless steel.

   It is also important that methods of joining the wire to other parts of the appliance are readily available.

STAINLESS STEEL

Although a few different metals have been used for orthodontic wires, the material in most widespread use is 18–8 stainless steel. The basic character-istics of this steel have been discussed in Chapter 10 in relation to its use in dentures, from which it will be recalled that the alloying elements present in addition to the iron are 17–19 per cent chromium, 8–10 per cent nickel, and less than 0·15 per cent carbon. This composition is sufficient to ensure an austenitic structure when the steel is in the undeformed state.

*Mechanical properties.* The elastic modulus of stainless steel is approximately 200 GN/m². Bearing in mind the conflicting requirements outlined above, this represents a reasonable compromise.

The elastic limit, ultimate tensile strength, and ductility are very much dependent on the amount of work hardening that has taken place. Stainless steel is particularly susceptible to work hardening. This arises because, in addition to the disruptive effects of dislocation movement, as described in Chapter 1, a phase transformation takes place as some of the austenite transforms to martensite under stress, the latter phase being harder and more brittle. A fully annealed 18–8 austenitic stainless steel (that is, in the fully softened state) may have an elastic limit of less than 300 MN/m², an ultimate tensile strength of about 600 MN/m², and a ductility of 50 per cent. In the work-hardened condition, the corresponding figures may be 1500 MN/m² 1700 MN/m², and less than 5 per cent.

Work hardening takes place both when the wire is drawn by the manu-facturer and when it is deformed during fabrication of the appliance. It is important that the material in its final form should have a high elastic limit, and this is usually achieved by using a hard-drawn wire, that is, one which has been work-hardened to a considerable extent during manufacture. Soft-drawn wires are available if extensive manipulation, resulting in further work hardening, is necessary. Since the work hardening results in a very significant reduction in the ductility, some manufacturers give the wire a stress-relieving anneal after drawing in order to restore a little ductility, at the expense of a slight softening. A wire that is too brittle may fracture during fabrication of the appliance. Annealing is a very critical process, however, and either a temperature that is too high, or an excessive time at high temperature can completely soften the material and cause it to lose its resilience and also adversely affect the corrosion-resistance.

*Welding of stainless steel.* Most joining operations in orthodontic appliances are carried out by welding. This is the direct bonding of two materials by either heat, pressure, or a combination of both, where there is no intermediate material. Stainless steel is readily welded by the use of mechanical pressure at high temperature in a process known as spot welding. In this technique, an electric current is passed directly through the components to be joined, the electrical resistance of the steel causing sufficient heat to be generated to produce localized fusion. The bonding is enhanced by the pressure that holds the two components together.

The heat generated in the wires is proportional to the square of the current, the electrical resistance of the wires, and the time for which the current is passed. Since, in order to retain the ideal properties in the steel wire, the time it is held at the high temperature has to be a minimum, it is desirable that high currents are used. The electrical resistance is kept high by using electrodes that are tapered to a fine point, as shown in Figure 13.4, which localizes the area over which the current passes. This also minimizes the area of metal which is affected by the rise in temperature. The use of bulky electrodes made of materials with high electrical and thermal conductivity, such as copper alloys, also reduces the effect of the heat on the rest of the wire by conducting much of the heat away rapidly. These electrodes are usually clamped firmly against the wires to ensure adequate pressure is maintained when the current is passed. A timing device is used to carefully control the duration of the pulse of current.

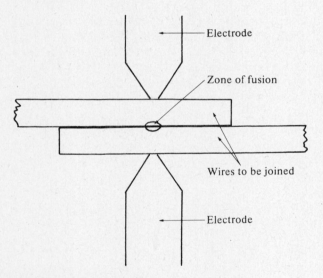

**Fig. 13.4** Spot welding of stainless steel.

*Soldering of stainless steel.* Soldering may also be used to join stainless steel components, and this does have the advantage of involving lower temperatures, thus minimizing the problems associated with heating these wires. With soldering, a low melting-point alloy is used as an intermediary to bond the two components. The solders most commonly used with stainless steel are the silver solders, which contain 45–65 per cent silver, up to 25 per cent copper, and varying quantities of cadmium and zinc. Their melting range is typically 630–650 °C. As noted in Chapter 1, stainless steel has a passive oxide layer, and this has to be removed before any bonding can take place.

This is achieved through the use of a fluoride flux, such as that based on potassium fluoride and boric acid.

The soldering may be done either free-hand or by using a cast to hold the parts in place. A gas–air torch is normally used to melt the solder. The presence of a zone of silver–copper rich alloy between the stainless steel components is, of course, detrimental to the corrosion-resistance, but in practice this does not seem to be too important.

*Corrosion-resistance of stainless steel.* As noted in Chapters 1 and 10, stainless steel is a reasonably corrosion-resistant alloy, relying on the passivating effect of chromium. Although it is possible to select alloys of greater corrosion-resistance, stainless steel seems to be adequate for this purpose, bearing in mind the relatively short periods of time the appliances are left in the mouth and the regularity with which they may be examined.

The one important point about the corrosion behaviour of austenitic stainless steel is the detrimental effect of heating the alloy. If the steel is heated to the range 650–1050 °C there is a tendency for chromium carbides to form. If this occurs and a large amount of the chromium becomes tied up with the carbides, there may be too little chromium in the regions around the carbides to afford complete passivation, resulting in a lower corrosion-resistance. This is the reason why high temperatures must be avoided whenever possible.

### ALTERNATIVE ALLOYS

Among the alloys that have occasionally been used as alternatives to stainless steel are nickel–chromium, cobalt–chromium and nickel–titanium alloys. The first two are variations on the compositions described in Chapter 10 for casting alloys in denture construction, certain elements being added to increase the ductility. An alloy known as Elgiloy, including about 40 per cent cobalt, 20 per cent chromium, and 15 per cent nickel is particularly useful as it can be fabricated in a soft and relatively ductile condition and then heat-treated to improve the elastic properties, thus overcoming some of the problems associated with the conflicting requirements discussed earlier.

## Orthodontic elastics

Elastic bands, usually referred to as elastics or elastic modules, are used to produce tooth movements in some specific situations where, for example, inter-maxillary traction is necessary or in the retraction of prominent incisors where an aesthetic appliance is considered important. The materials used are either derived from natural rubber, giving the latex elastics, or from synthetic elastomers. Details of synthetic products are not available from the manufacturers, although it is known that they are derived from polyester–urethane elastomers.

Since these materials are highly viscoelastic, it is necessary to consider the time factor in the force-extension relationship. As elastomers they deform readily under small forces, and conversely should be able to exert a low force on teeth over a large distance. However, because of stress relaxation within the elastomer, the force exerted on the tooth after the elastic has been stretched will decay, sometimes fairly rapidly. After 24 hours, the force may have dropped to about 50 per cent of the original value, while at four weeks only about 33 per cent may remain. Generally the synthetic elastics lose force at a slower rate than the latex elastics. Also as the rate of tooth movement increases, the rate of force decay increases. The viscoelastic nature of the materials also implies that the force loss will be greatest when the elastic is stretched rapidly. The elastics are normally considered to be effective for 4–6 weeks.

### Screws, bands, and brackets

Most of the commercially available screws, hooks, pins, and other pre-fabricated components are made from the same type of stainless steel used in the wires. Occasionally some other alloy may be employed, but the choice of material does not significantly affect the performance of the appliance.

As noted earlier, the wires in fixed appliances have to be attached to the teeth by the use of either bands or an adhesive via a bracket. The material used for the bracket depends to a certain extent on the method. They are usually made from stainless steel when the banding method is used, so that welding to the bands, also made of stainless steel, is readily achieved. These brackets are preformed and available commercially, having a suitable design for accepting and retaining the wires. The bands may be either preformed or made individually from thin strips of steel. They are usually secured to the teeth by the use of cements such as those discussed in Chapter 3.

If direct bonding is employed, the brackets may be made from either stainless steel or the plastic polycarbonate. The stainless steel brackets are either perforated or have a metal mesh on their back to faciliate bonding to the enamel, as discussed below. Polycarbonate is a clear plastic and this material is used in an attempt to improve further the aesthetics associated with the bandless, direct-bonding technique. While this objective is certainly achieved, these brackets are mechanically inferior to those made of steel. Distortion and fracture of the brackets may occur and since, in addition, the polycarbonate tends to discolour, the metal brackets are usually preferred.

### Adhesives for the direct bonding of orthodontic appliances

The direct bonding of orthodontic appliances to teeth offers several advantages over the banding technique. These may be grouped as follows:

**a** the aesthetics are improved, since bands are not required;

**b** bands take up a large amount of interdental space, which may be a dis-advantage in some cases;

**c** it is often difficult to maintain good oral hygiene with bands; and

**d** bands may irritate the soft tissue.

Several different types of adhesive have been used, including poly-carboxylates, acrylic resin, and diacrylate resins. The polycarboxylate cements, discussed in Chapters 2 and 3 display specific adhesion to enamel and to stainless steel. They have therefore been used in orthodontics, although generally the bond strength to enamel is not as great as that produced with the other resins described below.

The acrylic and diacrylate resins are basically similar to those used as filling materials and fissure sealants, and, since they do not display any significant specific adhesion to enamel, they have to be used in conjunction with the acid-etch technique. The acrylic resins are cold-cured, being activated either chemically or by ultraviolet light. The diacrylate resins are based on the BIS–GMA system and they may or may not contain fillers. Several important points relate to their effectiveness as adhesives:

**a** As mentioned above, the enamel has to be etched with an acid prior to application of the resin. This technique has been described in Chapter 5.

**b** A low viscosity, unfilled resin, sometimes referred to as a sealant, is usually applied first to penetrate the etched surface.

**c** The bracket is bonded to this sealant, usually with a higher viscosity, filled resin.

**d** Acrylic resins can bond directly to polycarbonate brackets. These brackets cannot be bonded with the diacrylate resins but acrylic resin can be used as a coupling agent in this system.

**e** Direct bonding to stainless steel is not possible with these resins. The brackets therefore either have perforations around their periphery or have a mesh backing to allow their gross mechanical retention by the resin. This mesh has to be firmly fixed to the bracket.

**f** Moisture contamination is a principal cause of bond failure. Thorough washing and drying of the etched enamel surface is essential.

Generally, the filled diacrylate resins, with a low viscosity resin sealant, bonded to a mesh backed stainless steel bracket appears to provide the best results.

# 14

## Materials in oral surgery and periodontology

There are a small number of conditions encountered by the oral surgeon and prosthetist where the treatment may involve the insertion of a synthetic material in oral tissues rather than into the tooth itself. These uses include the following:

**a** to assist in the retention of dentures;

**b** to stabilize mobile teeth;

**c** for the purpose of facial reconstruction following trauma, resection of tumours, or congenital abnormalities; and

**d** to assist in the repair of facial fractures.

In this context the term 'implantation' refers to the surgical transfer of non-living tissue or the insertion of synthetic materials into tissue, in contrast to transplantation which involves the surgical transfer of living tissues or organs. The parts that are involved in these cases are referred to as implants and transplants respectively. In relation to bone, autogenous grafts, being taken directly from the same individual and isogenous grafts, taken directly from an individual of the same species and who is genetically related to the recipient, may be classed as transplanted tissue. Allogenic grafts, originating from an individual who is not genetically related to the recipient, xenogenous grafts, obtained from a donor of another species, and alloplastic materials, which are completely synthetic, are classed as implants. Generally the term 'implant' is used to convey the meaning of implantation into living tissue, but in dental and oral surgery there is some confusion over this terminology, as many materials are inserted into teeth. Conventionally, however, in this situation, the term is reserved for those cases where the material penetrates bone or soft tissue, either with or without attachment to teeth.

### Implants for denture retention

There are a number of patients for whom conventional dentures are unsuccessful. While the difficulties encountered in many of these are of psychological or social origin, a significant proportion can be the result of abnormalities of soft or hard tissues, which make denture retention difficult. In such cases, preprosthetic surgery may be performed in an attempt either to create a more suitable alveolar ridge for denture bearing, or to provide some artificially created support for the denture superstructure.

ALVEOLAR RIDGE AUGMENTATION

In the edentulous patient with atrophy of the alveolar ridge, two commonly used surgical procedures are vestibuloplasty and alveoloplasty. In the former, the alveolar sulcus is extended by surgical displacement of the muscle attachments and mucosa from the crest of the ridge to a deeper point in the sulcus. Alveoloplasty involves reshaping the alveolar ridge to give better support characteristics.

Since it is now accepted that the alveolar ridge need not necessarily be smooth and uniformly shaped, and since removal of alveolar bone can be detrimental to long-term denture stability, alveolectomy is performed only very conservatively and it is becoming more common instead to extend the alveolar process to achieve a good denture-bearing area. Bone grafts are frequently used for this purpose, autogenous grafts being the most suitable, obtained either from the ribs or iliac crest. One major problem with bone grafts is that they themselves may suffer from resorption, with a significant proportion of the graft height being lost within a few years. For this reason, alloplastic materials have been used to give a non-resorbable ridge augmentation.

Clearly there are no proprietary ridge augmentation implants, since they have to be shaped according to the anatomy of the individual ridge, and indeed there are only a few materials available in a form suitable for this use. While many different types of material have been tried, those currently preferred are porous rather than solid, so that tissue may grow into the pores of the implant and give extra stabilization. This is important since the implant that has no continuity with the surrounding tissue will be unstable and will lead to a mobile or flabby ridge. Examples of materials utilized include alumina or aluminate ceramics. Certain ceramics may be prepared with a controlled porosity, calcium aluminate and alumina (aluminium oxide) being two examples. One difficulty with ceramics is that their hardness prevents accurate trimming of the implant at insertion. This same hardness may also cause erosion of the relatively soft overlying tissue. Both these problems are obviated by the use of a proprietary composite material consisting of a dispersion of pyrolytic graphite fibres in PTFE (polytetrafluoroethylene), with a 70–90 per cent porosity and 100–500 $\mu$m pore size. This is soft enough to carve and has a resilience more compatible with soft tissue. Both this and the ceramics appear to possess those properties of tissue compatibility that are necessary for implantation and which are discussed later.

SUBPERIOSTEAL IMPLANTS

In cases of marked alveolar bone resorption and in patients who have attempted to wear removable dentures but found them intolerable, a subperiosteal implant is sometimes employed. This may be either a full arch or, less frequently, a unilateral implant, with mandibular implants being more common than those in the maxilla. The implant consists of a metal framework which is seated on solid cortical bone beneath the periosteum, with a small number of posts protruding through the mucosa to support the denture superstructure. Apart from tissue compatibility, the material used must possess the properties of good strength and rigidity to allow thin sections in the framework, and good castability, since the implants have to be shaped to the contour of the bone. Thus, cobalt–chromium alloys have been universally used in this application. Traditionally a two-stage procedure, some weeks apart, is used, although some prefer immediate casting after the impressions are taken in the first stage, so that the procedure is completed in one day.

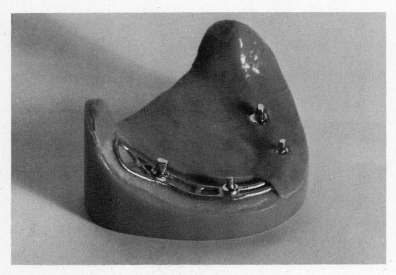

**Fig. 14.1** Full arch mandibular subperiosteal implant.

Technique and implant design vary according to the operator's preference, but typically a full arch mandibular subperiosteal implant will look like that shown in Figure 14.1. Clearly the framework must be closely adapted to the bone over a wide area, with thin sections to reduce the bulk of material. Obvious exposed anatomical features, such as blood vessels and nerves have to be avoided. The first stage is the preparation of an accurate bone impression, usually necessitating the fabrication of an acrylic special tray following a preliminary soft tissue impression. The impression of the bone is taken, preferably with an elastomeric impression material, after reflecting the periosteum. The tissues are then sutured. A mould is cast and a wax framework prepared, taking care to utilize the areas of soundest compact bone for support, those in the mandible, for example, including the genial tubercles and mylohyoid ridges. Appropriate posts are added, usually four for a complete arch, and the casting made in the normal way. A removable metal superstructure is then cast, which will locate directly on the abutments and which will be incorporated into the denture base.

The framework is implanted during the second stage utilizing the same line of incision, and then the overlying tissues are sutured over it. A temporary overlay dressing may be used until the sutures are removed. The denture itself may be constructed with the superstructure processed into the base.

Interpretation of success with this type of device is very subjective, but general opinion is that subperiosteal implants, especially full-arch mandibular implants, are quite successful when used selectively, over 60 per cent giving adequate function for more than ten years.

### ENDOSSEOUS DENTAL IMPLANTS

As their name implies, endosseous implants are partially buried in the bone itself as opposed to lying on the bone surface; as such they are sometimes referred to as 'intraosseous' or 'endosteal' as well as endosseous implants. In contrast to the subperiosteal implant, which can be used in cases of marked resorption of the ridge and which require good solid compact bone for seating, the endosseous implant can only be used where there is sufficient vertical height in the alveolar ridge, requiring cancellous rather than compact bone for support.

There are a number of different types, which, although of varied shape and size, have the same objective of directly supporting a denture, single crown, or bridge by mechanical fixation to the underlying bone. Although again they may be employed for full arches and quadrants, they are generally used for, and give better results with, a small number of crowns. Since these implants do not have to fit a bone surface, they are not individually cast and are available commercially in a series of sizes and forms. The necessity for good mechanical properties, especially adequate strength, rigidity, and impact strength has again led to the prominent use of metals.

A very widely used design is the blade-vent implant, a typical example being illustrated in Figure 14.2. Most commonly, titanium is used for the construction of these implants. The essential features are a large mesio-distal length to give good stability, vents in the structure to allow bone to grow through, again maximizing stability, a thin section to minimize bulk and to facilitate insertion with little bone loss, and a thin neck to reduce the risk of epithelial downgrowth. The insertion is simpler than with subperiosteal implants as a small hole or slot is prepared with an appropriate bur and the implant tapped into place.

For single tooth replacements, especially in the mandible and in patients with good oral hygiene, these implants give quite satisfactory results. Their widespread use, especially in more extensive cases, is not yet recommended, however. The main reasons for failure lie in the type of tissue that forms around the implant, and especially at its neck. Ideally, the implant should be held firmly in the bone, either by direct bony attachment, effectively giving

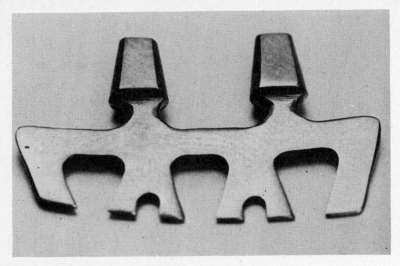

**Fig. 14.2** Blade-vent endosseous implant.

ankylosis, or by a pseudo-periodontal membrane of the correct collagen orientation.

Neither an abundance of epithelium nor a capsule of fibrous tissue with collagen oriented parallel to the implant surface is required, since these are unlikely to give stability.

In many cases, however, either of these two latter events may occur, especially with epithelial invagination of the space immediately around the implant. This situation predisposes the tissues to infection, since bacteria are able to penetrate between epithelium and implant. Because of this, attempts have been made to produce alternative materials to the titanium, which promote a more favourable tissue response. This has resulted in experimentation with a series of porous materials, including porous titanium, cobalt–chromium alloy, alumina, and polymethyl methacrylate, which achieve stability through bony ingowth, and a selection of materials based on carbon, which appear to be highly compatible with tissues.

ENDODONTIC STABILIZERS

Teeth which have lost some of their bony support through disease and are inadequately supported may be stabilized by endodontic endosseous stabilizers. These are metallic implants which are placed through the root-canal and extend beyond the root apex into the bone. The implants may be used alone or utilized in a post-crown technique. They are especially useful where the bony loss is mainly in the apical region of the tooth, since in such cases there is a greater chance of healthy gingival tissue, and the extension of the implant beyond the deficient bone provides a much needed additional fixation. The implant posts are prepared from standard wire of a nickel–chromium alloy, titanium, or cobalt–chromium alloy and may be shaped as a conventional post and core if necessary. This procedure appears to be very successful, the main advantage over endosseous implants lying in the absence of a gingival crevice adjacent to the implant.

## Facial reconstruction

Certain parts of the maxilla, mandible, and face may be missing, either partially or completely, as a result of congenital or developmental abnormalities, trauma, pathological conditions, or surgical removal. Reconstruction of these areas may be possible and the procedures frequently utilize maxillofacial prostheses. These can be classified as intra-oral implanted prostheses, intra-oral non-implanted prostheses, and extra-oral non-implanted prostheses.

### IMPLANTED MAXILLOFACIAL PROSTHESES

The most significant type of implanted maxillofacial prosthesis is the mandibular replacement, frequently used after excision of a tumour. Reconstruction of the mandible is a very difficult procedure, especially as the successful treatment in many cases of head and neck tumours necessitates removal of much of the mandible and associated soft tissue. Interference with the attachment of genio-hyoid and genio-glossus muscles may affect the function and integrity of the lower part of the face and tongue. A further problem is that the remaining tissue may have already received irradiation therapy, giving a poorer prognosis for immediate reconstructive surgery.

Autogenous bone has been used widely for mandibular reconstruction, in the form of either cancellous bone from the iliac crest or rib grafts, but in recent years there has been a greater emphasis on alloplastic reconstruction, either by implant alone or in conjunction with cancellous bone. One successful type of rigid alloplastic prothesis is the Bowerman–Conroy plate, made of titanium. These are available, as illustrated in Figure 14.3a, as straight body sections and separate ramus and angle sections. The straight sections are sufficiently malleable to allow bending at the time of operation to the correct curvature, using contouring tools. These prostheses may be used in cases of complete mandibulectomy or hemimandibulectomy, an example of the latter construction being shown in Figure 14.3b.

While these plates appear to be successful, even in cases of considerable irradiation damage to the already poor soft-tissue coverage, there is an alternative approach which makes use of the osteogenic potential of cancellous bone chips.

These have been placed in perforated trays, made from either tantalum, titanium, cobalt–chromium alloys, or a variety of polymers, including a polyether urethane–polyethylene terephthalate composite contoured to the shape of the mandible. The use of these implants is, at this stage, still only experimental.

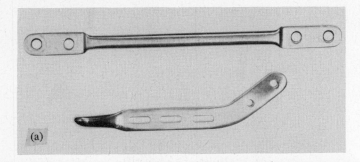

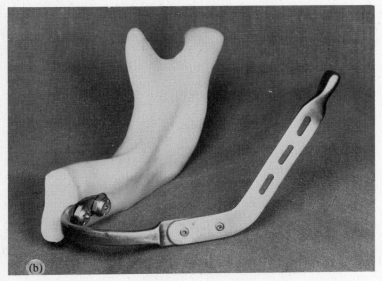

**Fig. 14.3** Mandibular replacement prostheses (a) body and ramus sections; (b) hemi-mandibulectomy prosthesis (courtesy of Mr B. Conroy, Queen Mary's Hospital, Roehampton).

EXTERNAL MAXILLOFACIAL PROSTHESES

The desired characteristics of materials for extra-oral maxillofacial prostheses are necessarily a little different from those for implanted prostheses, since the emphasis is turned away from biocompatibility to aesthetics, ease of preparation, and durability. While the prostheses should not irritate the adjacent tissues, the really important requirements are the reproduction of the colour and texture, detail of moulding, and resistance to weathering and handling.

The choice of materials depends to a certain extent on the particular application. Some prostheses require fairly rigid materials while others demand more flexibility. Most situations requiring rigidity utilize acrylic polymers, very similar to the denture base material. The advantages of this material are the ease of colour matching and moulding and environmental stability. The rigidity may, however, lead to little freedom of movement to accommodate facial expression, and also there may possibly be mechanical irritation of the tissue.

Flexible materials generally give better adaptation to tissue and greater comfort to the patient. Plasticized polyvinylchloride, flexible acrylics, silicone rubber, and certain polyurethanes are all used to some extent. Silicone rubber, widely known under proprietary name 'Silastic', is a particularly good material from the performance point of view, although colouring and shading are more difficult.

IMPLANTS IN THE TREATMENT OF MANDIBULAR FRACTURES

The treatment of fractures of the mandible depends on the class of fracture and type of patient. As with fracture fixation in any bone, accurate reduction of the fracture, to ensure good alignment and good immobilization is essential. In the jaws, the immobilization may be achieved by interdental eyelet wiring, where pairs of teeth in both jaws are connected by eyelet wires. Alternatively, and especially if fewer teeth are available, either an arch bar or cap splints, constructed with the aid of plaster models may be used. In all these cases, the immobilization is maintained only until union occurs, typically in about six weeks. This relatively short period, together with the supra-gingival location, implies that the biocompatibility characteristics of the material are not too critical.

Standard stainless steel is used for arch bars and wiring while silver is commonly used for cast splints.

More complex fractures, and also fractures in edentulous patients, may require some type of internal fixation. A convenient method in edentulous patients utilizes the lower denture, which is fixed to the jaws by means of wire passed around the mandible. If dentures are not available, an acrylic splint may be used for the same purpose. Here the wiring is located within tissue and, although removed after 5 or 6 weeks, should be made of a surgical grade metal, usually surgical stainless steel.

Open reduction and fixation may be used. For example, internal wire fixation of both lower and upper borders of the mandible is frequently performed, either from an intra-oral or extra-oral approach. The use of implant-grade stainless steel obviates the necessity for removal. Finally more secure fixation can be obtained by means of bone plates, which, if properly located, can prevent shearing displacements at the fracture line as well as preventing distraction. Small bone plates, similar to those used in ortho-paedics for fixation of metacarpal fractures, are commercially available, made from either implant-grade stainless steel, titanium, or cobalt–chromium alloy. They are secured to the bone by means of screws, as illustrated in Figure 14.4. Again these implants need not necessarily be removed, although this

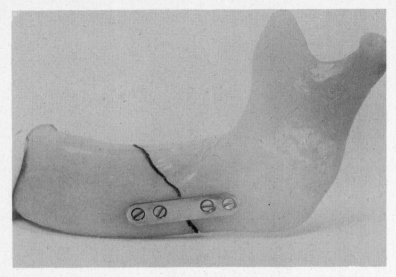

**Fig. 14.4** Bone plate and screws used in treatment of fractured mandible (courtesy of Mr B. Conroy, Queen Mary's Hospital, Roehampton).

is advocated by many surgeons. A further feature has been applied to these fracture plates. This is the ability, achieved by specially-designed screw holes in the plates, to compress the bone across the fracture line, rather than simply holding it together. This increases stability and appears to promote more efficient fracture healing.

### Materials for implantation

The properties desired in a material for permanent or semi-permanent implantation in living tissue fall into two basic categories, the first relating to the performance of the implant and the second to its compatibility with tissues. Most implants used in oral surgery, being either a replacement or support for hard tissue, have to transmit the fairly high forces that are associated with the function of the mouth. Therefore, the materials must have adequate strength, especially as it is often desirable for the section of the implant to be as thin as possible. This is the case, for example, in the framework of subperiosteal implants, the neck of endosseous implants, and mandibular fracture fixation plates. For the same reason, a degree of rigidity, implying a reasonably high elastic modulus, is required, although this does depend on the application. Also the conditions of impact loading which are often encountered usually necessitate a tough rather than a brittle material. Metallic materials, which offer the best combination of mechanical properties, are therefore frequently chosen for oral implants. For those cases which require individual moulding, cobalt–chromium alloy is the most suitable because of its castability. Prefabricated or proprietary products are most often made of stainless steel, titanium alloy, cobalt–chromium, or, very occasionally, tantalum.

TISSUE RESPONSE TO IMPLANTS

Compatibility with the tissue presents a more difficult problem. For short-term contact with tissue, the main requirement is that there should be no allergic response to the material and no obvious, immediate cytotoxicity effects. With long-term implantation, more subtle effects become important. The normal response of tissues to an implanted foreign body, after the trauma induced by its insertion has subsided, is to wall off the implant by a capsule or sheath of fibrous connective tissue. With an extremely inert material, this capsule may be very thin, but as the degree of irritation to the tissue produced by the implant increases, so the thickness may increase, and indeed, various types of inflammatory tissue may take its place, involving macrophages and foreign body giant cells. Irritation may take the form of chemical toxicity, arising, for example, from corrosion of a metal or degradation of a polymer, or mechanical irritation due to movement of the implant. Ideally, therefore, an implant should be immobile to avoid mechanical irritation and be made of a chemically stable and biologically inert substance. This implies the use of highly corrosion-resistant metals, high molecular weight non-degradable polymers, and stable ceramics, all of which must be sufficiently pure and well characterized in terms of toxicity. An excessive response by the tissue may involve oedema, tenderness, and pain, sometimes necessitating removal of the implant. In extreme cases, necrosis of the tissue will occur. An important complicating factor is that the presence of a foreign body increases the risk of infection.

With sufficient care over materials selection, implant design, and operative technique, the tissue response can be kept to a minimum with totally implanted structures, but far greater problems arise with transcutaneous or transgingival devices and this is the major reason, as indicated above, why endosseous implants are not always successful.

## Extraction wound dressings

There are some situations where it is necessary or desirable to place a dressing in an extraction socket, the two most commonly encountered indications being to aid haemostasis and to treat infection in the dry socket.

When haemorrhage occurs from the bony walls of a tooth socket rather than from the soft tissue margin, pressure packs and sutures do not help in its control. Provided bleeding is not from a single prominent vessel, a socket dressing may be of value. These generally act as a matrix to stabilize the blood while it clots, and are usually presented in the form of a foam or sponge. Gelatin, fibrin, oxidized cellulose, and oxidized regenerated cellulose have all been used. They all undergo fairly rapid resorption, with the possible exception of oxidized cellulose. Fibrin foam is often preferred as it is a natural material present in human tissue and directly aids the clotting mechanism.

The dressing of extraction sockets has been criticized since it allows the collection of debris and may lead to infection and delayed healing. It is interesting, therefore, that the treatment of an established infected socket often involves the placement of a pack in the socket.

This pack is generally in the form of a ribbon gauze, and sometimes cotton wool, impregnated with some antibacterial agent. Zinc oxide/eugenol may be used, which has the advantage of producing an obtundent effect, thus reducing the patient's pain, which may be severe. It also has an anti-bacterial action. The main disadvantage is that it tends to delay healing, and treatment may be protracted.

## PERIODONTOLOGY

The only dental material used widely in periodontal surgery is the periodontal dressing, or pack, which is used post-surgically to cover the exposed wound surface. There are a few other situations in which materials have been used experimentally or on a limited basis, such as the use of the adhesive cyanoacrylate, which can be employed as a protective film on wound surfaces, and the use of alloplastic materials in the repair of infra-bony pockets, but these are not yet of widespread interest.

### Functions of periodontal dressings

The periodontal dressing does not intrinsically alter the rate of healing after surgery; exposed tissue will heal irrespective of its presence. Instead, its purpose is to protect the wound in order to ensure uneventful healing. The following factors may be important in providing this function.

**a** A dressing may physically protect the wound surface from direct mechanical trauma during healing.

**b** A closely adapted dressing may prevent the formation of excessive granulation tissue by reducing the space available.

**c** It may provide a physical barrier to salivary and bacterial contamination, reducing the risk of post-operative infection.

**d** When containing suitable antimicrobial agents, it may be bactericidal and bacteriostatic.

**e** It may reduce the tenderness and give increased comfort to the patient.

Since the periodontal tissues do not easily provide retentive features for dressings, and since it is usually desirable for the dressing to remain in place for up to 7 days, the principal requirements specific to this situation relate to the flow, adhesive, and mechanical properties of the material. Ideally the dressing should be prepared as a mass of sufficient plasticity for it to be pressed through the interproximal spaces and of sufficient cohesiveness for individually placed parts to hold together as a single unit after adaptation to the tissue. On setting, the material should be strong but not brittle, bearing in mind the relatively thin sections present in the interproximal spaces and the need to avoid fracture at these points. A smooth, non-irritant surface is also desirable.

There is some controversy over the virtues of bactericidal or bacteriostatic properties. However, the presence of dressings covering the wound area is itself responsible for a change in the balance of the flora under it, so that some anti-bacterial activity is probably desirable. Naturally, the use of any substance for this purpose should not compromise the low degree of tissue irritation and lack of hypersensitivity reactions that are desirable in wound dressings.

## Materials for periodontal dressings

At least three classes of periodontal dressing materials are available. These are:

**a** a two-component zinc oxide/eugenol based system;

**b** a two-component zinc oxide/fatty acid based system;

**c** a one–paste calcium sulphate system.

### ZINC OXIDE/EUGENOL DRESSINGS

The material used in these dressings is basically the same as that used in the zinc oxide/eugenol preparations for impressions and linings, as discussed in Chapters 6 and 3. Presentation is in the form of a powder and a liquid of the following basic formulations.

*Powder*. This contains zinc oxide and resin in proportions varying from 2 : 1 to 1 : 1. The resin is usually pine resin, which enhances the zinc oxide–eugenol reaction and increases the strength of the product. Various other substances may be present. Zinc acetate or stearate (1–2 per cent) act as accelerators in the usual way. Tannic acid and asbestos fibres have also been included in some formulations, at about 3 per cent of each, the former for its apparent beneficial effect on wound healing and the latter to increase the cohesiveness of the dressing. Neither constituent is really suitable, however, and their inclusion is not normally recommended. Any fibrous component on the surface can only increase the irritation of the tissues, since the dressing itself has a tendency to strip superficial cell layers from the epithelium; furthermore asbestos is a particularly harmful substance in tisuues. Tannic acid may also be absorbed through the mucosal surface in sufficient quantity to induce liver damage.

*Liquid*. The liquid is basically eugenol, (up to 85 per cent) in a diluent of an oil, such as cotton seed, olive, or pine oil. It may also contain isopropyl alcohol and colouring agents, as well as thymol (about 1 per cent).

*Properties.* The powder and liquid are mixed in a manner similar to that used for zinc oxide/eugenol impression paste, to give a material of a fairly firm, putty-like consistency which is pressed into the form of strips. These are applied to the wound surface and kneaded into the interproximal spaces so that buccal and lingual segments join together. It may be trimmed if necessary. The material sets quite hard, giving a fairly rough surface and potentially sharp edges, which may irritate adjacent mucous membranes.

Although these dressings have been in use for many years, they do have some disadvantages, relating especially to the presence of eugenol. The taste is persistent and not very pleasant and the dressing may produce a burning sensation on initial contact with the tissues. The actual effect of the set dressings on the tissue is not clear. The absorption of eugenol into the tissue and its penetration of nerve tissue gives a mild analgesic effect. However, it has been claimed that this can produce tissue necrosis. Any such effect would be continuous, since the zinc oxide–eugenol reaction does not go to completion so that there is always free eugenol present. Although some studies have shown no apparent difference between these and eugenol-free dressings, it is generally believed that they do elicit a more marked inflammatory response than the latter. Even though they may contain thymol, these dressings do not have a very significant anti-bacterial effect, any such activity in a freshly made dressing being rapidly lost. It is also known that the dressing encourages yeast growth.

ZINC OXIDE/FATTY ACID SYSTEM

This material relies on a saponification reaction (see Chapter 1) for its setting; in this case the zinc oxide reacts with a weak organic acid to produce a zinc-based soap. It is commonly presented as a two-paste system.

*Paste compositions.* One paste consists largely of zinc oxide, to which has been added a suitable oil to give the required plasticity, a gum to give cohesiveness, and an anti-microbial agent. This is typically lorothidol, a hexachlorophane-type of fungicide or tribromosalicyl anilide, although the antibiotic zinc bacitracin has been used in some cases.

The second paste contains the appropriate fatty acid, details of which are not divulged by the manufacturers, mixed with a resin, such as pine resin, for thickening purposes and an antimicrobial substance, such as chloro-thymol. The setting time may be controlled by retarders supplied with the pastes.

*Properties.* Mixing of the two pastes is readily achieved, a more plastic mix being produced than with the zinc oxide/eugenol material, giving better adaptability to the tissue. Initially it is tacky, but remains workable for up to 20 minutes and sets slowly to give a smooth surface which is less irritant to the tissues. There is no unpleasant taste or odour associated with these dressings. The presence of the lorothidol and chlorothymol gives stronger bacteriostatic properties, although the material is selective, depressing the growth of gram positive rods more than gram negative rods, for example. Whilst many would claim that these materials are less irritant than the eugenol-containing dressings, they still cause some degree of inflammatory response, possibly due to the quantities of antimicrobial agents they contain.

CALCIUM SULPHATE SYSTEMS

At least one proprietary periodontal dressing material does not rely on a zinc oxide reaction at all, but is based on the chemistry of calcium sulphate. This is presented as a pre-mixed paste, consisting largely of calcium sulphate with small amounts of zinc oxide and sulphate which influence strength and setting characteristics, acrylic-type resin, and a glycol which acts as a solvent to form the paste. On exposure to air or moisture, the glycol is extracted and the calcium sulphate reacts with water molecules to give a hard mass when set. By setting in this way, the material is not very cohesive and it is, therefore, relatively difficult to join together pieces or build up layers. No antimicrobial agents are added to the paste so there is only a slight bactericidal effect and this is soon lost when the paste has set.

# Index